Progress in Pediatric Surgery

Volume 20

Historical Aspects of Pediatric Surgery

Volume Editor

P. P. Rickham, Zurich

With 119 Figures

Springer-Verlag
Berlin Heidelberg New York Tokyo

Professor Dr. P. P. Rickham, M.D., M.S.,
F.R.C.S., F.R.C.S.I., F.R.A.C.S., D.C.H., F.A.A.P.
Universitäts-Kinderklinik
Chirurgische Abteilung
Steinwiesstraße 75
CH-8032 Zürich

Volumes 1–17 of this series were published by Urban & Schwarzenberg, Baltimore–Munich

ISBN-13: 978-3-642-70827-5 e-ISBN-13: 978-3-642-70825-1
DOI: 10.1007/ 978-3-642-70825-1

Library of Congress Cataloging-in-Publication Data. Historical aspects of pediatric surgery. (Progress in pediatric surgery; v. 20). Includes index. 1. Children – Surgery – History. I. Rickham, P. P. (Peter Paul) II. Series. [DNLM: 1. Surgery – history. 2. Surgery – in infancy & childhood. W1 PR677KA v. 20 / WO 925 H673]
RD137.A1P7 vol. 20 617'.98 s [617'.9809] 86-6691
ISBN 0-387-15960-6 (U.S.)

2123/3130-543210

Preface

At first sight it may appear strange that a volume of *Progress in Pediatric Surgery* should be devoted to the history of our specialty. One assumes that *progress* is concerned primarily with recent developments whilst *history* deals with matters of the past. However, in the past there has also been considerable progress in the development of our understanding of paediatric surgical problems, otherwise we would not have progressed to our present achievements. The editors, therefore, do not apologize for compiling this volume but, on the contrary, feel that the publication of this volume is most timely.

Modern paediatric surgery has now been practised for three generations. The handful of pioneers who were the founders of our specialty worked mainly before the last world war. A few dozen of the intermediary generation started work immediately after the war, while the new generation who are now dominating our specialty must be counted in thousands. Two factors have radically altered paediatric surgery as practised by the intermediary and the present generation of surgeons. Firstly, there has been an enormous increase in the number of men and women working in our specialty, resulting in a drastic reduction in the number of patients seen by each surgeon. Secondly, the fact that whilst practically every problem studied by the surgeons of the intermediary generation was new and unknown, most of these problems have now been largely solved. The new generation of paediatric surgeons is thus confronted with a well-studied subject, and progress will only be achieved in relatively small, well-defined areas. This lies in the nature of progress of a surgical specialty. The change, however, calls for a different attitude towards progress. The pioneering spirit which was still so dominant in the intermediary generation has, I believe, somewhat abated, and painstaking, detailed research has taken its place.

The modern paediatric surgeon, being two generations removed from the beginning of his specialty, has not had the same knowledge of these beginnings as surgeons of my, the intermediary generation. He is, however, aware of the fact that the enormous development of our specialty during the last fourty years was to a large extent brought about by improvement in techniques and materials rather than by the quality of the surgeons. In addition, the establishment of paediatric surgery as a specialty in its own rights has stimulated the interest into the roots of our specialty.

It is not accidental that the World Association of Paediatric Surgeons and the British Association of Paediatric Surgeons have both this year established a study group for historical questions. This volume was planned in order to further stimulate these interests. In previous volumes we have occasionally published historical contributions, for instance, on malformations of the anus and rectum. In the present volume we do not attempt to provide the reader with a complete history of paediatric surgery. This is a volume in a specialised series, not a textbook, and we have included articles on a variety of historical subjects. These are broadly divided into four sections: firstly, biographical sketches of some of the most important pioneers of the first generation of paediatric surgeons; secondly, brief accounts of the development of paediatric surgery in some countries or institutions; thirdly, biographies of some of our predecessors of the dim distant past; and fourthly, and perhaps most important, descriptions of the progress in our understanding of the pathophysiology of certain malformations and the improvements in treatment. Research in these historical subjects is time-consuming and necessitates working through a large volume of relevant and irrelevant literature. It is, therefore, a source of pride that so many authors have submitted their contributions to this volume.

This will be the last volume which I personally edit, and it gives me great pleasure to present the reader with a sample of the history of our great past which will, I hope, lead to an even better future.

P. P. Rickham, Zurich

Contents

List of Editors and Contributors

Editors

Angerpointner, T. A., Dr., Kinderchirurgische Klinik im Dr. von Haunerschen Kinderspital der Universität München, Lindwurmstraße 4, D-8000 München 2

Hecker, W. Ch., Prof. Dr., Kinderchirurgische Klinik im Dr. von Haunerschen Kinderspital der Universität München, Lindwurmstraße 4, D-8000 München 2

Rickham, P.P., Prof. Dr. M.D., M.S., F.R.C.S., F.R.C.S.I., F.R.A.C.S., D.C.H., F.A.A.P., Universitätskinderklinik, Chirurgische Abteilung, Steinwiesstraße 75, CH-8032 Zürich

Prévot, J., Prof., Clinique Chirurgical Pédiatrique, Hôpital d'Enfants de Nancy, F-54511 Vandœvre Cedex

Spitz, L., Prof., PhD. FRCS, Nuffield Professor of Pediatric Surgery, Institute of Child Health, University of London, Hospital for Sick Children, Great Ormond Street, 30 Guilford Street, GB-London WC1N 1EH

Stauffer, U. G., Prof. Dr., Universitätskinderklinik, Kinderchirurgische Abteilung, Steinwiesstraße 75, CH-8032 Zürich

Wurnig, P., Prof. Dr., Kinderchirurgische Abteilung des Mautner Markhof'schen Kinderspitals, Baumgasse 75, A-1030 Wien

Contributors

You will find the adresses at the beginning of the respective contribution

The History of Pediatric Surgery in Germany

W. Ch. Hecker[1]

The present has developed from the past, and the future will go forth from the present. Thus yesterday, today, and tomorrow constitute a dynamic whole. If the direction of future developments is to be recognized correctly, it is not only necessary for the present to be interpreted correctly, but also necessary to realize how the present has grown out of the past. Hence, the course of medical history indicates the foundation of future medicine.

Surgery, including surgery on children, has been performed in some form as long as mankind has existed. One of the oldest instructions in neonatal surgery is written in the Bible in the First Book of Moses:

"Every male among you shall be circumcised. You shall be circumcised in the flash of your foreskins .... He that is eight days old among you shall be circumcised" (Genesis 17.10–12).

According to today's opinion, this was a hygienic, prophylactic operation, and the discussion on indication and technique for circumcision has still not come to an end.

Pediatric surgery as defined today is a fairly young specialty; it has developed only since the middle of the last century. Its initial growth took place exclusively in the newly established children's hospitals throughout Europe, yet it was not until 100 years later that pediatric surgical units were established at surgical clinics in Germany. Its general development can be divided into four periods.

Four Periods of Development

Pediatric Surgery in Children's Hospitals

Stage 1: The Pediatrician as Operating Surgeon. We want to describe the four-stage development by means of a few examples. In the first stage we find the pediatrician Dr. von Hauner, an operating surgeon (1846–1850) who founded the University Children's Hospital in Munich. In Heidelberg the founder of the children's hospital Luisenheilanstalt, Prof. Dusch, also performed operations. He

[1] Kinderchirurgische Klinik der Universitäts-Kinderklinik München, Lindwurmstr. 4, D-8000 München 2, FRG

Progress in Pediatric Surgery, Vol. 20
Ed. by P. P. Rickham

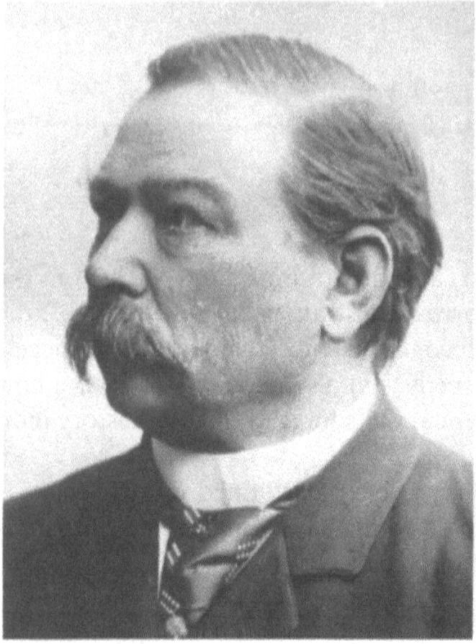

Fig. 1. Prof. Hermann Lossen

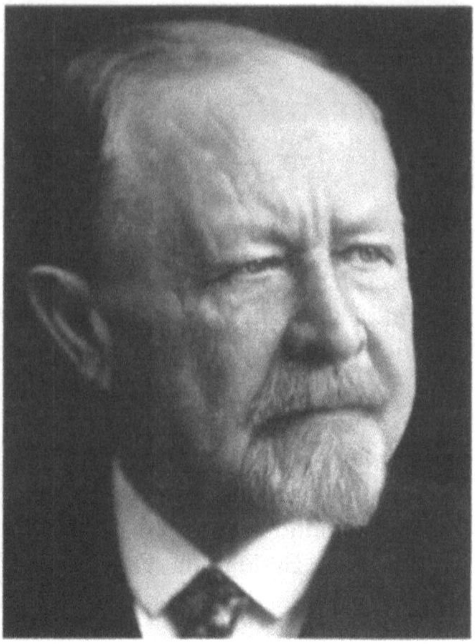

Fig. 2. Prof. Benno Schmidt

had previously been surgical assistant to Prof. Chelius. Similarly, the founder of the children's hospital in Hamburg-Altona, Dr. Grünberg, was an operating surgeon around 1860.

Stage 2: The Surgeon as Consultant. These operating pediatricians soon recognized that more extensive surgery on children required specially trained surgeons. The second stage was introduced in Munich with the appointment of Prof. Karl Thiersch in 1850 and shortly later of his successor Prof. Johann Nepomuk Ritter von Nußbaum. In Munich this stage lasted until 1886. Nußbaum was the pediatric surgeon at the Dr. von Haunersches Kinderspital for 32 years. In Heidelberg Prof. Hermann Lossen (Fig. 1) was appointed surgeon in 1864. He was succeeded by Prof. Benno Schmidt (Fig. 2). In Heidelberg this stage lasted until 1935.

Stage 3: Pediatric Surgical Hospitals at Children's Hospitals. The third stage of establishment of pediatric surgical departments at children's hospitals was introduced at the Hannover children's hospital in 1867. The department there was directed by Dr. Hüpeden until 1890; he was even director of that children's hospital in 1879.

A pediatric surgical unit was established at the Dr. von Haunersches Kinderspital in Munich in 1886 under the direction of Prof. Otmar von Angerer. The post was permanently established by the Ministery of Education upon application of

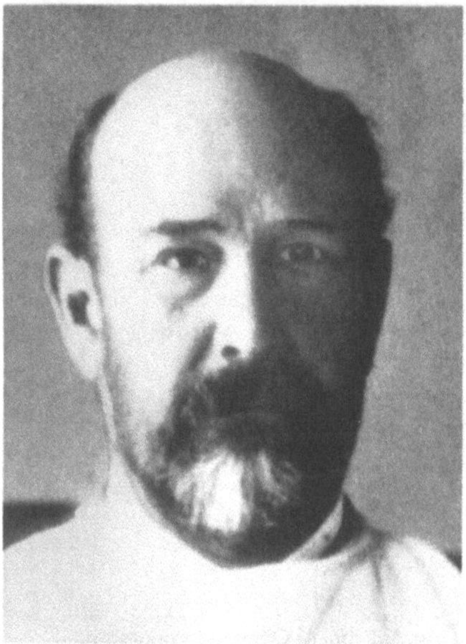

Fig. 3. Prof. W. Herzog

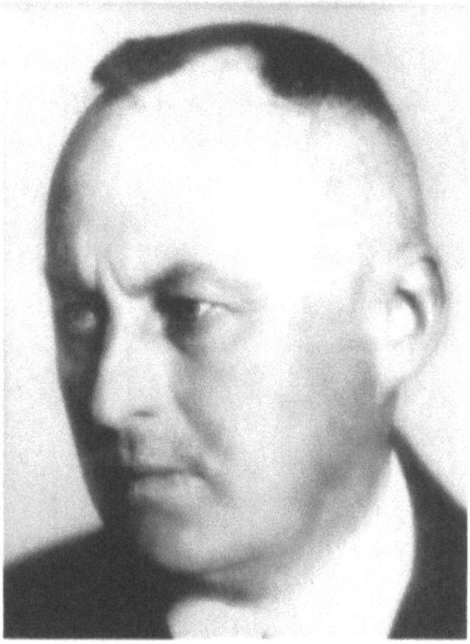

Fig. 4. Prof. R. Drachter

the medical faculty of the University of Munich. Von Angerer was the chief of this department from 1886 to 1891. Thereafter he was appointed full professor of surgery at the University of Munich. Prof. Wilhelm Herzog (Fig. 3) joined the pediatric surgical department of the Dr. von Haunersches Kinderspital in 1891 and was its director for 23 years. He became special professor of surgical diseases in childhood and their treatment. By the beginning of the war in 1914, Prof. Richard Drachter (Fig. 4) was appointed surgeon at the University children's hospital in Munich, but not to the chair as special professor, which was suspended. Prof. Sauerbruch, full professor of surgery at that time, had achieved a transfer of this chair to the surgical outpatient clinic. Drachter was chief surgeon for 21 years and died tragically of an unrecognized appendicitis. From 1936 to 1969 Prof. Anton Oberniedermayr (Fig. 5) was director of this department. In 1959 he was given a special chair for pediatric surgery upon the initiative of the pediatrician Prof. Wiskott and the surgeon Prof. Zenker. This post was transformed into a full professorship in 1966.

In 1882 a pediatric surgical department was established at the Olga-Kinderhospital in Stuttgart, which was directed by Prof. von Köstlin.

Stage 4: Pediatric Surgery as an Independent Discipline. The fourth stage of the development of pediatric surgery began after Prof. Oberniedermayr became professor emeritus. The University of Munich became the first university in Germany to create a chair in pediatric surgery, appointing me to this position in 1969.

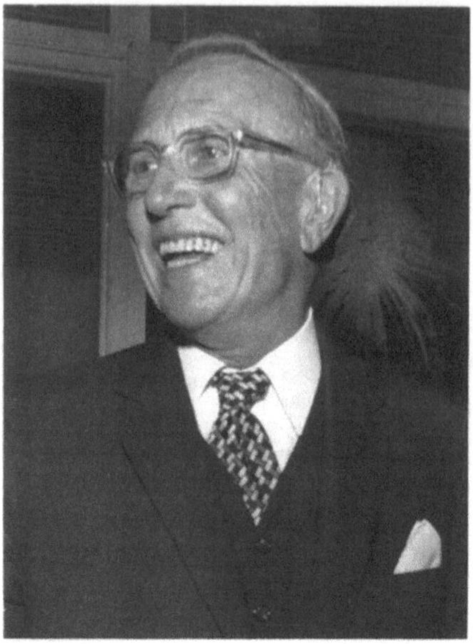

Fig. 5. Prof. A. Oberniedermayr

Pediatric Surgical Units at Surgical Clinics

The second period in the development of pediatric surgery consisted in the establishment of pediatric surgical units at surgical clinics. It was the surgeon Prof. Fritz Linder who called for the creation of a pediatric surgical department at the surgical clinic of the University of Heidelberg in 1962. In 1966 this unit was provided with a professorship, which I was appointed to. In 1973 the University of Heidelberg appointed Prof. Roland Daum to a newly created chair of pediatric surgery.

Further pediatric surgical units were installed at the surgical clinics of the universities of Düsseldorf, Mainz, Berlin-Steglitz, Homburg, Erlangen, Würzburg, Tübingen, and Hamburg as well as at the surgical clinics in Augsburg, Göppingen, Landsberg, and Braunschweig. These were led by surgeons who had already been employed at these hospitals for some years.

Pediatric Surgeons in Pediatric Surgical Units

The third period in the development of pediatric surgery was marked by the appointment of pediatric surgeons to newly established pediatric surgical units. We can distinguish three variants:

1. At a pediatric surgical unit of a surgical clinic, as was the case in Mannheim and Krefeld
2. At a pediatric surgical unit of a pediatric clinic, as happened in Esslingen, Lübeck, Bonn-St. Augustin, Siegen, Hamm, Pforzheim, Kassel-Parkschönfeld, Trier, Hamburg-Walddörfer and Landshut

3. At a university pediatric surgical hospital, as was the case in Hannover, Bochum and Münster

Pediatric Surgeons in Private Practice

The most recent period in the development in pediatric surgery is characterized by pediatric surgeons in free practice, as is the case with four pediatric surgeons in Munich. They operate partly in their practice and partly in hospitals where they have reserved beds.

Professional Organization of Pediatric Surgery

The history of the German Society of Pediatric Surgery started with the establishment of a workshop of German pediatric surgeons by Prof. Anton Oberniedermayr in 1958. He initiated its transformation into the German Society of Pediatric Surgery in 1963. Prof. OBERNIEDERMAYR was its first president and today is its honorary president. Further presidents have been Prof. FRITZ REHBEIN, Dr. WERNER VON EKESPARRE, Prof. WALDEMAR HECKER, Prof. HEINZ SINGER, Prof. ANDREAS FLACH, and Dr. WOLFGANG MAIER.

Prof. ANTON OBERNIEDERMAYR was the first who applied for the establishment of pediatric surgery as an independent discipline in 1962. Regrettably, this was refused and the German Medical Council installed pediatric surgery as subdiscipline of general surgery in 1967 instead. That this specialty is a subdiscipline is unique to Germany and is not found anywhere else in the world. However, the suggestions for advanced training in pediatric surgery made by the German Medical Council did not meet the approval of pediatric surgeons since they made pediatric surgery very dependent on general surgery. Thus I initiated a second application for pediatric surgery to be recognized as an independent discipline in 1973; at the time I was president of the Society. This application was renewed for the third time in 1977. From then on exhaustive, tedious, and often controversial discussions with general surgeons ensued, until agreement about training in pediatric surgery was reached in 1982. Advanced training in pediatric surgery now consists of 3 years' training in general surgery, 3 years' in pediatric surgery, and 1 year's in pediatrics. This form of advanced training was ratified by the German Medical Council in the spring of 1984; the Bavarian Government was the first federal state of Germany to official recognize this agreement, in October 1984. The articles of the section of pediatric surgery within the German Society of Surgery were set up in this sense. Further conferences with general surgeons guaranteed the position of pediatric surgery as a completely independent discipline. The independent development of pediatric surgery is therefore secure.

A sign of the appreciation of German pediatric surgery was the award of the Paracelsus Medal to Prof. Fritz Rehbein; it is the highest award given by the German Medical Council.

Pediatric Surgery at Universities

Chairs in pediatric surgery have now been established at the Ludwig-Maximilians-University in Munich and the Technical University of Munich as well as at the Universities of Tübingen, Heidelberg, Hannover, Mainz, Düsseldorf, Bochum-Herne, Münster, and Lübeck.

University pediatric surgical units with professorships exist in Mannheim, Berlin-Steglitz, Erlangen, Homburg/Saar, Würzburg, Frankfurt/Main and Kiel.

The following pediatric surgical hospitals and units are teaching institutions of medical faculties:

Pediatric surgical teaching institution	*University*
Karlsruhe	Freiburg
Munich-Schwabing	Technical University of Munich
Berlin-Wedding	Free University of Berlin
St. Augustin	Bonn
Cologne (Amsterdamer Straße)	Cologne
Siegen	Marburg
Krefeld	Düsseldorf
Bremen	Göttingen
Stuttgart	Tübingen
Hannover-Kinderheilanstalten	Medical School of Hannover
Augsburg	Munich
Dortmund	Münster

There are a total of 55 pediatric surgical units in the Federal Republic of Germany, 17 which are at universities and 38 at urban or social institutions. There were only 32 pediatric surgical units in 1973 (5 at universities) and 43 units in 1977 (7 at universities). We can therefore state that the claim made in 1874 by A. Steffen, the founder of the German Society of Pediatrics, that a pediatric surgical unit would be established at each greater pediatric center has nearly been satisfied 110 years later.

The advancement of a discipline can also be seen in the publication of textbooks and journals. In Germany, surgery in childhood was first discussed in Gerhard's *Handbuch der Paediatrie* in 1860. A textbook of pediatric surgery diseases, edited by Ferdinand Karewski, was published by Enke Publishers of Stuttgart in 1894. Fritz Lange and Hans Spitzi published their textbook in 1910, followed by that by Gohrbandt, Karger, and Bergmann in 1928, and then by the internationally acclaimed *Lehrbuch der Chirurgie des Kindesalters* by Drachter and Gossmann in 1930. After the war the textbooks by Oberniedermayr, Hecker, Helbig, and Pompino as well as the contributions on pediatric surgery to *Breitner's Operationslehre* written by Hecker, Daum, and Maier were published. Feer's *Lehrbuch der Kinderheilkunde, Zenker's Operationslehre* as well as Heberer's

Lehrbuch der Chirurgie contain chapters on pediatric surgery written by Hecker and Holschneider.

In Germany the *Zeitschrift für Kinderchirurgie* has been edited by Fritz Rehbein since 1964. The journal, which has meanwhile been given the additional English title *Surgery in Infancy and Childhood,* has become practically the European counterpart of the *Journal of Pediatric Surgery.* Upon my initiative the series *Progress in Pediatric Surgery,* edited by Rickham, Prevot, and myself, has been published since 1970.

Furthermore, it deserves to be mentioned that the German Society of Pediatric Surgery in 1962 instituted the biannual Anton Oberniedermayr Lecture in honor of its honorary president Anton Oberniedermayr and first awarded the Richard Drachter Prize, given annually for the most outstanding scientific work in pediatric surgery. Previous prize winners were Prof. Stauffer, Prof. Engert, Prof. Holschneider (twice), Prof. Halsband, Dr. Bolkenius, and Dr. Zimmermann.

Summary

Pediatric surgery as defined today is a very young specialty, and it was not until the middle of our century that pediatric units were established at surgical clinics in Germany. Pediatric surgery in Germany developed first in children's hospitals. The author distinguishes four stages:

Stage 1: The pediatrician as operating surgeon;
Stage 2: The surgeon as consultant;
Stage 3: Pediatric surgical hospitals at children's hospitals;
Stage 4: Pediatric surgery as an independent discipline in its own right.

This chapter then relates the history of the German Society of Pediatric Surgery and the coming of age of pediatric surgery as a completely independent discipline, in which there are now 55 pediatric surgical units in the Federal Republic of Germany. The publications, textbooks, and journals listed at the end of this chapter show the advance of this discipline.

Résumé

La chirurgie infantile, au sens moderne du terme, est une discipline toute récente et ce n'est qu'au milieu de notre siècle que des services de chirurgie des enfants commencèrent à être installés dans les cliniques chirurgicales.

La chirurgie infantile évolua d'abord dans le cadre des hôpitaux pour enfants. L'auteur distingue quatre phases de cette évolution:

1ère phase: le pédiatre est l'opérateur;
2ème phase: le chirurgien est le consultant;
3ème phase: services de chirurgie infantile dans les hôpitaux pour enfants;
4ème phase: la chirurgie infantile est devenue une discipline indépendante.

Ce chapitre relate ensuite l'histoire de l'Association Allemande de Chirugie Infantile et insiste sur le fait qu'il s'agit maintenant d'une spécialité parfaitement indépendante qui compte à l'heure actuelle 55 services de chirurgie infantile en République Fédérale d'Allemagne. Enfin, l'auteur traite des publications, manuels et journaux qui apportent la preuve de l'indépendance et du dynamisme de la chirurgie infantile.

Zusammenfassung

Kinderchirurgie, wie wir sie heute verstehen, ist eine sehr junge Fachrichtung, und es wurden erst in der Mitte unseres Jahrhunderts Abteilungen für Kinderchirurgie an chirurgischen Kliniken eingerichtet.

Die Kinderchirurgie entwickelte sich anfangs innerhalb der Kinderkrankenhäuser. Der Autor unterscheidet 4 Entwicklungsphasen:

Phase 1: der Kinderarzt als Chirurg;
Phase 2: der Chirurg als Konsiliarius;
Phase 3: kinderchirurgische Abteilungen an Kinderkrankenhäusern;
Phase 4: Kinderchirurgie als selbständiges Fach.

Es wird dann über die Geschichte der Deutschen Gesellschaft für Kinderchirurgie und die Anerkennung als völlig selbständiges Fach mit jetzt 55 kinderchirurgischen Abteilungen in der BRD berichtet. Am Schluß werden Veröffentlichungen, Lehrbücher und Zeitschriften erwähnt, die alle von der Selbständigkeit und der Vitalität des Faches zeugen.

The History of Pediatric Surgery in France*

J. PRÉVOT[1]

As surgeons knew of neither anesthesia nor resuscitation, and as adequate materials and techniques of operating visceral lesions were unknown, the first developments in pediatric surgery only concerned the treatment of congenital or acquired orthopedic lesions.

In 1741, Nicolas Andry, counsellor of King Louis XV, lecturer and teacher at the Royal College, regent and first dean of the medical faculty of Paris, published a book entitled *Orthopedics or the Art of Preventing and Correcting the Deformities of the Body in Children by Means that Are Within the Father's and the Mother's Capabilities as well as Any People who Bring Up Children* [1] (Figs. 1–3).

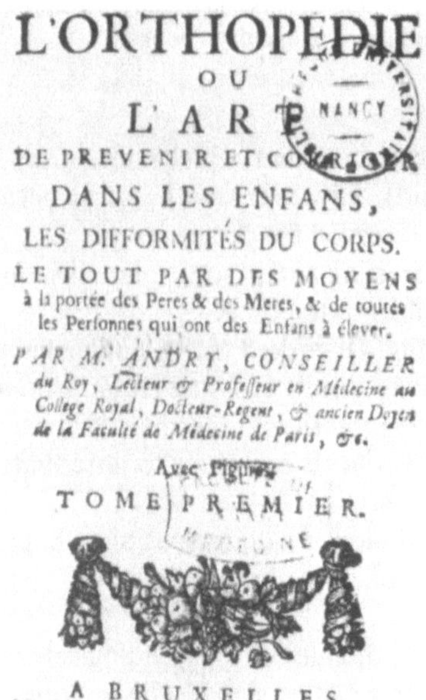

L'ORTHOPEDIE
OU
L'ART
DE PREVENIR ET CORRIGER
DANS LES ENFANS,
LES DIFFORMITÉS DU CORPS.
LE TOUT PAR DES MOYENS
à la portée des Peres & des Meres, & de toutes
les Personnes qui ont des Enfans à élever.
PAR M. ANDRY, CONSEILLER
du Roy, Lecteur & Professeur en Médecine au
College Royal, Docteur-Regent, & ancien Doyen
de la Faculté de Médecine de Paris, &c.
Avec Figures.
TOME PREMIER.
A BRUXELLES,
Chez GEORGE FRICX, Imprimeur de
Sa Majesté. 1743.
Avec Privilege de Sa Majesté.

Fig. 1. Title page of Andry's book

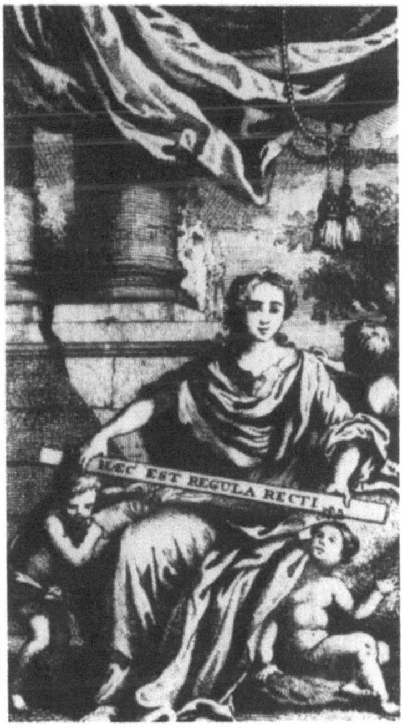

Fig. 2. Frontispiece of Andry's book

* Based on a lecture given at the Greek Pediatric Surgical Association, Chios, 1983

[1] Hôpital d'Enfants, F-54511 Vandeouvre Cédex, France

Progress in Pediatric Surgery, Vol. 20
Ed. by P. P. Rickham

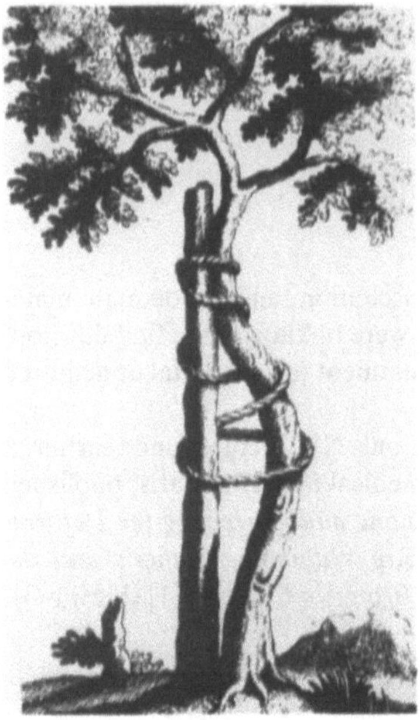

Fig. 3. The famous illustration of the correction of the crooked tree from Andry's book

It was therefore Andry who invented the word orthopedics, which comes from the Greek words *orthos* (straight) and *pais* (child). However, as the term became more and more widespread, it was no longer reserved for pediatrics.

The two volumes of Andry's book are interesting and in some places picturesque. The author often refers to beliefs and habits of the time.

More than a century later Guersant [4] (Fig. 4) worked along similar lines in Paris, publishing in 1864 a work 398 pages in length entitled *Notes About Pediatric Surgery* (Fig. 5). This book was translated into English and German and was accepted as an authorative work in the medical world. It is curious to note that the English translation is 30 pages shorter than the original French work!

Guersant's book is not another collection of picturesque recipes of orthopedic customs, as Andry's work was, but a real textbook on pediatric surgery, the larger part concerning itself with visceral affections.

The author already refers to the importance of children's psychological training and to ways to immobilize them in order to practice short interventions. He stresses the importance of an anesthesia by chloroform. This type of anesthesia was used in France until 1946, that is to say for more than a hundred years. Concerning postoperative care, he recommends giving water or mother's milk to the patient rapidly after the operation. The interventions were carried out at home rather than in a hospital. At that time the conditions of hospitalization were very bad and interventions carried out at home gave better results.

The pathology studied in Guersant's book is vast and various. He describes the use of tracheotomy for croup and recommends draining cervical adenitis and

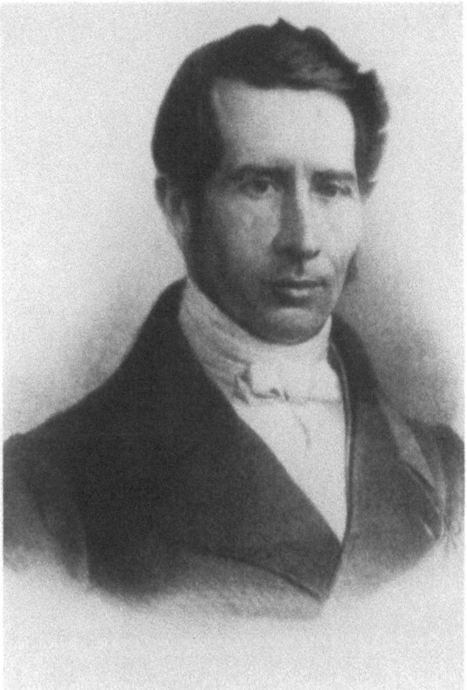

Fig. 4. P. Guersant

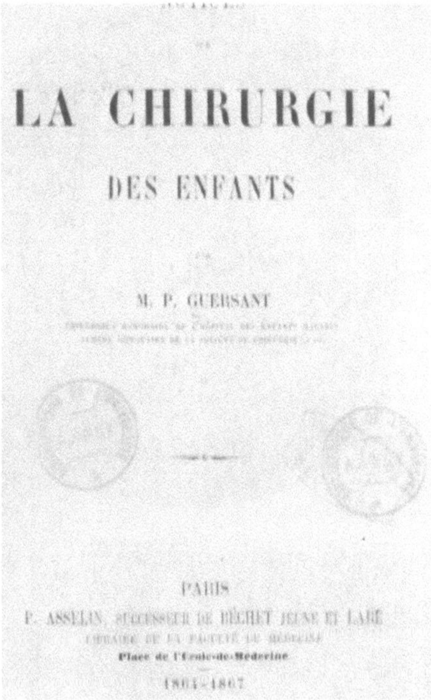

LA CHIRURGIE

DES ENFANTS

M. P. GUERSANT

PARIS

P. ASSELIN, SUCCESSEUR DE BÉCHET JEUNE ET LABÉ

1864–1867

Fig. 5. Title page of Guersant's book

extracting stones from the bladder by lithotrity after the age of five; before this age it was necessary to incise the perineum. Complications such as peritonitis must be treated by applying leeches and Neapolitan ointment. An infusion of roses in wine is used to treat hydroceles. Cleft lip is operated using needles for approximation, and rectal prolapse is treated by cauterization with red hot irons.

The classification of bone affections is still confused in Guersant's book. Tuberculosis and syphilis already have an important place. The expressions "vertebral caries" and "necrosis of the bones" are used for all infections, from osteomyelitis to a cold abscess. Hypospadias is not treated by surgery for, according to the author, "some congenital malformations must be left without trying to attempt dangerous cures."

Although without radiology, knowledge of bacteria or any idea of asepsis, Guersant was a pioneer in pediatric surgery and the translation of his book into several languages pays homage to his genius.

Pediatric Surgery Studies is the title of a book published in 1905 and authored by Froehlich from Nancy [3] (Fig. 6; see also Fig. 7). It dealt exclusively with visceral surgery. This book shows some progress compared with Guersant's. It recommends early surgical treatment of inguinal and strangulated hernia, but it still does not recognize intestinal intussusception.

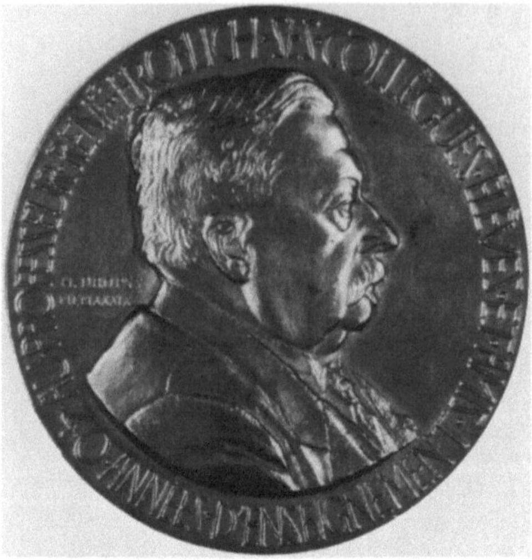

Fig. 6. A. Froehlich

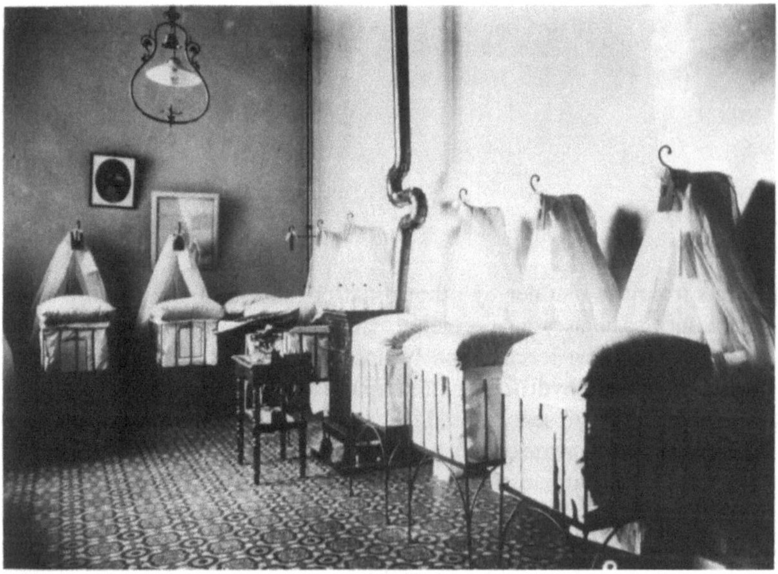

Fig. 7. A children's ward in 1905

In 1906, Kirmisson [5] (Fig. 8; from Paris) published his pediatric surgical textbook. In this book the first appearance of radiology can be found. The pathology of the omphalomesenteric duct and some other congenital malformations is described (Figs. 9 and 10), and osteomyelitis is given its proper name. A logical explanation is given explaining cervical fistulas. Kirmisson achieves real progress, which was continued in 1914 by Auguste Broca [2] (Fig. 11) who, in a pediatric surgical textbook more than one hundred pages in length, gathered all that was

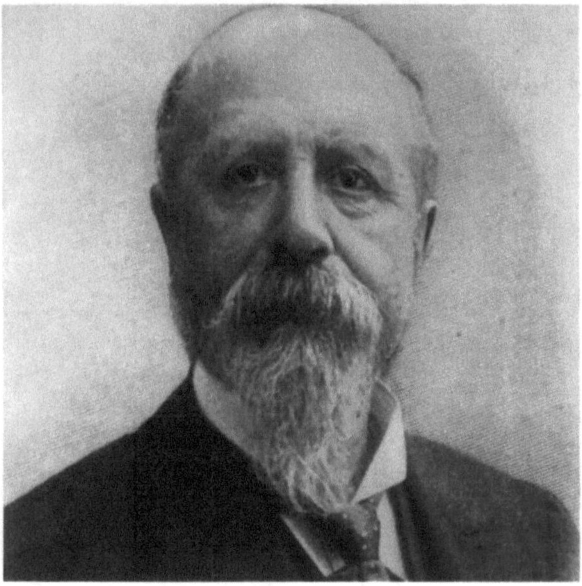

Fig. 8. E. Kirmisson

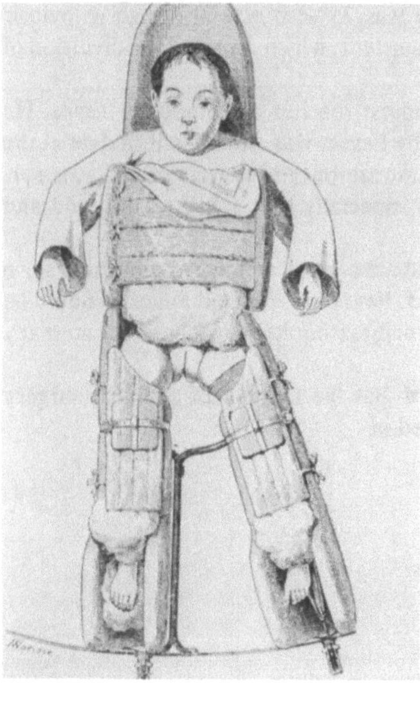

Fig. 9. Splinting of a child with Pott's disease (from Kirmisson's book)

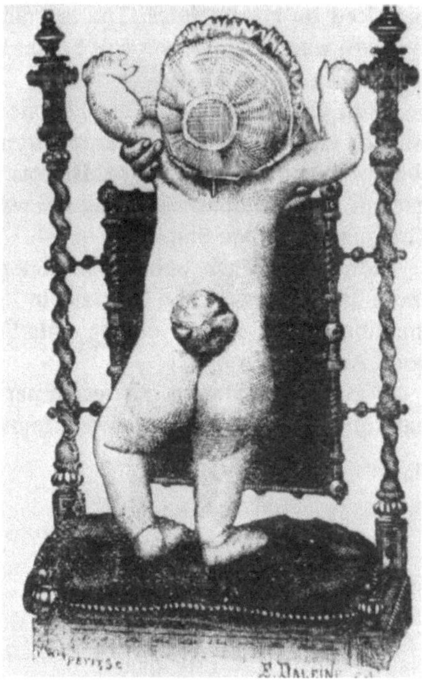

Fig. 10. Spina bifida (from Kirmisson's book)

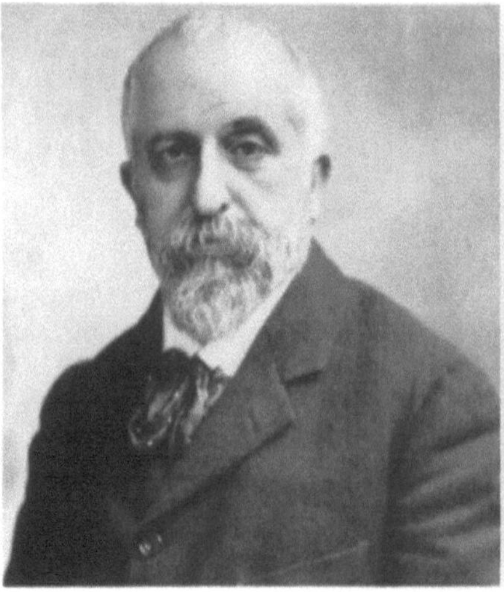

Fig. 11. A. Broca

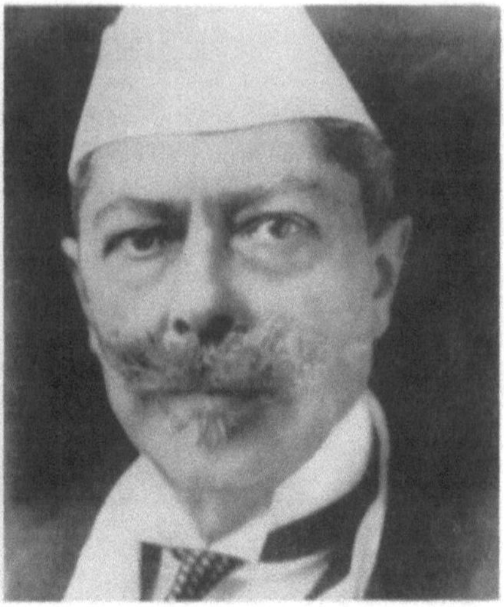

Fig. 12. L. Ombredanne

known in the world on this subject. The description of past treatments of megacolon is enlarged upon, intussusception is described with many details as is its treatment with hydrostatic enemata which, according to the author, was already practiced by Hyppocrates. The mortality was 75%; it was also high in pyloric stenosis, where the operation of Fredet Ramstedt, which replaced the divulsion of Loreta, is referred to.

With Ombredanne [6] (Fig. 12) one almost reaches contemporary times. He was self taught. His book, later rewritten by Fevre, was already out of date at the time of its publication in 1944. He was unaware of the progress in pediatric surgery in foreign countries during the war, especially that achieved by Ladd and Gross in the United States.

Although French publications on pediatric surgery have diminished since those times, the works by Duhamel in 1953, Fevre in 1958, and Pellerin should be mentioned. It is a pity, yet why write French textbooks when there are so many good American books?

It is precisely during this recent period that the number of pediatric surgery have grown in France. Chairs were founded in:

Paris	1901	Kirmisson
Bordeaux	1907	Piechaud
Lille	1907	Phocas
Montpellier	1908	Forgue
Lyon	1912	Nove Josserand
Nancy	1919	Froehlich

Many have followed. Rich with its past, proud in the present, French pediatric surgery must go on trying to find a precise identity.

Summary

In 1741, Nicolas Andry, counsellor of King Louis XV, published a book about "orthopedics," inventing this word. The book is interesting as the author refers to beliefs and habits of the time. In 1864, Guersant published *Notes About Pediatric Surgery,* a real textbook which was translated into English and German and dealt with the importance of children's psychological training, anesthesia, and water or mother's milk after the operation, and also described tracheotomy, draining of cervical adenitis, and lithotrity. The classification of bone affections was still very confused. Tuberculosis and syphilis have an important place; hypospadias is not treated by surgery.

In 1905, Froehlich published *Pediatric Surgery Studies* dealing exclusively with visceral surgery and demonstrating progress compared to Guersant's study. In 1906, Kirmisson published *Pediatric Surgical Textbook,* containing the first discussion of radiology and the description of the pathology of the omphalomesenteric duct and of other congenital malformations. Osteomyelitis was given its proper name, and cervical fistulas were explained. In 1914, A. Broca achieved further progress describing treatments of megacolon, intussusception, and the operation of Fredet Ramstedt. The book by Ombredanne, already out of date at the time of its publication, showed that he was not aware of the wartime, progress achieved by Ladd and Gross in the USA. French publications have diminished since then, and French pediatric surgery is still trying to find a precise identity.

Résumé

En 1741, le conseiller du roi Louis XV, Nicolas Andry, publia un ouvrage intitulé "Orthopédie". Le terme est resté. Cet ouvrage est d'un grand intérêt et informe le lecteur sur les croyances et coutumes d'alors. En 1864, Guersant publia les "Notices sur la chirurgie des enfants". Cet ouvrage a été traduit en anglais et en allemand et traite des sujets suivants: importance de la préparation sur le plan psychologique des enfants devant subir une intervention, anesthésie, alimentation des jeunes opérés après l'opération, eau et lait maternel, trachéotomie, drainage des lymphadénites, lithotritie. La classification des maladies osseuses reste vague. Tuberculose et syphilis jouent un grand rôle. Pas de traitement chirurgical de l'hypospadias. En 1905, Froehlich publie "Etudes de chirurgie infantile". Cet ouvrage traite uniquement de la chirurgie du mésentère et constitue un progrès par rapport à l'ouvrage de Guersant. En 1906, Kirmisson publie son "Précis de chirurgie infantile". Pour la première fois, il est question de radiologie. Il y traite aussi de la pathologie du canal omphalomésentérique et d'autres malformations. L'ostéomyélite est bien définie et on y trouve des explications sur les fistules congénitales. En 1915, A. Broca réussit à traiter le mégacolon, l'invagination et la sténose du pylore. Le livre publié par Ombredanne était déjà dépassé lors de sa parution et prouve que son auteur n'était pas au courant des progrès réalisés aux Etats-Unis par Ladd et Gross. Depuis, les publications françaises sont rares et la chirurgie infantile en France est encore à la recherche d'une identité propre.

Zusammenfassung

1741 veröffentlichte der Berater Königs Ludwigs XV., Nicolas André (engl. auch: Andry), ein Buch über *Orthopädie* und prägte somit das Wort. Das Buch ist sehr interessant, denn es gibt Auskunft über die damaligen Überzeugungen und Bräuche. 1864 erschienen Guersant's *Notices sur la chirurgie des enfants.* Das Buch wurde ins Englische und ins Deutsche übersetzt; folgende Themen wurden darin behandelt: Bedeutung der psychologischen Vorbereitung von Kindern vor den Eingriffen, Anästhesie, Verabreichung von Wasser oder Muttermilch nach dem Eingriff, Tracheotomie, Drainage der Halslymphadenitis und Lithotripsie (frz. „lithotritie“). Die Klassifizierung der Knochenkrankheiten war immer noch recht verworren. Tuberkulose und Syphilis spielten eine große Rolle. Hypospadie wurde nicht chirurgisch behandelt. 1905 publizierte Froehlich *Études de chirurgie infantile;* darin wurde ausschließlich die Mesenteriumchirurgie behandelt. Das Werk stellte aber einen Fortschritt gegenüber Guersant dar.

In dem *Précis de chirurgie infantile* von Kirmisson (1906) wurde zum ersten Mal die Radiologie behandelt. Die Pathologie des Ductus omphalomesentericus und andere angeborene Mißbildungen wurden beschrieben, die Osteomyelitis richtig bezeichnet, und Halsfisteln wurden erklärt. 1915 gelangen Broca weitere Fortschritte: Behandlung von Megakolon, Invagination, Pylorusstenose. Das (bekannte) Buch von Ombrédanne war beim Erscheinen schon überholt und bewies, daß er von den Fortschritten von Ladd und Gross in den USA nichts wußte. Seitdem sind die französischen Veröffentlichungen noch seltener geworden, und die französische Kinderchirurgie ist noch auf der Suche nach einer eigenen Identität.

References

1. Andry N (1741) L'orthopédie ou l'art de prévenir et de corriger dans les enfants, les difformités du corps. La Veuve Alix, Paris
2. Broca A (1914) Chiurgie infantile. Steinheil, Paris
3. Froehlich R (1905) Etudes de chirurgie infantile. Maloine, Paris
4. Guersant PLB (1861) Notices sur la chirurgie des enfants. Asselin, Paris
5. Kirmisson E (1906) Précis de chirurgie infantile. Masson, Paris
6. Ombredanne L (1944) Précis clinique et opératoire de chirurgie infantile. Masson, Paris

100 Years of Pediatric Surgery in Stockholm, with Personal Memories from the Last 50 Years

T. Ehrenpreis[1]

Recognition of the specific nature of children's diseases dates back to the middle of the 18th century. Nils Rosén von Rosenstein (1706–1773), the "Father of Pediatrics", was one of the two professors of medicine at the University of Uppsala. In 1764 Rosén published the first comprehensive textbook in Swedish on *Diseases in Childhood and Their Treatment.*

In 1802, the first children's hospital (Hôpital des Enfants Malades in Paris) was founded by Napoleon. During the mid-nineteenth century a number of children's hospitals were established, e.g., Nicolai Children's Hospital, St. Petersburg, St. Annenspital, Vienna, The Children's Hospital, Budapest, The Hospital for Sick Children, Great Ormond Street, London, and The Children's Hospital, Boston. The majority of these hospitals were later subdivided into medical and surgical departments. The first textbooks on surgical problems in childhood were published around the middle of the nineteenth century in England and France.

In Sweden the first hospital for children, Kronprinsessan Lovisas Children's Hospital, was established in Stockholm in 1854. This was a small hospital comprising 30 beds, which soon proved to be quite insufficient, and in 1859 the hospital was enlarged to 60 beds. No surgical beds or facilities for surgery were available. The professor of general surgery at the nearby University Hospital served as a surgical consultant.

In 1885, the "Lovisa Hospital" was divided into separate medical and surgical units. This constituted the birth of pediatric surgery in Sweden. The professor of general surgery continued to serve as consultant surgeon. In 1892 an independant head of pediatric surgery was appointed. In 1899 entirely new buildings for the Lovisa Hospital, comprising about 75 medical and 75 surgical beds, were completed (Fig. 1). This hospital served its purpose for 70 years. In 1970 the hospital was transferred to separate buildings at the St. Göran's Hospital in Stockholm (Fig. 2).

A second children's hospital was established in Gothenburg in 1859. Originally consisting of a small unit of 12 beds, it was later considerably enlarged and subdivided into medical and surgical departments. More than 50 years elapsed before a third department of pediatric surgery was established. In 1952, the children's clinic at the Karolinska University Hospital in Stockholm was opened (Fig. 3). In 1960, pediatric surgery was introduced as a subdivision of the surgical department at the University Hospital of Uppsala, later (1968) to be converted into an inde-

[1] Ljuskarrsv 92, S-13300 Saltsjobaden, Sweden

Progress in Pediatric Surgery, Vol. 20
Ed. by P. P. Rickham

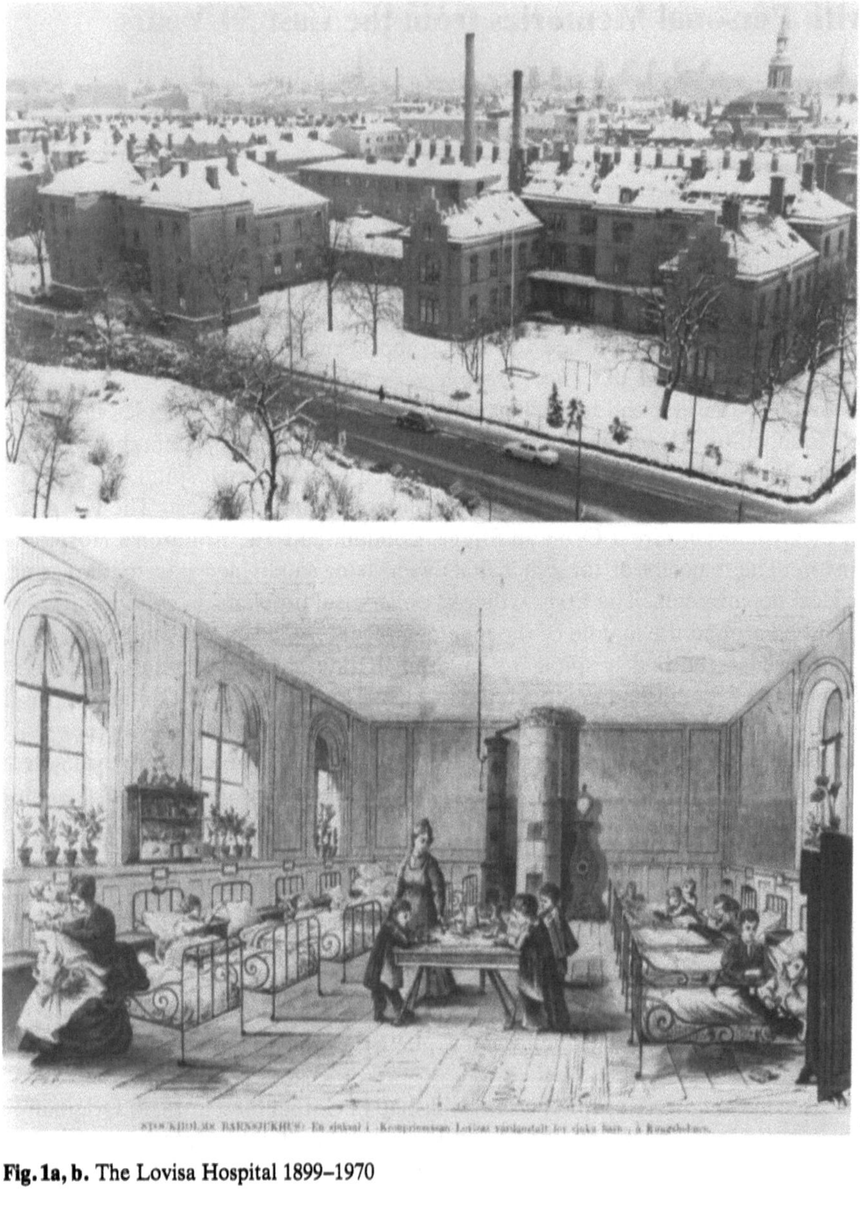

a

b

Fig. 1a, b. The Lovisa Hospital 1899–1970

pendant department. In 1969, a fourth department of pediatric surgery was established at the University Hospital of Lund. Subdivisions for pediatric surgery instituted at the University Hospitals of Malmö and Linköping increased the number of pediatric surgical units in Sweden (population 8.3 million) to seven. No further units have been planned for the near future.

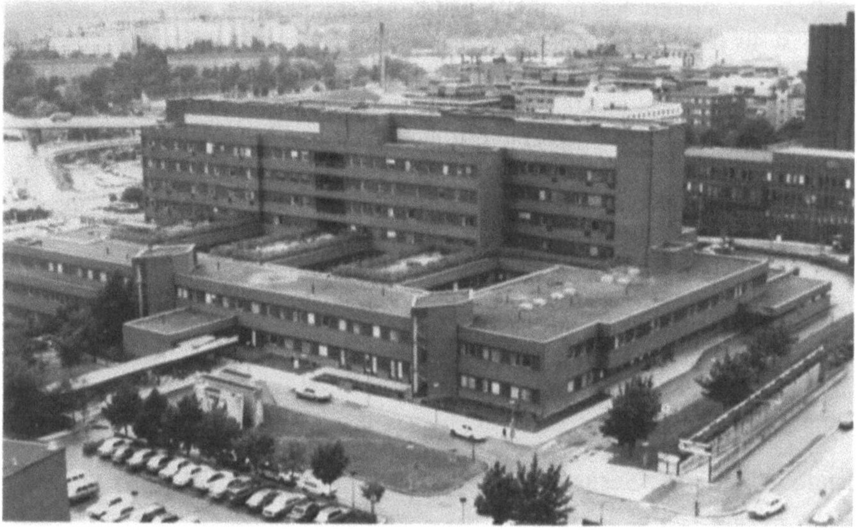

Fig. 2. Children's Clinic, St. Görans Hospital

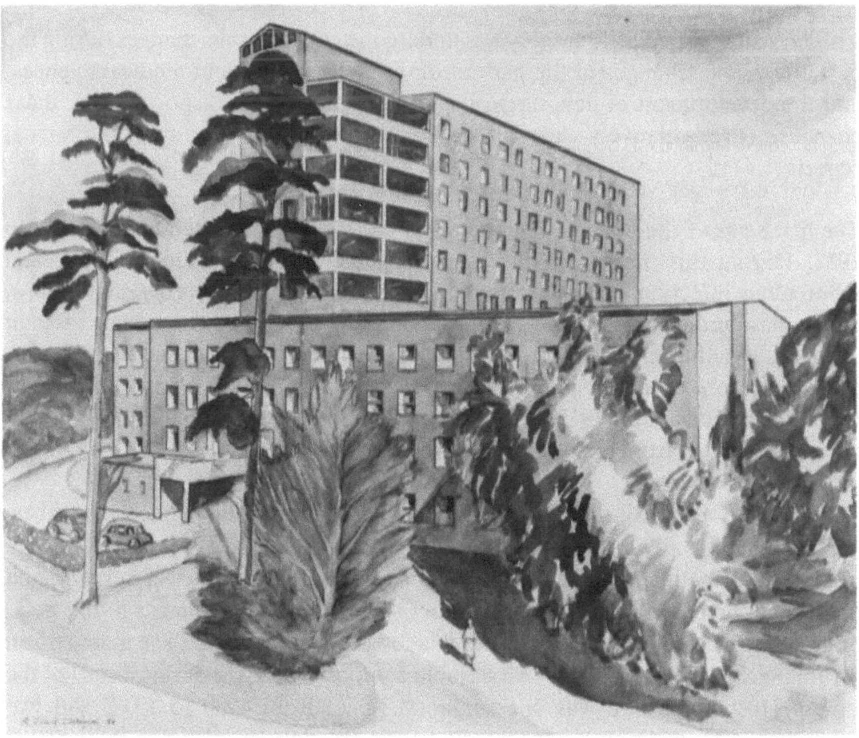

Fig. 3. Children's Clinic, Karolinska Hospital

Pediatric Surgery has been included in undergraduate teaching programs for the past 40 years. Comprehensive chapters on pediatric surgery have been included in Scandinavian textbooks on pediatrics and surgery.

In the late 1950s, a personal associate professorship in pediatric urology was instituted for N. O. Ericsson at the Karolinska Medical School in Stockholm. Following his retirement in 1976, this personal chair was converted into an established professorate in pediatric surgery – the first in Scandinavia. In addition to this full-time appointment, about 15 pediatric surgeons in Sweden have an affiliation with medical schools as assistant professors.

Pediatric surgery has been recognized as an independent specialty by the Swedish Medical Association since 1947.

These are, in brief, some of the significant milestones in the development of our specialty in Sweden.

Scope of Pediatric Surgery in Sweden

In order to study the development of pediatric surgery in Sweden over the years, a survey was made of the annual reports of the Lovisa Hospital from 1885 to 1969. The developments at the children's hospital in Gothenburg have followed a similar pattern.

The scope of pediatric surgery has undergone considerable changes during the past 100 years. Changes in the pattern of diseases, progress in medical sciences, and the development of new surgical specialities have been responsible for these changes. Three relatively clear-cut stages emerge from the study of the annual reports.

The first stage – the birth and "infancy" of our specialty – extends from 1885 to 1932. During this period the disease panorama was dominated by septic and tuberculous infections of bones, joints, lymph glands, and the urogenital organs, empyemas, and diseases of the ear, nose, and throat (ENT). Only a few cases of congenital malformations were reported, mainly cleft lips and palates, club feet, and dislocations of the hip joint. The first successful operation for an intestinal atresia was performed in 1913. The bulk of general surgery in childhood was still performed in departments of general surgery.

The second stage (1932–1945) is characterized by a decreasing incidence of tuberculous infections, by a successive transfer of orthopedic and ENT patients to the newly established (1912–1913) departments of orthopedic and ENT surgery, and by a rapid increase in the volume of general surgery. These changes in the trend of activities started in the 1920s but took a long time to develop. The main reason for this seems to have been the very stable composition of the surgical staff of the Lovisa Hospital. There was one surgeon-in-chief from 1900 to 1932, and two associate surgeons, who seem to have been very slow in changing their accustomed routines. With a new chief surgeon, Einar Perman, appointed in 1932, the earlier trend changed into a rapid development. A marked increase also occurred in the volume of malformation surgery, mainly cleft lips and palates, and abdominal neonatal surgery. This was enhanced by the organized centralization of the treatment of congenital anomalies from a major part of Sweden at the Lovisa Hospital, by the excellent work of pediatric consultants at the major maternity units, and by the increasing attendance (more than 90% of all infants and small children) at the child welfare centers.

Having achieved his aim to convert the Lovisa department into a purely surgical department, Perman returned to general surgery in 1939. His successor was another promising general surgeon, James Hindmarsh who led the department on along the course set by his predecessor. His particular interest was Hirschsprung's disease. He introduced lumbar sympathectomy in Sweden, which brought new hope to many parents and doctors, and the number of patients referred to the department from all over the country rapidly increased. Unfortunately, the results soon proved to be very disappointing. The career of this excellent man was ended by his untimely death in 1945.

Hindmarsh was succeeded by a very promising general surgeon, Philip Sandblom, as chief surgeon of the department. The year was 1945, the war had ended, and the 6 years of isolation from the rest of the world were finally broken. This brought about a rapid and dramatic development of pediatric surgery in Sweden – the third stage, which is still in progress.

Sandblom started his work by acting as an assistant for the first 3 months of his appointment. He attended ward rounds, assisted at operations, and read a lot of the literature, which began to inundate Sweden after the end of the war. He then went to the U.S.A. for 3 months, visiting the leading centers of pediatric surgery, before returning to take up his appointment. The main advance was the possibility of opening the thoracic cavity for surgery. Congenital anomalies of the heart and great vessels, the esophagus, and the diaphragm now became accessible to surgical repair. Another important addition to our armamentorium was the introduction of experimental surgery, for scientific as well as practical purposes. Before using the new intrathoracic operations on patients they were tried and trained on a number of dogs. These new operations soon became an important part of our work.

A couple of years later, rectosigmoidectomy was introduced for the treatment of Hirschsprung's disease, again increasing the volume of surgery in neonates and infants.

The Sandblom era – the most dynamic and stimulating in the history of pediatric surgery in Sweden – unfortunately was of short duration. In 1950, Sandblom was offered the Chair of General Surgery at the University of Lund, which he accepted after some hesitation – he had enjoyed the dramatic development of pediatric surgery as much as his staff.

He was succeeded by the present author, which marked a new milestone in the recognition of pediatric surgery in Sweden. All previous heads of the Lovisa department had been general surgeons. From then on, only pediatric surgeons have been considered qualified for these posts.

In 1952, I was appointed as head of the surgical department of the new children's clinic at the Karolinska University Hospital and was succeeded at the Lovisa Hospital by Gunnar Ekström, who had acted as an associate head of the department for 5 years. In order to maintain the experience needed for treatment of complicated and relatively rare anomalies, a subdivision of activities in such fields between the two departments was organized. During the Sandblom period, a well-functioning team of surgeons, cardiologists, roentgenologists, and anesthesiologists had been established at the Lovisa Hospital. It was thus obvious that cardiovascular anomalies should be concentrated at that hospital. For administrative reasons, the Lovisa Hospital, being a county hospital, had to take the major responsibility for patients from the Stockholm area. The Karolinska Hospital was a state hospital serving a minor part of the Stockholm area, but also admitting specific cases from a major part of Sweden, with a population of approximately 5 million. We thus had to take care of the load of neonatal surgery, cleft lip and palate surgery, and specific abdominal surgery (Hirschsprung's disease, ulcerative colitis, Crohn's disease). In order to improve the rather under-developed situation of pediatric urology, a qualified general surgeon and urologist, Nils Olof Ericsson, was offered the position as associate head of the department of pediatric surgery at the Karolinska Hospital and also served as a consultant to the Lovisa Hospital (Figs. 4–5).

The period of the three E's (Ehrenpreis, Ekström, Ericsson) came to extend over nearly 25 years, the three of us retiring in 1974, 1974, and 1976 respectively. Development during this period was not as dramatic as during the Sandblom period. the most spectacular progress was achieved by Ericsson in the field of pediatric urology, bringing this specialty into the frontlines of international standards with the close cooperation with pediatric nephrologists and roentgenologists [1]. Progress was further achieved by the establishment of a team of pediatricians, pediatric surgeons, and radiologists from the Karolinska Oncology Center for the total care of pediatric malignancies.

A new principle for the treatment of cleft lips and palates was elaborated by Carl-Erik Nordin [2], an orthodontic surgeon, in collaboration with pediatric and plastic surgeons. The concept presented to us by Nordin was that it should be easier to prevent constriction and underdevelopment of the maxilla and palate by preoperative expansion and stabilization than by postoperative correction of the deformity. This proved to be the case, and the results achieved were spectacular [3].

An important contribution in the field of neonatal surgery was made by Ludvig Okmian [4]. In order to prevent the development of a sometimes fatal hypoxia during prolonged respirator anesthesia and postoperative artificial respiration in neonates and infants, extensive experimental, clinical, and laboratory studies were undertaken. This resulted in the adaptation of a new shunt and valve mechanism and a new monogram for the Engström respirator, suitable for this age group. A new and sensationally simple method for bridging long gaps between the two ends of the esophagus in esophageal atresia was devised by Alexander Livaditis on the basis of a large series of animal experiments [5]. The method [6] con-

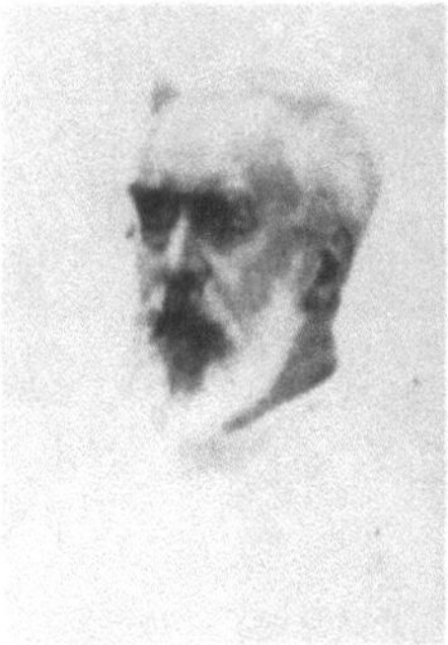

John Berg
1886–1892

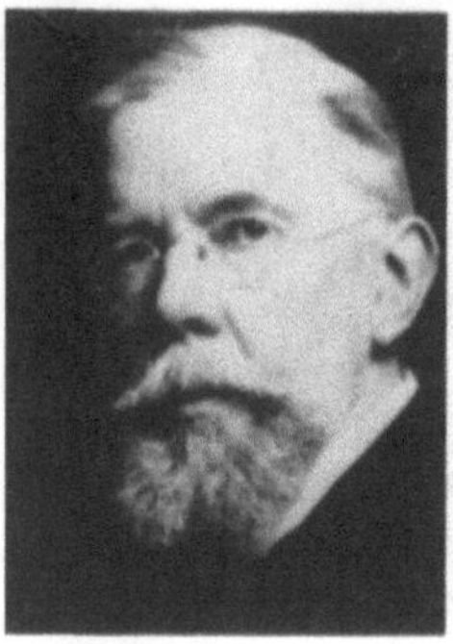

Emil Perman
1892–1899

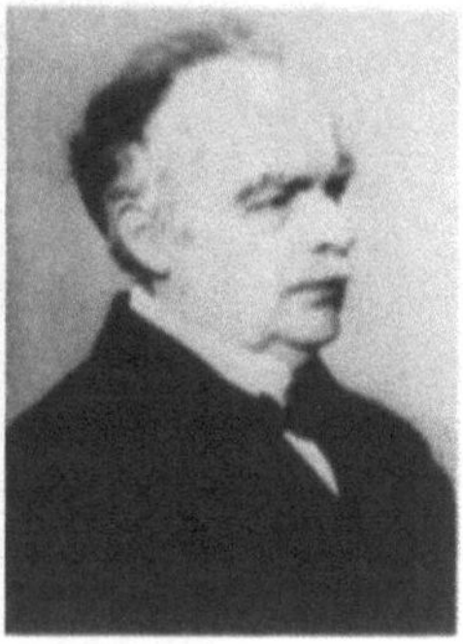

B. Floderus
1900–1932

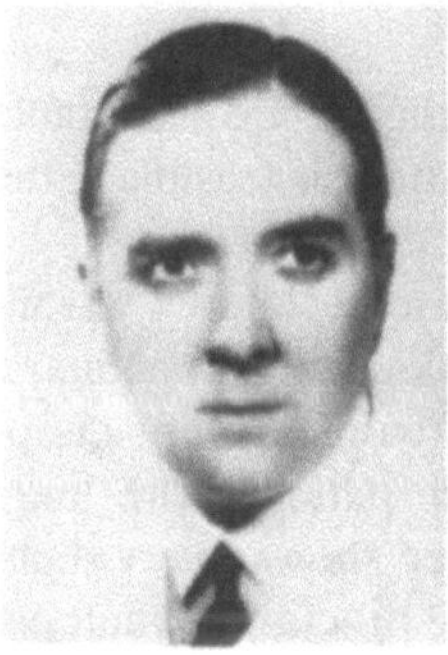

Einar Perman
1932–1939

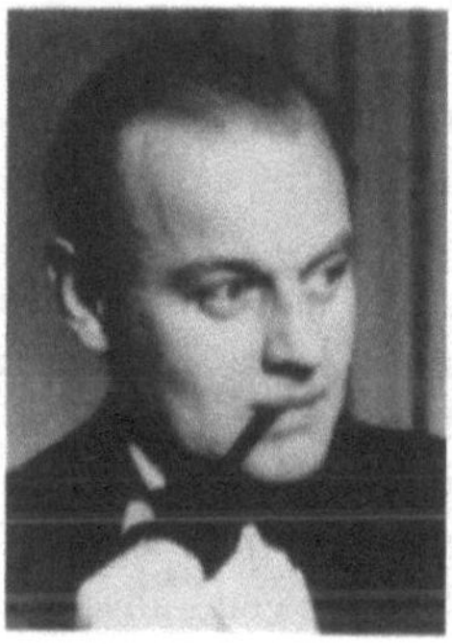

J. Hindmarsch
1940–1945

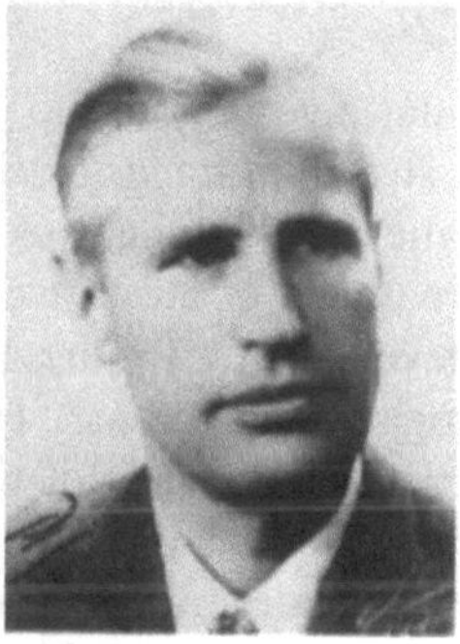

P. H. Sandblom
1945–1950

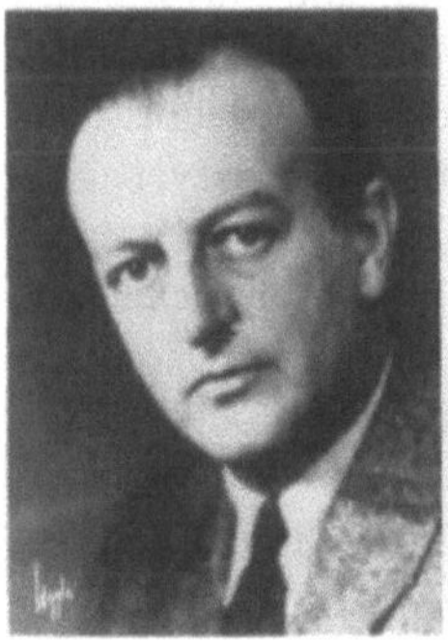

T. Ehrenpreis
1950–1951

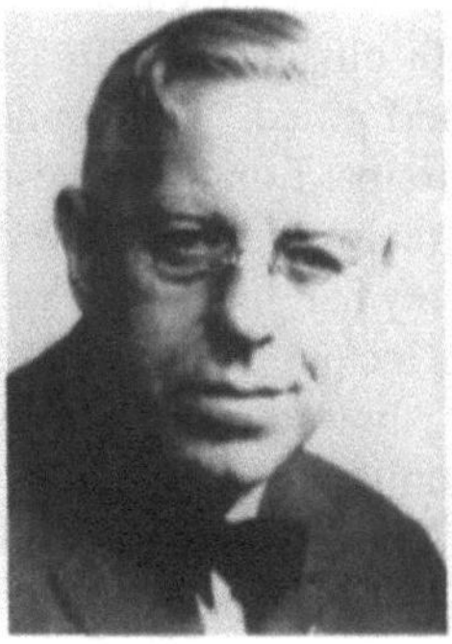

G. Ekström
1952–1974

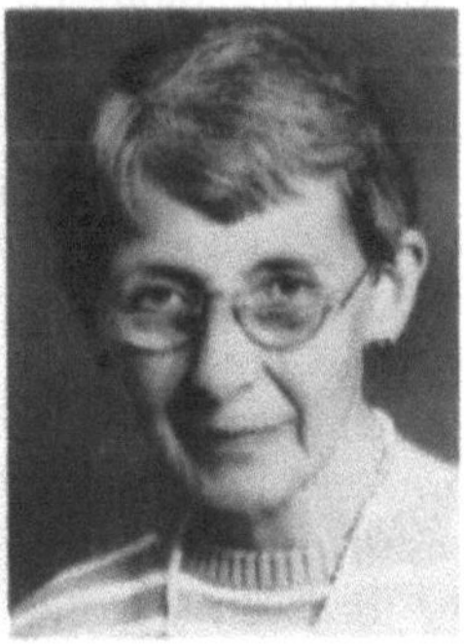

S. Söderlund
1974–

Fig. 4. Chief surgeons, Lovisa/St. Görans Hospital

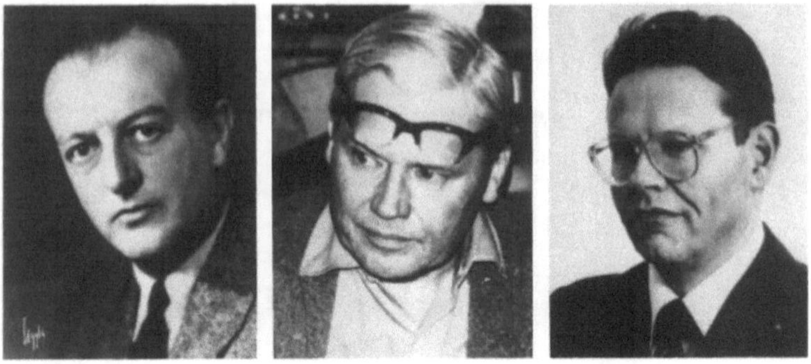

T. Ehrenpreis 1952–1974 | N. O. Ericsson 1974–1976 | B. Thomasson 1976–

Fig. 5. Chief surgeons, Karolinska Hospital

sists of a circular myotomy of the proximal segment, allowing for a considerable increase in its stretching capacity, thus making a direct anastomosis feasible in the majority of patients with long gaps.

Surgical treatment of ulcerative colitis and Crohn's disease in children was instituted and developed by T. Ehrenpreis [7] in close cooperation with our pediatric gastroenterologist, Lagercrantz. He had found medical treatment very disappointing, particularly in view of the incidence of cancer in patients with longstanding disease. He had also observed that the rectum often showed very slight or no changes in children, in contrast to the generally severe proctitis in adult patients. Our starting point was, therefore, to remove the entire colon and perform an ileorectal anastomosis in patients with minimal changes in the rectum; when in doubt, we removed the colon, left the closed rectum behind, and performed a temporary ileostomy. In patients with obvious proctitis, a pan proctoedectomy with a permanent ileostomy was performed. The immediate and short-term results were promising in all three groups. Long-term results [8], however, convinced us that the rectum should be removed in all these patients; those treated by a pan proctoedectomy and ileostomy had fared very well, both physically and psychologically, while those where the rectum had been left, whether anastomosed to the ileum or "temporarily" closed, showed progressive signs of proctitis, forcing us to perform secondary proctectomies.

At the Lovisa Hospital (since 1970 at St. Görans Hospital) the main interest continued to be focused on cardiovascular surgery. Improved surgical and anesthesiological methods permitted operations on infants and even neonates, when required. The number of patients increased, and results improved over the years.

Much of the history of pediatric surgery in Sweden is reflected in the writings of its surgeons. In the early years, G. Holmgren [9] (1908) and H. Waldenström [10] (1910) published important contributions in the fields of otolaryngology and orthopedic surgery, respectively, based upon studies of their patients at the Lovisa Hospital. Both authors eventually became professors of their recently introduced specialties at the Karolinska Medical School. More recently, increasing interest has been focused on the specific surgical problems in childhood. A number of pediatric surgical monographs and other major studies have been published [11–25]. The subjects of these studies are evident from their titles, given in the reference list.

In 1955, a major investigation of all childhood accidents occurring in the Stockholm area during one year was undertaken. This was a joint venture of the two departments of pediatric surgery. The results, published (in Swedish) in 1957 [26], constituted the first analysis ever made concerning incidence, age and sex distribution, place of accident, types of injuries, etc. and proved to be of great value in the planning of preventive measures [27]. Surgeons from both departments took active part in the work of the Swedish Joint Committee for the Prevention of Childhood Accidents, established in 1954. This proved to be a very rewarding exercise and resulted in a decrease in children's accident mortality by 50% between 1954 and 1980 [28].

The British Association of Pediatric Surgeons (BAPS)

It would be utterly wrong to finish this short survey of the development of pediatric surgery in Sweden without acknowledging the enormous stimulus derived from the founding and continued activities of the BAPS. In November 1953, a meeting was held at the Hospital for Sick Children in London with Denis Browne as chairman. It was decided "to form a Society of Surgeons in Great Britain interested in pediatric surgery" and to include overseas members. In the early 1950s there were only 50–60 pediatric surgeons in the entire world (Fig. 6). They were all approached, and the majority of them became members from the start. In 1981, the Association had grown into a large international body consisting of some 650 members, a hundred of whom worked in the United Kingdom, the rest being overseas members from about 60 different countries. From 1961, the annual meetings were held outside the U.K. every third year. We were greatly honored in being invited to arrange the first of these overseas meetings in Stockholm in 1961.

Prior to the establishment of the BAPS, pediatric surgeons in each country were rather isolated in medical surroundings which were only moderately interested in our problems and could offer little help in their solution. At the annual meetings we were suddenly surrounded by a big family, talking the same language and both willing and able to help – a wonderfully stimulating feeling. The contacts and friendships made during these meetings virtually opened the doors to pediatric surgeons all over the world for studies and for exchange of experiences.

The founding and the successful development of the BAPS has been a strong stimulus for the institution of national associations of pediatric surgeons in many countries. A Swedish Association was formed in 1952 and a Scandinavian Association in 1964.

This brings me to the end of this history. The present and the future – that is another story which will have to be told by our "children" or "grandchildren" in pediatric surgery.

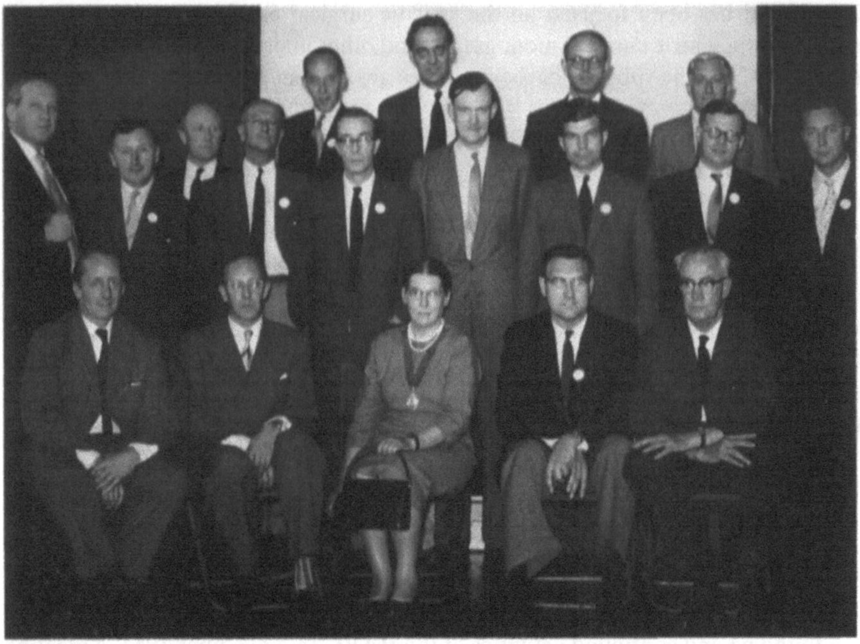

Fig. 6. Council Meeting of the BAPS, Liverpool 1959. *Sitting* (left to right): David Waterston (London), Max Grob (Zürich), Isabella Forshall (President, Liverpool), Chick Koop (Philadelphia), Denis Browne (London). *Standing* (left to right): Peter Rickham (Liverpool), Bob Zachary (Sheffield), Ian Kirkland (Edinburgh), T. Ehrenpreis (Stockholm), W. M. Dennison (Glasgow), John Johnston (Liverpool), Andrew Wilkinson (Edinburgh), A. Jolleys (Manchester), J. F. R. Bentley (Glasgow), B. T. Smyth (Belfast), V. A. J. Swain (London), H. H. Nixon (London), Barry O'Donnell (Dublin)

Personal Memories and Reflections

In 1934, a couple of years before my graduation, I was accepted as a voluntary assistant at the Department of Pediatric Surgery of the Lovisa Hospital during my three months summer vacation. I wrote the records of admitted patients, attended ward rounds, and assisted at operations. Toward the end of the summer I was allowed to perform an appendectomy under the guidance of one of the junior surgeons – a great moment in the life of a prospective surgeon.

The next summer I returned as a voluntary assistant for 6 weeks, and then replaced the junior surgeons as a locum tenens during their vacations for three months. One evening, while waiting for an appendectomy, I was sitting in the hospital library looking through a number of recent pediatric journals. I found an annual report from the Boston Children's Hospital with an introduction on the scope of pediatric surgery by William E. Ladd. This report stuck me like a revelation; it was written with such gusto and reflected such profound knowledge and understanding of our speciality and of the specific requirements of infancy and childhood that I suddenly perceived the immense possibilities and the challenge of pediatric surgery. I believe that it was there and then that I decided to go on with my training in this field – a rather adventurous enterprise, since at that time there were only two permanent positions in pediatric surgery in Sweden.

Looking back from present standards, surgical routines were rather primitive. The importance and techniques of pre- and postoperative treatment were poorly understood. Anesthesiology had not been introduced as a specialty in Sweden. Open ether narcosis was administered by nurses, as a rule providing adequate anesthesia. Facilities for isolation of children with infectious diseases were scarce. Antibiotics had not been introduced. Visiting hours were restricted to 1–2 hours on Sundays.

Prolonged periods of hospital care were the rule. Uncomplicated appendectomies were kept in bed for 2 weeks (today 2–3 days), hernia repairs 2 weeks (today 2–3 days if uncomplicated). The average time of hospital care was reduced from 17 days in 1934 to 6.5 days in 1969. In spite of poor conditions, we somehow managed to achieve fair results. The overall mortality rate successively decreased from 3% in 1934 to 0.75% in 1969. Similar improvements occurred in the more complicated fields as evidenced by two examples:

Diagnosis	*Period*	*Cases*	*Deaths*
Esophageal atresia	1952–1962	101	45 (45%)
	1963–1973	82	15 (18%)
Hirschsprung's disease	1948–1958	69	4 (5.8%)
	1959–1966	51	1 (2.0%)

Soon after my return from Great Ormond Street in 1950 I was appointed chief surgeon at the Lovisa Hospital and 1 year later to the corresponding post at the new children's clinic at the Karolinska Hospital. After 10 years service under highly respected and competent chiefs, always ready to give advice in difficult situations, I felt a bit worried to be left on my own. I soon realized that I was not alone – I was surrounded by a staff of intelligent and experienced colleagues, contributing substantially to the solutions of our problems.

Moving to the Karolinska was a challenge. This was the first unit of pediatric surgery in Sweden to be part of a large University Hospital. This opened new possibilities for cooperation with specialists in other fields as well as in research projects. We had to discuss and define border lines between pediatric surgery and other surgical specialties. ENT patients and "purely" orthopedic cases (club feet, congenital dislocations of the hip joint, etc.) were no problem. These patients had left pediatric surgery 20–30 years ago, while traumatology remained with pediatric surgeons. Cleft lips and palates remained with us for a number of years. With the introduction of preoperative orthodontic treatment these patients had to stay in our wards for prolonged periods of time, up to 6–7 months. The simultaneous development of pediatric urology and pediatric oncology, other groups of long-term patients presented us with a serious problem. Our waiting lists for elective procedures grew. Patients with hernias, cryptorchism, etc. had to wait 18–24 months for their operations. The plastic surgeons were very eager to take over the cleft lips and palates and we finally relented. Cardiac surgery was concentrated to the Lovisa Hospital while operations requiring the use of a heart-lung machine were referred to the thoracic clinic of the Karolinska Hospital. Neurosurgery was performed by the neurosurgeons with the exception of myelomeningoceles and shunt operations for hydrocephalus.

Several pediatric surgeons of my own and the previous generation (for instance, Denis Browne and my associate N. O. Ericsson) were of the opinion that a pediatric surgeon should do everything surgical in children. I have never shared this view, and I believe that the enormous development in all fields of medicine and surgery in recent decades is making it impossible for any single surgeon to cover the entire field.

We also have problems within our own specialty. The greatest challenge is presented by neonatal surgery. We now have relatively firmly established standards for diagnostic procedures, pre- and postoperative treatment (including total parenteral nutrition), and operative techniques for the various surgical emergencies in the newborn. The problems we are faced with are posed by prematurity, multiple anomalies, and complications. There are no standard solutions to these problems; they have to be dealth with on an individual basis. One standard possibility is to resort to staged procedures, which we have done in the more or less desolate cases of extreme prematurity and/or critical complications. There is no doubt that this has saved lives. There are, however, two factors which have made the use of staged procedures a rare exception in our practice. One is the fact that Sweden is a small country with a highly developed medical care and social welfare program, favoring early diagnosis and immediate transfer of neonatal emergencies to centers for adequate treatment. These patients are, as a rule, admitted within 24–48 h after birth, without pulmonary complications. The second factor favoring primary repairs is the amazing tolerance of neonates to starvation, dehydration, and prolonged major surgical procedures. Two examples:

In the late thirties, a newborn baby was admitted from a maternity hospital with an esophageal atresia. The reason was psychological but there was nothing we could do at that time. This baby took 15 days to die, very quietly, from extreme starvation and dehydration, without signs of complications.

In the mid-sixties, a full-term male baby was admitted about 10 h after birth with an esophageal atresia, a duodenal atresia, and an anal atresia with a recturethral fistula. After the repair of his esophageal atresia I asked the anesthetist how he felt about going on and he said O.K. We then performed a duodenojejunostomy for his duodenal atresia. Again I asked if we could go on. He said everything was just fine, and we agreed that it would be better to have everything done within one session than to postpone the repair of his anal atresia. We thus concluded the operation by an abdominoperineal repair, finishing about 7 h after having started on the esophagus. The condition of the baby was excellent throughout the procedure, and the postoperative course quite uneventful.

This may sound like surgical acrobatics, but I still feel that the patient was better off this way than he might have been after a number of staged procedures. The prerequisites were, of course, a perfect anesthesia and adequate pre- and postoperative treatment.

The question whether or not to perform a life-saving operation for a myelomeningocele with gross neurological defects or for a surgical emergency at birth combined with Down's syndrome has not been a problem. We decided at an early stage that we are not judges over life or death, and that we, accordingly, should confine our efforts to the surgical problem at hand.

A long life as a surgeon cannot be free from disappointments, caused by mistakes by oneself, by other members of the staff, by failed hopes for good results of a surgical method (ulcerative colitis!), or by patients not responding to adequate treatment the way we would have expected. My most macabre experience in this context: A boy of 10, the son of a diplomat from a foreign embassy in Stockholm, was admitted with a diffuse peritonitis from a perforated appendix. His postoperative course after appendectomy was stormy. During the next 4 weeks an intra-abdominal abscess was drained, another intra-abdominal abscess was drained, a pelvic abscess was drained, a subphrenic abscess was drained, and, finally, a low intestinal obstruction was relieved. At long last he recovered. Upon his discharge from the hospital, his father told me that he had been sitting at his son's bedside every night with a loaded gun in his pocket, for fear of a terrorist action. I couldn't believe that something like this could happen inside a quiet Swedish hospital, but he was serious about his fears and was not a nervous or hysterical type. Here was a boy, whose life we had been fighting to save for 4 weeks – even the slightest suspicion of someone trying to take this life was sickening.

However, the moments of disappointment are by far outweighed by the enormous satisfaction derived from the practice of childhood surgery. The expectations evoked in 1935 in a young surgeon-to-be by a report by William E. Ladd have been more than fulfilled by a development of pediatric surgery which not even Ladd could have anticipated.

Summary

The first children's hospital in Sweden (Kronprinsessan Lovisa's Children's Hospital) was established in Stockholm in 1854. In 1885 it was divided into a medical and a surgical department. This constituted the birth of pediatric surgery in Sweden.

Pediatric surgery has been included in undergraduate teaching programs since 1945. A personal Associate Professorate in Pediatric Urology was instituted at the Karolinska Medical School in Stockholm for N. O. Ericsson in the late fifties. Upon his retirement in 1976 this personal chair was converted into an established Professorship in Pediatric Surgery.

Pediatric surgery has been recognized as a specialty by our Medical Association since 1947.

A survey of the Annual Reports from the Lovisa Hospital from 1885 to 1969 shows three phases in the development of our specialty in Sweden.

The first stage extends from 1885 to 1932. During this period the disease pattern was dominated by septic and tuberculous infections, by empyemas, and by ENT diseases. Few cases of congenital malformations were reported. The bulk of general surgery in childhood was performed in the departments of general surgery.

The second stage (1932–1945) was characterized by a decreasing incidence of tuberculous infections, by a successive transfer of orthopedic and ENT patients to the Departments of Orthopedic and ENT surgery respectively. During this period, a marked increase occurred in the volume of malformation surgery. This was due to the centralized treatment of congenital anomalies.

The third stage started in 1945. The war had ended and we became acquainted with the dramatic development of pediatric surgery in other countries, in particular in the USA. The main advance was the possibility of opening the chest for repair of congenital anomalies of the heart and the great vessels, of the esophagus, and of the diaphragm. Soon afterwards, rectosigmoidectomy was introduced for the treatment of Hirschsprung's disease.

In 1952, a second department of pediatric surgery was opened in Stockholm as a part of a new Children's Clinic at the Karolinska University Hospital. The major part of general surgery from the Stockholm area and all of the cardiovascular surgery stayed with the "Lovisa Hospital", while the major part of neonatal surgery and specific abdominal surgery was performed at the Karolinska Hospital. In order to improve the rather underdeveloped situation of pediatric urology, N. O. Ericsson was appointed to the post of Associate Head of the Karolinska Department, soon bringing this field to the frontlines of international standards.

This historical review ends with some of the author's personal memories from the last 50 years.

Résumé

Le premier hôpital pour enfants en Suède, "Kronprinsessan Lovisa Klinik" fut fondé en 1854 à Stockholm. En 1885 il fut partagé en un service médical et un service de chirurgie. Ce fut le début de la chirurgie infantile en Suède.

Depuis 1945, la chirurgie infantile fait partie du programme des examens. A la fin des années 50, N. O. Ericsson fut nommé professeur sans chaire d'urologie des enfants à l'École de Médecine Karolinska à Stockholm. Quand il se retira en 1976, on créa pour le remplacer une chaire de chirurgie infantile.

En 1947, l'association médicale suédoise avait reconnu la chirurgie infantile comme discipline indépendante.

Les rapports annuels de l'hôpital Lovisa entre 1885 et 1969 font l'historique de la chirurgie infantile en Suède. On distingue trois phases:

La première va de 1885–1932. Les maladies les plus fréquentes à l'époque étaient les septicémies, la tuberculose, les empyèmes et les affections ORL. Il n'est pas question de malformations. Les interventions chirurgicales se faisaient dans le service de chirurgie générale.

La seconde phase (1932–1945) est caractérisée par une diminution des cas de tuberculose et le traitement des cas orthopédiques et ORL dans le services respectifs. A cette époque on corrige de plus en plus de malformations. Cela tient au fait que la plupart des cas sont envoyés à cet hôpital.

La troisième phase commence en 1945. La guerre est finie et la Suède se rend compte des progrès énormes faits à l'étranger et en particulier aus Etats-Unis. Le progrès le plus considérable était alors la thoracotomie qui permet de traiter les malformations cardiaques et des grands vaisseaux, de l'œsophase et du diaphragme. Peu après on y ajouta la rectosigmoïdectomie pour le traitement de la maladie de Hirschsprung.

En 1952, un second service de chirurgie infantile fut installé à Stockholm, à l'Hôpital des Enfants de l'Université Karolinska. La plupart des cas de chirurgie générale et toutes les affections cardiovasculaires continuèrent à être traités à l'Hôpital Lovisa tandis que l'Hôpital Karolinska était réservé aux nouveaux-nés et à la chirurgie abdominale. Pour accélérer les progrès dans le domaine de l'urologie pédiatrique, N. O. Ericsson fut appelé à diriger le Service d'Urologie à l'Hôpital Karolinska. En peu de temps, son service avait acquis une solide réputation sur le plan international.

Le chapitre se termine sur les souvenirs personnels de l'auteur qui passe en revue les 50 dernières années.

Zusammenfassung

Die erste Kinderklinik in Schweden (Kronprinsessan-Lovisa-Klinik) wurde 1854 in Stockholm gegründet. 1885 wurde sie in eine innere und eine chirurgische Abteilung aufgeteilt. Dies war die Geburtsstunde der Kinderchirurgie in Schweden.

Kinderchirurgie ist seit 1945 Prüfungsfach. Ende der 50er Jahre wurde Ericsson zum außerordentlichen Professor für Kinderurologie an der Karolinska Medical School in Stockholm ernannt. Als er 1976 emeritiert wurde, wurde sein Lehrstuhl in eine ordentliche Professur für Kinderchirurgie umgewandelt.

Die schwedische Gesellschaft für Medizin hat 1947 Kinderchirurgie als selbständiges Fach anerkannt.

Die Jahresberichte des Lovisa-Krankenhauses 1885–1969 zeigen eine Entwicklung der Kinderchirurgie in Schweden in 3 Phasen:

Die 1. Phase erstreckt sich von 1885 bis 1932. In dieser Zeit waren die häufigsten Krankheiten septische Erkrankungen, Tuberkulose, Empyem und HNO-Erkrankungen. Es wird über wenige angeborene Mißbildungen berichtet. Die meisten chirurgischen Eingriffe bei Kindern wurden in der allgemeinen Chirurgie durchgeführt.

Die 2. Phase (1932–1945) ist gekennzeichnet durch einen Rückgang der Tuberkulose und eine allmähliche Verlagerung der orthopädischen und der HNO-Fälle in die jeweiligen Abteilungen. Während dieser Zeit nahmen die chirurgischen

Korrekturen von Mißbildungen deutlich zu. Dies ist darauf zurückzuführen, daß die meisten Fälle in dieses Krankenhaus überwiesen wurden.

Die 3. Phase begann 1945. Der Krieg war zu Ende, und Schweden erfuhr von den dramatischen Fortschritten dieses Fachs im Ausland (insbesondere in den USA). Der größte Fortschritt war die Thorakotomie, die es erlaubte, angeborene Mißbildungen des Herzens, der großen Gefäße, des Ösophagus und des Zwerchfells zu behandeln. Kurz danach wurde die Rektosigmoidektomie zur Behandlung der Hirschsprung-Krankheit eingeführt.

1952 wurde in Stockholm eine 2. Abteilung für Kinderchirurgie eingerichtet, und zwar in der Kinderklinik des Karolinska-Universitätskrankenhauses. Die meisten allgemeinchirurgischen Fälle des Einzugsbereichs Stockholm und alle kardiovaskulären Fälle wurden weiterhin im Lovisa-Krankenhaus behandelt, während fast alle Eingriffe bei Neugeborenen und in der Bauchregion am Karolinska-Hospital durchgeführt wurden. Um den Fortschritt in der pädiatrischen Urologie zu beschleunigen, wurde Ericsson zum Karolinska-Krankenhaus berufen. Bald hatte seine Abteilung ein im internationalen Vergleich sehr hohes Niveau erreicht.

Dieser geschichtliche Überblick endet mit den persönlichen Erinnerungen des Autors aus den letzten 50 Jahren.

References

1. Kjellberg SR, Ericsson NO, Rudhe U (1957) The lower urinary tract in childhood. Year Book Medical, Chicago
2. Nordin KE (1957) Treatment of primary total cleft palate deformity. Preoperative orthopedic correction of the displaced components of the upper jax in infants followed by bone grafting to the alveolar process clefts. Trans Europ Orthod Soc, The Hague
3. Nordin KE, Larson O, Nylén B, Eklund G (1983) Early bone grafting in complete cleft lip and palate cases following maxillofacial orthopedics. Scand J Plast Reconstr Surg 17:33
4. Okmian L (1966) Artificial ventilation by respirator for newborn and small infants during anaesthesia. A method for predicting and determining the volume of pulmonary ventilation and a clinical evaluation of the application of the method during surgery. Acta Anaesthesiol Scand [Suppl] XX
5. Livaditis A, Rådberg L, Odensjö G (1972) Esophageal end-to-end anastomosis. Reduction of anastomotic tension by circular myotomy. Scand J Thorac Cardiovasc Surg 6:206
6. Livaditis A (1973) Esophageal atresia: a method of overbridging large segmental gaps. Z Kinderchir 13:298
7. Ehrenpreis T (1969) Ulcerative colitis. In: Pediatric surgery, vol 2, 2nd edn. Year Book Medical, Chicago, p 940
8. Lindham S, Lagercrantz R (1980) Ulcerative colitis in childhood: should the rectum be preserved at surgery? Scand J Gastroenterol 15:123
9. Holmgren G (1908) Om innerörats variga sjukdomar. Stockholm
10. Waldenström H (1910) Die Tuberkulose des Collum Femoris im Kindesalter. Stockholm
11. Nyborg S (1943) Intussusception in children. Acta Chir Scand [Suppl] 80
12. Holmberg L (1945) Fractures in the distal end of the humerus in children. Acta Chir Scand [Suppl] 103
13. Ehrenpreis T (1946) Megacolon in the newborn. A clinical and roentgenological study with special regard to the pathogenesis. Acta Chir Scand [Suppl] 112

14. Ekström G (1952) The surgical treatment of patent ductus arteriosus. Acta Chir Scand [Suppl] 169
15. Ericsson NO (1954) Ectopic uroterocele in infants and children. Acta Chir Scand [Suppl] 197
16. Söderlund S (1959) Meckel's diverticulum. Acta Chir Scand [Suppl] 248
17. Ehrenborg G (1962) The Osgood-Schlatter lesion. A clinical and experimental study. Acta Chir Scand [Suppl] 288
18. Ehrenpreis T (1964) Omphalocele. In: Nelson LM (ed) Hernia. Lippincott, Philadelphia, p 322
19. Livaditis A (1969) End-to-end anastomosis in esophageal atresia. A clinical and experimental study. Scand J Thorac Cardiovasc Surg [Suppl] 2
20. Gierup J (1970) Micturition studies in infants and children. Scand J Urol Nephrol [Suppl] 5
21. Ehrenpreis T (1970) Hirschsprung's disease. Year Book Medical, Chicago
22. Svensson J (1979) Hypospadias. Etiological studies and clinical follow-up. Stockholm
23. Karpe B (1983) Cryptorchidism. Testicular function and effect of treatment. Stockholm
24. Pettersson BA (1983) Idiopathic hydronephrosis in childhood. A clinical pathological and experimental study. Stockholm
25. Molander ML (1984) Anal sphincter reflexes. Investigation in healthy children of different ages and a follow-up study in adults, operated for imperforate anus. Stockholm
26. Berfenstam R, Ehrenpreis T, Ekström G, Garsten P, Myrin SO (1957) Barnolycksfallen i Stockholm år 1955. Svenska Läkartidn 54:1950
27. Ehrenpreis T (1973) Prevention of childhood accidents in Sweden. The Swedish Institute, Stockholm
28. Ehrenpreis T (1983) Verhütung von Kinderunfällen in Schweden 1954 bis 1980. Sozialpäd Praxis Klin 5:352

The Cradle of Pediatric Surgery*

D. Anagnostopoulos and D. Pellerin[1]

The progress of pediatric surgery is undoubtedly due to the fact that it achieved autonomy from adult surgery and that all the surgical diseases of children were treated in clinics specially designed for this purpose.

When did this happen for the first time anywhere in the world? According to our sources it happened in Paris while Napoleon was consul; the date of the appropriate decree was 18 floréal of the year X, that is to say on the 8th of May 1802.

In accordance with the decree the monastery of Dames hospitalières de Saint Thomas de Villeneuve in the rue de Sèvres was turned into a hospital and it was given the name Enfants-Jesus. Later it changed its name to Enfants-Malades. Following the decree, Petitbau was appointed director of the clinic of pediatric surgery, which consisted of 14 beds. This first pediatric surgeon was not a well-known doctor, but he was very hardworking. One can imagine the difficulties he had to face in such a troubled period for France and Europe. He managed to keep the clinic on a decent level while having only two doctors as interns. He tried to separate the surgical diseases of children [1] from the pediatric ones which were the responsibility of two famous doctors of that time, Jadelot and Eusèbe de Salle [4, 5].

In 1814, the French government appointed the surgeon Baffos to the position of pediatric surgeon. This appointment was made because of his excellence as a surgeon, as no competition was held. Baffos was a noble, sociable, and well-educated man. He also had connections with most of the famous people of that time. He was a friend of Chataubriand, Duchesse de Berry, Cardinal Fesch, and Laennec, the greatest doctor of that time who worked in the same hospital with Baffos [2].

Baffos stayed on as director for 30 years although his activity was trivial. Saint-Germain commented on Baffos in these words: "No director had ever been so sober minded, so kind, so hostile to violence during his long service in Enfants-Malades. His emblem was: 'abhoret sanguine'. So he rightfully can be characterized as the father of conservative surgery."

Every morning a gentleman with long white whiskers and an impressive look entered the hospital. He started to visit his patients right away. He was informed about the progress of his small patients and gave instructions. If by chance an intern suggested that the patient should not be given medicine but operated in-

* Based on a lecture given at the Greek Pediatric Surgical Association, Chios, 1983

[1] Hôpital des Enfants Malades, Berceau de la chirurgie infantile, Paris, France

Progress in Pediatric Surgery, Vol. 20
Ed. by P. P. Rickham

stead, Baffos' forehead wrinkled. He did not approve of operations because he did not believe that there would not be any probability of success. Generally the patients in his clinic healed or died with conservative treatment without being operated upon. Only emergency cases were operated upon and these were the only operations done in his clinic.

In the summer, however, Baffos took his vacation for two months. At this time the new surgeon, who substituted for him, took his chance to embark upon an impressive career in the clinic where operations were not practiced and which was filled with patients with necroses and abscesses. The massacre was carried out in Baffos' absence and lasted 2 months. When Baffos came back he was enraged by what he saw, and calmness reigned again until his next holidays.

During Baffos 30 years of service the average number of operations was eight a year. This is rather disappointing if one considers that in the other clinics of the same hospital real progress was achieved in all branches [4]. For example, in the same hospital René T. Laennec invented the stethoscope and carried out such a great number of investigations that he was rightfully considered one of the greatests medical personalities of the nineteenth century. But we had better restrict our comments to children. Jadelot and Eusèbe de Salle translated and completed Underwood's work *Diseases in Childhood* (1823). Breschet (1820) wrote about and studied jaundice in the newborn. Furthermore, Denis de Commercy wrote *Pathology of Diseases in Children,* Lébut wrote *Infection of Rhinitis in Children,* Billard wrote *Newborn Diseases,* Valleix founded the first neonatal clinic in Enfants-Malades, and Guersant and Blanche wrote articles about children in the first medical dictionary, consisting of 30 volumes.

Fortunately for pediatric surgery during the time of Baffos' service, there were many skilled doctors in the hospital, like J. Guérin, V. Duval and the famous Bouvier, who operated on children as well as adults. Their specialities were subcutaneous tenontotomies, amputations, deviations of the vertebral column etc. Their reputation was world-wide, even reaching America, as will be described below [8, 11].

In 1844 Guersant took over the clinic of pediatric surgery and managed to make it as important as the other clinics of the hospital Enfants-Malades. In Guersant's family there were numerous doctors and he himself was a friend of Trousseau and Blache's collaborator. In a short time he raised the level and the reputation of his department, which became one of the most famous clinics in France and Europe. Guersant himself became the first great man of the school of pediatric surgery. In 1840 his book had already been translated into English and was the first book on pediatric surgery.

He was very skillful and hardworking. His passion was the rapidity with which an operation could be performed. Rapidity was the ideal of that time when anesthesia had not yet been invented. Guersant used to time every operation and he was very pleased when an operation lasted less than a previous one. Nowadays surgeons would be considered very slow in comparison with Guersant.

A great number of doctors applied for an unpaid position in Guersant's clinic. Foreign doctors arrived at the Enfants-Malades in order to attend Guersant's work [9]. His collaborators were doctors of high reputation, including Barthez, Pilliet, Barrier, and Legendre, who later published Guersant's lectures.

One of the greatest problems of that time was tracheostomy. Exhorted by Trousseau, Guersant used tracheostomy in children because he believed that it was the only correct therapy for diphtheria. The first 17 children thus treated in the Enfants-Malades died. The only reason that tracheostomy continued to be used as a routine operation was Guersant's presence. He did not lose courage although these bad results occurred within six months. Guersant himself wrote: "I continue to do operations because all the children who came to the hospital were in a very bad condition and if they had not been operated upon they certainly would have died." His next efforts met with success. The great number of the patients treated caused Trousseau himself to work in the hospital from 1850 to 1853. Pediatric surgery at Enfants-Malades became famous all over the world [4, 5].

Whenever Guersant was teaching the amphitheater was crowded. People who wanted to attend his lectures had to go there very early in order to find a seat. Unfortunately today we have only very few notes describing these operations, written by his collaborators. One is surprised by their simplicity and clarity.

From 1848 onwards another great surgeon started to work in the Enfants-Malades. This was Guérin, who dealt with orthopedic diseases of children. He and Guersant raised the reputation of the hospital to a very high degree.

In 1862, Giraldès succeeded Guersant. He was small-built, thin, lame, and pale, and had bad eyesight. His incomparable strength, clearheadedness, and great knowledge counterbalanced these physical disadvantages. He loved his students and his friends but he hated his adversaries and never missed a chance to attack and humiliate them. He was a great orator and a scathing debater. He was pleasant and amazingly mindful. His brain was like a library. He could recall even the smallest details needed in order to humiliate his adversaries. The result was that his clinic was always dominated by scientific vigilance. Although he was a cripple, he could exhaust the staff with his liveliness caused by his visits to the patients, the great number of operations, and his day-to-day teaching. Nevertheless, his patients and his students loved and admired him. They loved him because they could feel that behind his behavior and cool manners there was hidden a sensitive man, a man who was devoted to his patients and to his work [4, 9].

In 1869 Bourneville and Bourgeois published their lectures. Their book contains original statistics, methods to fight infections which continuously invaded the wounds, and a description of the application of carbolic acid which was not generally used at the time. There are also comments about anesthesia with cloroform and ether and their influence on children, who often did not wake up after an anesthesia of this kind. They warned against and avoided great quantities of anesthetics and suggested new methods for reanimation in cases with cardiac arrest. From 1844 onwards, regular measurements of temperature were practiced by Andral, who served as a pediatrician to the hospital [8].

In 1872 Giraldès retired because he was 63 years old, i.e., he had to resign although he did not want to. Six months after he had left the Enfants-Malades he died in the library of the medical school of Paris where he spent most of his time [4].

In 1873 Giraldès was succeeded by De Saint-Germain, who was a very skillful surgeon and a writer of many books. Saint-Germain was also an amazing orator who fascinated his audience and his students. His studies covered all branches of surgery including anesthesia and its problems, metabolic diseases (obesity, starvation) as prognostic preoperative factors, cleft palate, and abdominal surgery which had first been started by Péan and Billard. Knowing many languages, he became a center of attraction, especially for English doctors who started to come to the Enfants-Malades [10].

He was greatly interested in pediatric orthopedics. He also wrote a book entitled *Chirurgie orthopédie* describing a great number of apparatus and operative techniques. He improved the rules for sterilization in pediatric surgery and understood their importance. He worked in the same hospital as Parrot, with whom he studied congenital syphilis, and tried to apply on children what Louis Pasteur had discovered in order to protect the children from the worst diseases found in hospitals, tetanus, diphtheria, and anthrax.

The Enfants-Malades had developed into a very modern hospital. However, people were troubled by doubts about Parrot's and Saint-Germain's methods because a great number of deaths occurred in hospital [8]. Practice at the hospital during the next 20 years was based on knowledge of microbial agents, infections, biochemistry, aftercare of the operated child, the quality of milk and the danger of the microbial agents it contained. Parrot and Saint-Germain also separated newborn infants from the rest of the children and studied the special pathology of pediatric diseases. However, it must be added that Rendu and Grancher, Louis Pasteur's close friends, helped a lot in this field. Both of them worked with Saint-Germain in Enfants-Malades.

In 1899 the town council of Paris founded a pediatric and an orthopedic clinic in Enfants-Malades. Kirmisson, appointed as the first professor, started the second glorious period of Enfants-Malades. Later on he was succeeded by famous doctors like Auguste Broca, Léon Ombredanne, Leveuf, and Marcel Fèvre. Fèvre was the best teacher of contemporary French and foreign pediatric surgeons. Together they managed to create what the so-called French school of pediatric surgery [11].

This second period of the Enfants-Malades was equally creative and fascinating as the first one. The two world wars, the German occupation, and other events did not prevent it from being one of the best institutes of pediatric surgery in the world and one of the best and most creative hospitals in France. The methods and the instruments which were described by Kirmisson, Leveuf, and especially Ombredanne and Fèvre were used not only in pediatric surgery but also in adult surgery for a long time. The clinic has acted as a vanguard of pediatric surgery for two centuries. Few clinics in the history of medicine managed to achieve such a success.

Summary

The nearly two hundred years history of the Hôpital des Enfants-Malades in Paris is described, with special emphasis on the development of pediatric surgery in this hospital. Described is also the work of the various surgeons-in-chief, who since 1899 were also appointed professors of pediatric surgery. Progress was slow during the first half of the nineteenth century, but after Guersant took over in 1844 the hospital became a center for this speciality.

Résumé

Ce chapitre traite de l'histoire de l'Hôpital des Enfants Malades, fondé il y a près de 200 ans et insiste sur la chirurgie des enfants et les travaux des différents chirurgiens qui s'y sont succédés depuis 1899, date à laquelle la première chaire de chirurgie des enfants fut instituée. Les progrès furent lents durant la première moitié du XIXe siècle mais, à dater de la nomination de Guersant en 1844, cet hôpital devint rapidement une clinique hautement spécialisée en chirurgie des enfants.

Zusammenfassung

Es wird die fast 200jährige Geschichte des Hôpital des enfants malades in Paris mit besonderer Berücksichtigung der Kinderchirurgie erzählt und über die Arbeit der verschiedenen Chirurgen berichtet, für die seit 1899 auch ein Lehrstuhl für Kinderchirurgie eingerichtet wurde. In der ersten Hälfte des 19. Jahrhunderts wurden nur langsam Fortschritte erzielt, aber bald nach der Berufung von Guersant im Jahre 1844 entwickelte sich das Krankenhaus zu einer spezialisierten Klinik.

References

1. Andry Nicolas (1743) L'orthopédie ou'l'art de prevenir et de corriger dans les enfants, les difformites du corps. Paris
2. Bariety M, Coury C (1963) Histoire de la Medecine. Fayard, Paris
3. D'Allaines Cl (1967) Histoire de la chirurgie. Press Univ de France, Paris
4. DeSaint-Germain LA (1883) Chirurgie orthopédique. Billière, Paris
5. DeSaint-Germain LA (1884) Chirurgie des enfants. Lauwereyns, Paris
6. Fèvre M (1970) La chirurgie infantile. Press Univ de France, Paris
7. Giraldès J (1869) Leçons cliniques sur les maladies chirurgicales des enfants. De la Haye, Paris
8. Marfan AB (1926) Maladies de la première enfance. Masson, Paris
9. Rochard Jules (1875) Histoire de la chirurgie française. Paris
10. Sayre Lewis (1887) Chirurgie orthopedique. Steintier, Paris
11. Villey R (1976) Histoire du diagnostic medical. Masson, Paris

Pediatric Surgery in Islamic Medicine from the Middle Ages to the Renaissance*

C. A. Montagnani[1]

"After finishing for you, my sons, this book which is the part of knowledge dealing with medicine in its entirety; and having made it as clear and explicit as possible, I thought it well to complete it for you by adding this treatise which concerns surgical operating. For the skilled practitioner of operative surgery is totally lacking in our land and time."

These words begin the introduction to the thirtieth and last volume, dedicated to surgery, of the largest and most complete medical encyclopedia written in the Middle Ages with the following title: *Kitāb at-Taşrīf li-man ᶜajiza ᶜan at-ta ᶜlīf,* which means the manual (or collection) for the benefit of those who need to know about remedies and cannot manage to compile one. Most of the translations refer to the name only as at-Taşrīf, the practice or a praxis, but collection or the modern term encyclopedia would fit the meaning and the characteristics of this exhaustive book better.

The author of such a ponderous work was Abū l-Quasim Khalaf b. al-ᶜAbbas al-Zahrāwī, better known to the historians of medicine by the distorted latin names of Albucasis, Abulcasis, Ezaharagui, or Alsaharavius, who was Arab by descent. His father, ᶜAbbas, may have worked at the court of Cordoba. Albucasis was born in Zahra, the royal summer residence of the Umayyad caliphs, rulers of conquered Spain (Fig. 1). Az-Zahra, which means flower, was located 5 miles west of Cordoba and was founded in 936 A.D. by ᶜAbd ar-Raḫmān according to the wish and bearing the name of his beautiful favorite Az-Zahra, who died young. The town was also named Madīna, which means large city. It became a royal city with hundreds of mosques, some of which were very beautiful, sumptuous palaces with fabulous gardens and fountains, and a harem of 6000 women. Today the town still bears the name of Madīna Zahra, but only part of a mosque and remnants of the palace's foundations and part of the gardens are left. Because the date his home town was founded is known, it is assumed that the date of Albucasis' birth was later. However, Leo Africanus gives 912 as the date of his birth and 1013 as the date of his death, stating that he lived 101 hijri years, which corresponds to 97 solar years. This may be quite likely true. One should, however, think that Albucasis was born in the outskirts of Cordoba 20 years before the foundation of Zahra and that az-Zharāwī was added later to his name when he became famous.

---

[1] P. za Ponte S. Angelo 31, 00186 Roma, Italy

* Based on a lecture given at the Greek Pediatric Surgical Association, Chios, 1983

Progress in Pediatric Surgery, Vol. 20
Ed. by P. P. Rickham

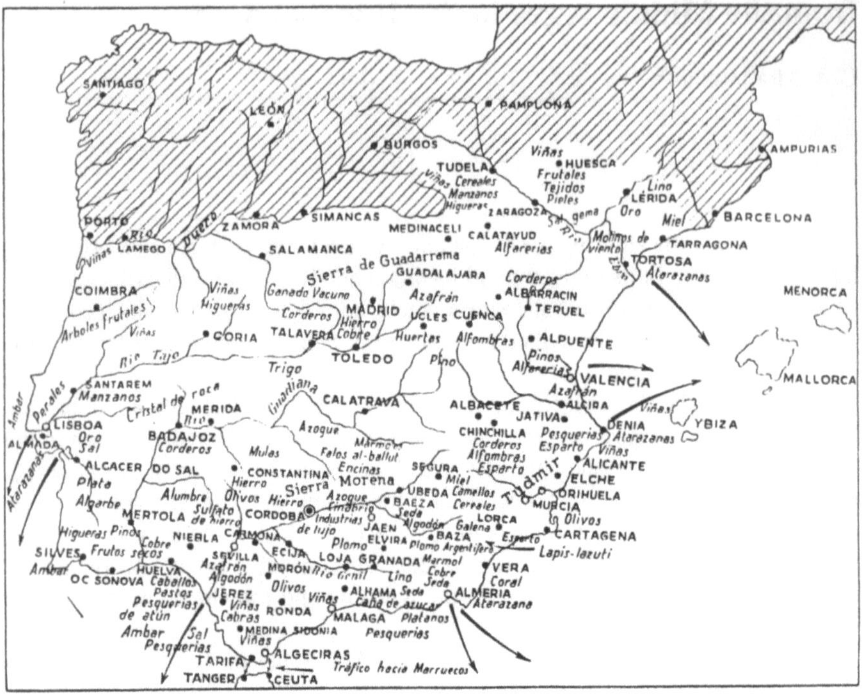

Fig. 1. Map of the territory of Spain under Islamic domination between 900 and 1000 A.D.

During his long and industrious life three caliphs ruled. The first was Abd ar-Raḥmān III, a clever politician, a determined man of war, and conqueror of Navarra and Saragoza. At his death almost the entire Spanish territory was under Arabic domination. He was succeeded by his son al-Ḥakam II. He was a wise ruler, a highly cultivated man, a great bibliophile, an enthusiastic reader of science, tolerant in racial and religious matters, and internationally oriented as a diplomat. His son Hišām was too young to reign, and after a short interlude of regency one of the Vizirs, Ibn Abī Amīr, a ferocious, impulsive, and vindictive warrior took over power and later assumed the name of al Manṣūr, which means "the victorious in the name of God."

This period of almost a century was the time of the greatest splendor of the Arabic-Hispano domination. In spite of an almost constant state of war at the northern borders of the country, illiteracy was eliminated and Cordoba, the capital, had half a million inhabitants, 300 mosques, many superb palaces, 300 public baths, 50 hospitals, 70 libraries, and 28 suburbs. The university of Cordoba was well established since the middle of the nineth century and became famous all over Europe for its teaching of Islamic religion, theology and philosophy, literature, poetry, algebra, chemistry, botany, pharmacology, astronomy, and of course medicine. Al-Ḥakam II kept sending copyists to Damascus, Alexandria, and Bagdad, and by the end of the tenth century the royal library was endowed with 600000 volumes. This was the period when Albucasis studied, practiced, and taught. One of the men copying his works said: "I have been told that Al-Zahrawi (God have mercy on him) lived an extremely ascetic life, that half of his daily work was done without fees, as an act of charity, and that he wrote this compendium for his sons over a period of forty years."

Albucasis' book on surgery was considered by the developing European medical world to be a basic work of reference for many centuries throughout the Renaissance and later on. That the book was considered an invaluable book of reference, almost a surgical "Bible," till the eighteenth century is shown by the numerous translations and editions of his "Surgery" and the quotations by other outstanding surgeons (Table 1). While cauterization for many pathological conditions, emergency surgery, and the treatment of fractures and joint dislocations are mainly discussed in his writings, pediatric surgery was known to Albucasis at least with regard to the more obvious congenital malformations.

It may be worthwhile mentioning some of the pediatric subjects in Albucasis' own words, as translated by Spink and Lewis from the Arabic manuscripts [8].

On Cauterization of Hare Lip [Chapter 18]

There often occur fissures in the lip to which are given the name of "hares"; they are particularly common in lips of boys. When you have ineffectually treated these clefts with those things that we have mentioned in their appropriate section, then heat a small edged cautery of this shape. The hollow should be as sharp as a knife. Then quickly place it when hot right on to the fissure till the burning has reached the depth of the lip. Then treat with wax plaster till healed.

Table 1. Translations and editions of Albucasis' book on surgery

1150–1200	Gerardo da Cremona (da Sabbioneta o Toledano) *Liber Alsaharavi de Cirurgia*
undated	Hebrew Spanish-Catalan Latin (University of Montpellier)
1300	Latin with Arabic text (National Library Paris) Jewish (Escurial Madrid) Latin (Marciana Library Venice)
1465	Turkish Sharaf ed-Din: *Surgery of Ilkhani* with 140 Turkish-Persian miniatures
1469	Latin (Ambrosiana Library, Milan)
1497	Latin First Edition in Venice, together with *Cyrurgia Parva* by Gui de Chauliac. Further editions 1499–1500, by Lucantonio Giunta Florentine
1519	Latin, Venice, together with *Chirurgia* by Rolando da Parma
1520	Latin, Venice, together with the *Chirurgia* by Pietro d'Argelata. Further editions 1532, 1540
1532	Latin (Strasburg)
1541	Latin (Basel)
1778	Latin with Arabic text. J. Channing, Oxford
1871	French with English-Arabic text. L. Leclerc, Paris
1973	English with Arabic text. M. S. Spink and G. L. Lewis, Oxford
Quoted by:	Ruggero di Frugardo da Parma (1180), Guglielmo da Saliceto (1200), Rolando da Parma (ca. 1240), Lanfranco da Milano (1200), Matteo Ferrari alias Matteo de Gradibus (1400), Sante de Ardoynis da Pesaro (1492), Guy de Chauliac (1497), H. Fabricii d'Acquapendente (1533–1619), Haller (1708–1780)

This attempt to promote the closure of the cleft lip by cauterization followed by healing and scarring is an original method previously not described by "the Ancients." Another personal and interesting contribution is the use of the wax plaster in order to protect the wound and possibly bring its edges together.

On the Cure of Hydrocephalus [Chapter 1]

This disease occurs most commonly in infants upon delivery when the midvife grasps the child's head roughly. It also sometimes happens from some hidden unknown cause. I have never seen this disease except in very small children, and death very quickly overtook all those I have seen; therefore I have preferred not to undertake operations in these cases.

Albucasis also classified the types of hydrocephalus according to the extent of the fluid collection and its location outside the bone and beneath the skin between the skull and the membrane. He also advocates the evacuation of fluid by one or multiple T incisions (Fig. 2). Moreover, he describes the knife to be used, which was slightly curved with a blunt end. It ought to be said that this last description is practically the verbatim translation of what was written by Paul of Aegina, although no mention is made of a H-shaped incision. Albucasis may have described this treatment for completeness and not from his personal experience, which was rather unfavorable. Another interesting point is that he did not mention spina bifida in association with hydrocephalus in the neonates he did observe.

Other conditions which are described along with their treatment are "the hydatid in the upper lid" (chapter 10), apparently a lipoma or a sebaceous cyst (Fig. 3), "the Nasal Polyp" and, we may add, "the Adenoids."

While the treatment of visible or prolapsing nasal polyps had already been described by Celsus and Paulus of Aegina, the treatment of the deeper polyps and adenoids is vividly and probably originally described by Albucasis:

You must take a linen thread, rather thick, and tie many knots in it with a space of a finger's breadth or less between each pair of knots; and let the patient try to get one end of the thread into his nose with a probe or anything he can. After making it into a form of a button, let him make a full inspiration till it reaches the cartilage and comes out through the throat. Boys at school often do this sort of thing and it is quite easy for anyone who wishes. Then hold together the two ends of the thread, one coming out through the mouth and the other remaining in the nose then saw off the polyps by means of the knots in the thread; continue doing this until you are sure that the growth has been cut off by the knotted thread.

He also advises the use of a lead tube to be inserted into the nostrils and the instillation of Egyptian oil or drying medicaments until healing was complete.

Two other headings are: "On Incising the Ligament Below the Tongue Which is an Impediment to Speech" and "On the Removal of 'Ranula' Beneath the Tongue" (chapter 35). About the latter he says:

Sometimes there occur under the tongue a swelling resembling a small frog, which hinders the natural movements of the tongue; sometimes it grows so as even to fill the mouth. The operation for it is to open the patient's mouth in the full light of the sun and inspect the tumor. If you see that it is dark or black and hard and the patient has no sensation in it, do not interfere with it for it is a cancer. But if it is inclined to be pale and has fluid in it, put a hook in it and incise it with a fine scalpel and free it all round; and if hemorrhage hinders you while operating apply pounded vitriol to it till the bleeding stops. Then proceed with your work till all is extracted; then let him rinse his mouth out with vinegar and salt. Then give all the suitable treatment until it is healed.

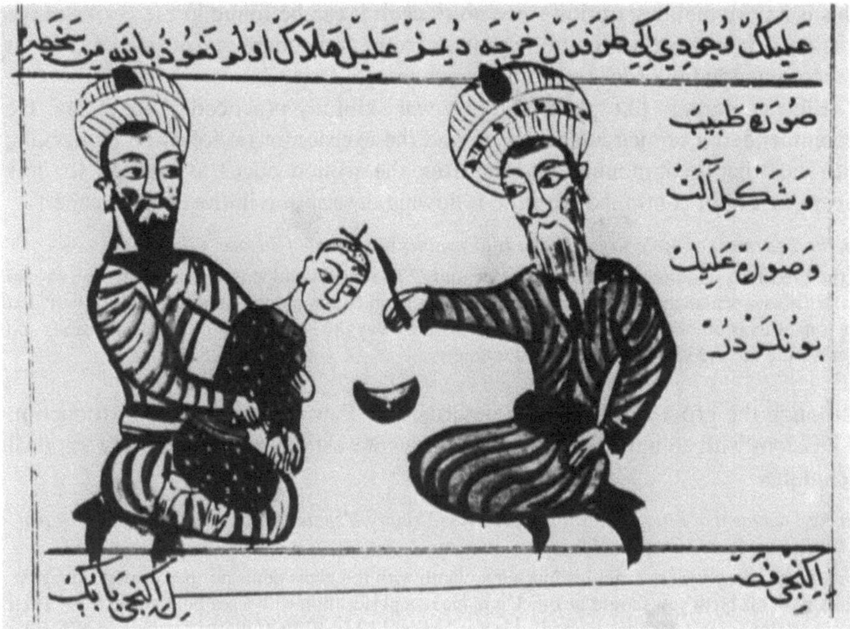

Fig. 2. Incision and evacuation of hydrocephalus

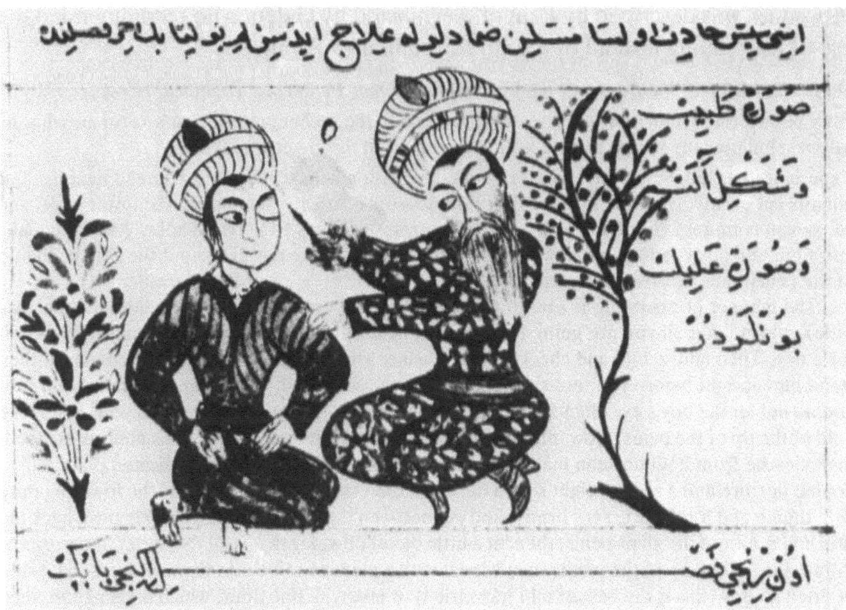

Fig. 3. Excision of a cyst or lipoma of the upper lid

This is an original description since no trace of it can be found in the books of the Ancients. It is worthwhile noting that a careful and complete excision of the cyst is recommended in order to avoid recurrence.

Elective surgery like plastic surgery was skillfully practiced at that time. He recommended a semicircular incision and the excision of fat followed by packing with cicatrizing compounds and suturing the wound edges as enough for less severe cases but continued with the following description in the chapter called

On the Treatment of Male Breast When It Resembles the Female [Chapter 47]

If the breast is pendulous and flabby on account of its size, as happens with women, you should make two semicular incisions on the upper side, the ends joining one another, in such way that the longer incision encircles the inner. Then dissect away the skin between the two incisions and remove the fat and sew up as described, etc. etc.

Although the procedure was fully described by Paul of Aegina, the introduction of incisions with an upper convexity is a very interesting example of a new surgical technique.

On the Treatment of Boys Born with Imperforate Urinary Meatus or with the Meatus Small or Not in the Proper Place [Chapter 55]

Sometimes a boy is born from his mother's womb with the glans penis not perforated. So at the moment of his birth you should be quick and make a perforation with a scalpel figured thus. Then put in the opening a slender leaden sound, tie it and keep it for three or four days. When he wishes to make water, it will be removed and he will do so and then put it back.

The treatment for hypospadias and meatal stenosis is just the same and consists in enlarging the meatus with an extremely fine small blade (Fig. 4). The procedure was described by Paul of Aegina and by Galen, who recommended the use of lead tubing instead of a solid rod similar to Albucasis.

On Circumcision of the Boys and the Correction of Their Erroneous Treatment [Chapter 57]

With regard to circumcision he says, after criticizing the technique of using a razor or what he calls a spindle-whorl (falka) as well as the fingernail, in the chapter called:

Experience has taught me the superiority of circumcision with scissors and a thread ligature. For scissors cut evenly, since the upper edge of the scissors is exactly the same as the lower edge; and so, as you compress your hand thanks to the correspondence of the two blades, you cut equally and simultaneously; and you make the girdle of the thread like a wall around the skin of the tip of the penis; thus no error can occur.

The manner of operating is first to make the boy (especially if he is one who understands a little) imagine that all you are going to do is tie a ligature round the tip of the penis and leave it for a day. Then amuse him and cheer him as much as you can according to his intelligence; then stand him upright before you, not sitting; and hide the scissors in your sleeve or under your foot and do not let the boy's eye chance upon that or any other instrument. Then with your hand take hold of the tip of the penis, blow into the foreskin, and draw it back till the glans penis is exposed; then cleanse from it all unclean matter that has collected. Then ligate the indicated place with a double ligature and a second right round beneath; then take hold at the site of the lower ligature with thumb and forefinger, very firmly, and cut between the ligatures; then quickly push back the skin and draw out the glans penis; then let a little blood flow, for that is all the better and prevents the swelling of the tip of the penis; then wipe it with a piece of soft cloth, then sprinkle on it ashes of dried gourds (this is the best of all I have tried) or else with fine flour, which is also good; then apply on top of the powders a piece of linen with egg-yolk cooked in rose-water, beaten up with fresh oil of roses of good quality.

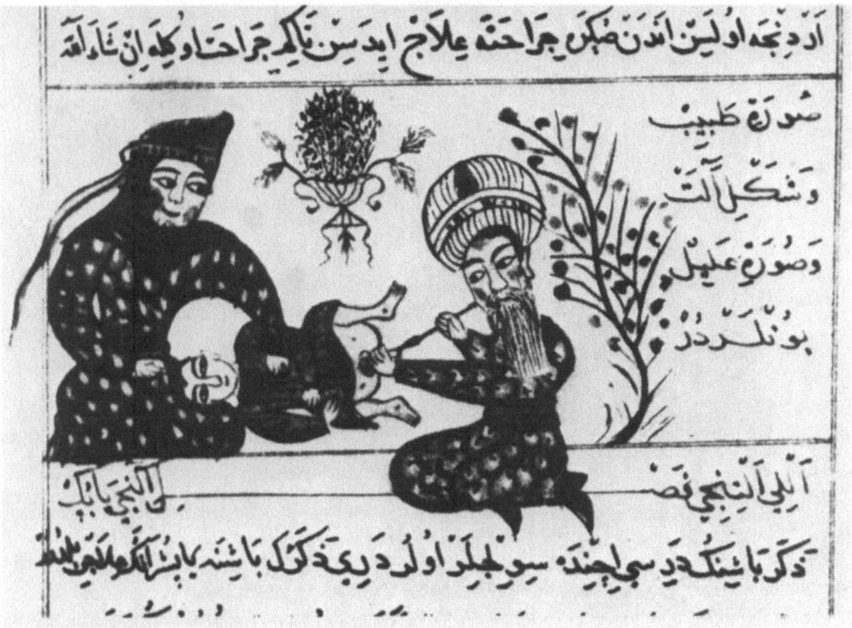

Fig. 4. Treatment of urethral meatal stenosis and hypospadias

He then describes the type of scissors to be used (Fig. 5).

This is the type of scissors most suitable for circumcision. They should be flat-nosed, sharp, with no bend in them, and with the pivot tempered; and the length of the handles should be equal to that of the blades.

The illustrations of different kinds of scissors reported in the arabic manuscripts leave no doubt that they are modern scissors and not shears as mentioned in the latest work of Celsus, Antyllius, and Paul of Aegina.

It is quite possible that scissors were first invented by the Arabs if not by Albucasis himself. They were large or small, pointed, or with the blades at right angles with the shaft or with a blunted tip as described here. It is also interesting to note the recommendation about the balanced length of shaft and blades which will transmit the right sensation to the fingers when thick and rather board tissues, as for instance the four layers of the prepuce have to be cut.

On the Treatment of Hermaphroditism [Chapter 70]

There are two kinds of male hermaphrodite: one has the appearance of female pudenta with hair in the region of the perineum; the other has the same lying in the skin of the scrotum between the testes. Sometimes urine is also excreted through that which is in the skin of the scrotum. There is also one type amongst women where there lies on the pubes, above the female pudenta, a structure resembling the male organ. These are small, but protuberant, one being like the penis and the other two like testicles.

The treatment of all three types, i.e., two males and one female, is as follows: "The superfluous growth must be cut away, so that every trace of it is destroyed;

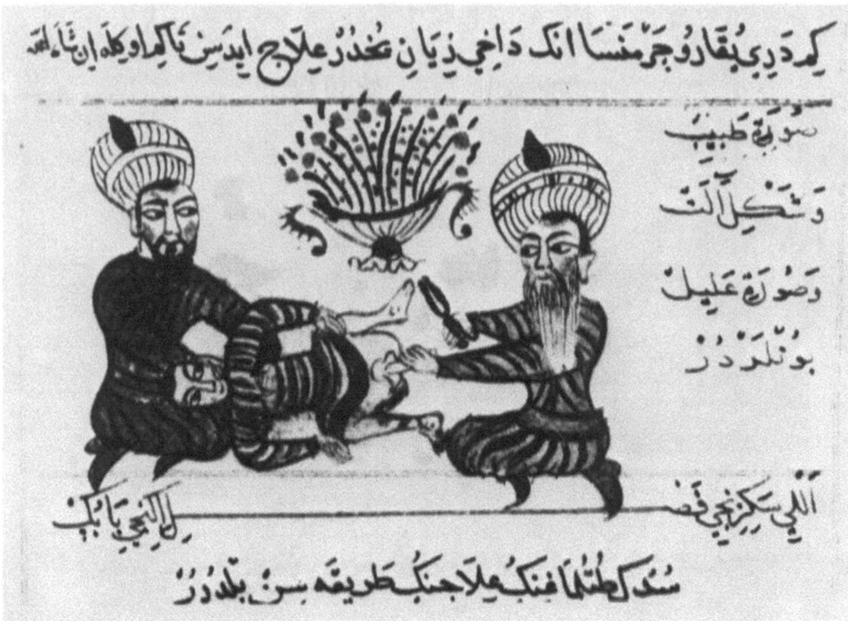

Fig. 5. Circumcision using scissors

then the usual treatment for wounds should be applied until they are healed".

Further, in chapter 71, he says:

The clitoris may grow in size above the order of nature, so that it gets a horrible deformed appearance; in some women it becomes erect like the male organ and achieves coitus. You must grasp the growth with your hand or a hook and cut it off. Do not cut too deeply, especially at the root of the growth, lest hemorrhage occurs. Then apply the usual dressing for wounds until healed (P). As to the second kind in man, where the opening is in the scrotum and the urine runs out of it, there is no operation for this, and no cure.

The conditions in the male may be a severe perineal hypospadias with a split scrotum associated either with undescended testicles or with descended ones. Female virilization is obviously the other condition.

Paul of Aegina had already described genital ambiguities.

On the Treatment of Imperforated Female Pudenda [Chapter 72]

This condition occurs when a woman's pudenda have no opening or have only a tiny opening; it may be either congenital or acquired. The acquired sort is due to some preceding disease; either to a fleshy growth or to a membrane, thick or thin. It may be in the fundus of the uterus or in its walls or in the upper part or in the lower part; and it prevents intercourse, conception and delivery; it often also hinders the menses. This is recognized on inspection by the midwife, if obstruction be obvious and low. But if it be not visible she should palpate with her finger or with a probe and when the obstruction is due to a thin membrane near the labia you should lose no time in breaking it down. This is done by applying some sort of pad to the labia; then put both thumbs upon it. The woman should be upon her back with her legs spread wide apart; then the labia are to be stretched strongly till the thin membrane is ruptured and the obstruction is laid open. Then

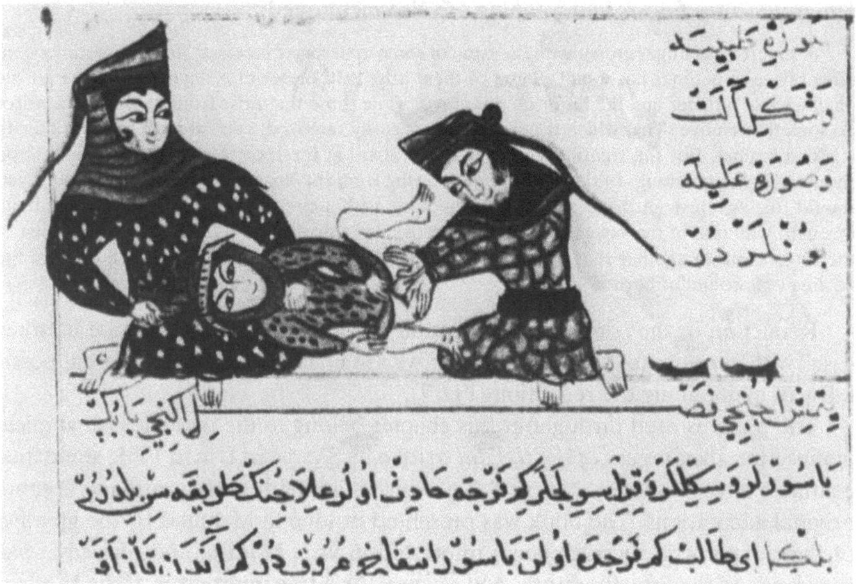

Fig. 6. Treatment of inperforated hymen

take wool soaked in oil and apply to the place, and let the woman engage in coitus every day lest the place close over. If the membrane be thick and strong you should incise it with a broad myrtle-leaf scalpel. But if the obstruction be due to a growth you should catch hold of it with two hooks and cut it away. And have at hand remedies for allying hemorrhage without pain, such as acacia and dragon's blood and olibanum, all mixed with egg-white. Then use a cannula of lead to prevent the wound healing up too quickly. She should keep it in position for some days and employ a bandage of dry linen. Then treat with usual healing dressing until it heals.

Although the possibility of a congenital condition is mentioned, the description seems to apply only to grown up females (Fig. 6). These conditions were dealt with by midwives like most of the female pathology; this was more strictly observed in Islamic medicine. It may be therefore possible that Albucasis was not very well acquainted with the subject and this chapter is taken directly from Paul of Aegina. Both Celsus and Soranus also mentioned different maneuvres, like grasping the obstructing membrane with a forceps and also using a speculum.

Treatment of anal fistula in children was carried out with a very fine cautery.

On the Treatment of Imperforate Anus [Chapter 79]

Infants are quite often born with the anus imperforate, closed by a fine membrane; then the midwife should perforate the membrane with her finger or pierce it with a sharp scalpel being careful not to touch the muscle. Then wool dipped in oil and wine should be applied, and treat it with ointments until healed. If you are afraid it may close up, put into the opening a leaden tube for many days, which will be removed when the child wants to evacuate the bowel.

This is a translation from Paul of Aegina.

Supernumerary fingers and *webbing* are also mentioned:

> A superfluous finger growing on the hand of some men sometimes is all flesh, sometimes contains bone, sometimes has a nail. Some of them arise at the root of a finger, or on one of the phalanges of a finger and the latter do not move, while those that arise from the root of a finger do sometimes move. That which is purely fleshy is easily removed; you cut it off at the root with a broad scalpel. But the treatment of that which arises at the root of a finger is difficult; you should avoid amputating. In the case of one growing from the finger at the phalangeal joint, you should first cut through the flesh down to the bone with a circular incision; then saw the bone through, with one of the saws that suit the purpose; then dress until it heals. As for webbing of the fingers one to another that occurs very frequently, it may be either congenital or from the healing of a wound or burn or the like.

Reduction of the congenital dislocation of the hip was practiced like in other cases with considerable manual skill but we are unable to evaluate the real possibility of maintaining the reduction (Fig. 7).

The pictures used throughout this chapter belong to the first Turkish surgical manuscript, the *Surgery of the Il<u>kh</u>āni* written by <u>Sh</u>araf ad Dīn in 1465, some four centuries after Albucasis' "Surgery," of which it is a faithful translation with some original adaptations. The book was presented in 1466 to Mehmed II, the greatest of the sultans who, besides being interested in war, politics, and pleasure, was very keen on the arts, literature, and science. As a free interpreter of the Moslem religious rules, which forbid the representation of the human figure, he had his portrait painted by the Gentile Bellini and for the same reasons he accepted and approved the first illustrated surgical manuscript. The Turkish-Persian miniatures

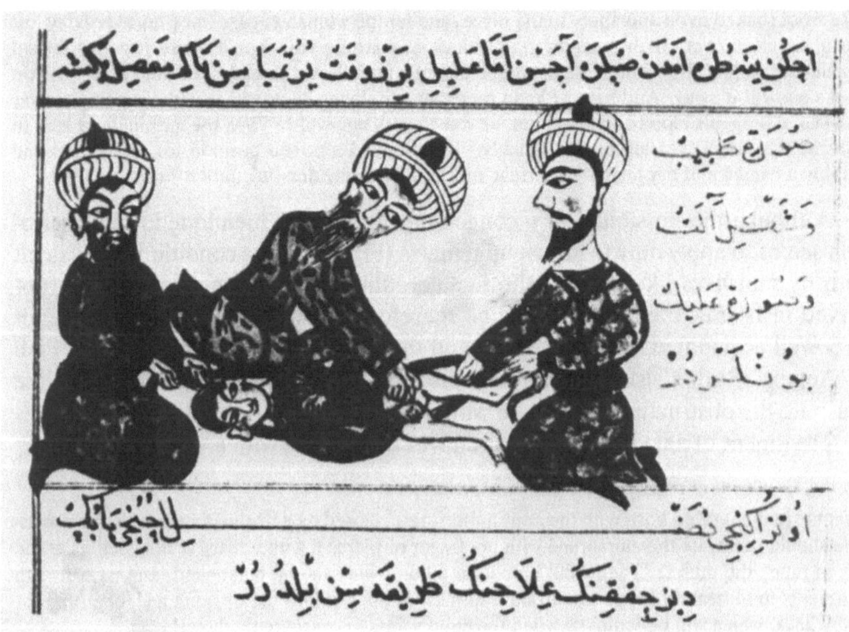

Fig. 7. Treatment of dislocated hip

are very instructive in spite of the gentle and unwordly attitude of the figures but somehow they cannot match the realism of the detailed descriptions of Albucasis – that great surgeon had indeed a perfect knowledge of the book of the Ancients from Hippocrates and Galen to Aetios of Amida, Alexander of Tralles (Ephesus), and especially Paul of Aegina. Many chapters of his "Surgery" are translations of the Aegina's book. We ought, however, to give him credit for his many original contributions, such as surgical procedures, postoperative treatments, and surgical instruments. He, and possibly other Arabic surgeons, probably developed the trocar for paracentesis, the tonsil guillotine, a full set of gynecological instruments, and the concealed knife or deceiver for incising abscesses. It is very likely that he invented surgical scissors, as mentioned above, as well as the syringe and the formula for a kind of compound plaster.

Albucasis knew of hemophilia and its transmissible character. He also gives what is very probably the first description of the use of catgut for suturing the wounded intestine. It reads as follows:

> The intestine may also be sewn up with the fine suture which is extracted from animals' gut and stick to it after being threaded in a needle. The method used is that the end is taken of this suture made of gut, well scraped; and to this end is fixed a fine linen thread, twisted, and then that thread is passed through the needle affixed to the suture of animal gut, with which the intestine is sewn and then replaced in the abdominal cavity.

Even in discussing the use of the cautery, to which an entire part is devoted, he is very sharp and objective in his analysis and judgement. While, according to the Ancients, the golden cautery was far superior to the bronze or steel ones, he points out that – because of the reddish color of the gold – this metal never gives assurance of the degree of heat that should be reached, it cools off too rapidly, and if overheated it may melt easily. Therefore, he states, the steel cautery is far closer to perfection.

How this important and comprehensive book, which combines the knowledge of Greek and Roman surgery with the practice and ingenuity of Arabic surgery, came to influence the development of European surgery is extraordinary. It occurred about the second half of the twelfth century. The Christians had already conquered Toledo, and Arab domination began to recede. The enormous treasure of an extraordinary culture and civilization was in danger of being destroyed and lost.

A benedictine monk from Cluny, Archibishop of Toledo, called upon a small group of brothers, Gerard of Moissac, Peter of Bourges, Peter of Agen, Peter of Palencia, Bernard and Jeronimus of Perigord, and Gerard of Cremona. The seven monks quickly learnt the Arabic language and went to live among the Arab population, driven as they were by their conscience to have a difficult and great task, namely to save for posterity the most significant works of Hispano-Arabic culture and civilization.

Gerard of Cremona, who was then also called Gerard Toledan, translated 70 scientifc works into latin, 21 of which were medical, and among these was Albucasis' "Surgery."

Summary

Albucasis lived throughout the tenth century, practicing medicine for more than 40 years in Zahra at the outskirts of Cordoba. This was the period of the greatest splendour of Arab domination of Spain. Albucasis taught medicine at the university of Cordoba and published an encyclopedia of medicine comprising 30 volumes, the last one dealing with surgery. This work was translated into all civilized languages and was the standard medical textbook right till the eighteenth century.

This paper deals with many pediatric surgical conditions as described in Albucasis' 30th volume. The pathology and treatment of harelip, hydrocephalus, the adenoids, ranula, gynecomastia, imperforated external urinary meatus, circumcision, hermaphrodites, imperforate anus, and supernumerary and webbed finger were all described by Albucasis, and his remarks are discussed here in some detail.

Résumé

Albucasis a vécu du début à la fin du Xe siècle et exerçait la médecine près de Cordoue. La domination arabe en Espagne était alors à son apogée. Il enseignait aussi la médecine à l'Université de Cordoue et il rédigea une encyclopédie de la médecine en 30 volumes. Le dernier volume était consacré à la chirurgie. Cet ouvrage fut traduit dans toutes les langues du monde civilisé et fit autorité jusqu'au XVIIIe siècle.

Ce chapitre traite aussi de différents cas: pathologie et traitement des fentes labiales, hydrocéphalie, adénoïde, ranula, gynécomastie, méat externe, circoncision, hermaphrodisme, imperforation, syndactylie.

Zusammenfassung

Albucasis lebte vom Anfang bis zum Ende des 10. Jahrhunderts und übte Medizin in der Nähe von Cordoba aus. Es war die Blütezeit der arabischen Herrschaft in Spanien. Albucasis lehrte Medizin an der Universität von Cordoba und verfaßte eine Enzyklopädie der Medizin in 30 Bänden. Der letzte Band war der Chirurgie gewidmet. Dieses Werk wurde in alle Sprachen der zivilisierten Welt übersetzt und blieb bis zum 18. Jahrhundert das Standardlehrbuch der Medizin.

Dieser Beitrag behandelt verschiedene Fälle aus der Kinderchirurgie: Pathologie und Behandlung von Hasenscharte, Hydrozephalus, Adenoiditis, (unechte?) Ranula, Gynäkomastie, Meatus externus, Beschneidung, Hermaphrodismus, Anus imperforatus, überzählige Finger und Syndaktylie.

Acknowledgements. The illustrations have been reproduced from P. Huard and M. D. Grmek (eds) *Le premier manuscript chirurgical turc rédigé par Sharaf ad-Din* (1465) by kind permission of Editions Roger Dacosta, Paris.

Passages of the English translation by M. S. Spink and G. L. Lewis from *Albucasis – On Surgery and Instruments* have been quoted through the kind permission of The Wellcome Institute for the History of Medicine.

References

1. Browne EG (1921) Arabian medicine. Cambridge University Press, London
2. Capparoni P (1936) La medinina araba nella Spagna fino a tutto il secolo XIII°. Boll Ist Naz Med Farm. Serono, Rome
3. Faludy A (1976) Medical illustrations of the Abulcasis manuscript. 24th International congress of history of medicine, Budapest, pp 854–872
4. Huard P, Grmek MD (1960) Le premier manuscript chirurgical turc rédigé par Chraf ed Din (1465). Dacosta, Paris
5. Leclerc L (1861) La chirurgie d'Abulcasis. Leroux, Paris
6. Leclerc L (1876) Histoire de la médecine arabe. Leroux, Paris
7. Said HM (1975) Traditional Greco-Arabic and modern Western medicine. Conflict or symbiosis. Hamdard 18: 1–59
8. Spink MS, Lewis GL (1973) Albicasis. On surgery and instruments. A definitive edition of the arabic text with English translation and commentary. The Wellcome Institute for the History of Medicine, London
9. Tabanelli M (1961) Albucasi. Un chirurgo arabo dell'alto medio evo. La sua epoca. La sua vita. La sua opera. Olshki, Florence

William E. Ladd, M.D.: Great Pioneer of North American Pediatric Surgery

H. Bill[1]

William E. Ladd (1880–1967) lived and worked in a time of an enormous development of medicine and surgery and yet a time when many of the new facts could be understood and utilized by one individual. He was born in the vicinity of Boston to a merchant family who had previously lived in northern New England. His education was at good preparatory schools and then at Harvard University, from which he received an A. B. in 1902 and an M. D. in 1906. During college he rowed on the Harvard crew, an activity which he continued for years, both as a rower and then as the doctor for the crew. Upon graduation from medical school, he received a general surgical training and embarked on a general surgical practice. His early hospital appointments included those at the Boston City Hospital and also the Infants and Children's Hospitals. He started as assistant in surgery at Harvard and advanced to instructor, assistant professor, clinical professor, and finally the Ladd Professor of Children's Surgery, a chair established in his honor 5 years before his retirement in 1945 (Fig. 1).

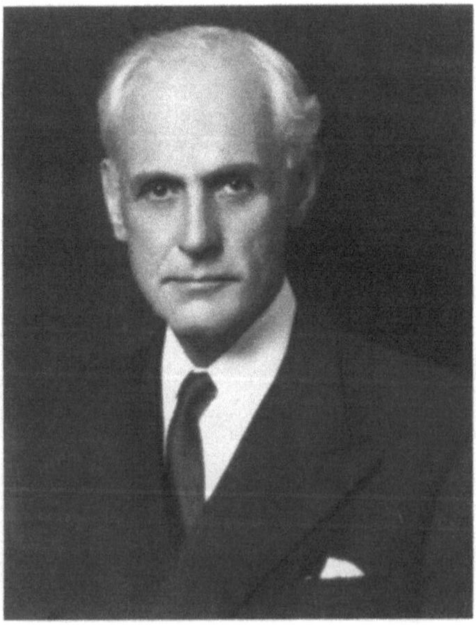

Fig. 1. William E. Ladd

[1] Children's Hospital, 4800 Sand Point Way, Seattle, WA 98105, USA

Progress in Pediatric Surgery, Vol. 20
Ed. by P. P. Rickham

The Medical Environment

The medical conditions which existed when Ladd graduated from Harvard Medical School in 1906 would be considered primitive by current standards. Tuberculosis, osteomyelitis, syphylis, yellow fever, typhoid, malaria, and many bacterial infections were rampant and without good means of management. There were few useful drugs beyond digitalis, aspirin, and the opiates. Insulin was unknown. Ether and chloroform anesthesia were available. Surgery was limited by the fact that intravenous fluid therapy was not yet understood and that there were no blood transfusions. When surgery was performed, speed was essential. Drainage of abscesses was the most frequently used procedure, although resections of tumors, hernia repairs, appendectomies, and other operations were well established.

Harvard University was then led by President Charles W. Eliot, who had been a chemist and who devoted himself to upgrading the Medical School. In the period between 1900 and 1920, steps were taken to encourage research and scholarship. These included the construction in 1906 of the large complex of laboratory and teaching buildings in the Medical School quadrangle, the construction and staffing of the Peter Bent Brigham Hospital in 1913, and the move of the Infants and Children's Hospitals to a location adjacent to the new Medical School buildings in 1914. Other medical facilities were soon to follow in the same area.

The new buildings accommodated a memorable group of medical scientists, including the physiologist Cannon, the chemist Folin, and the bacteriologist Zinnser. At Brigham were Wolbach in pathology, and Harvey Cushing and Henry Christian in surgery and medicine. Soon to appear at the Children's were James Gamble and L. J. Henderson, both of fluid balance fame. All of these great individuals and many more reinforced one another, each in his own way, and laid a basis for the many advances which were generated. Ladd entered this atmosphere through his activities at the Children's Hospital. He contributed to this same environment until his retirement in 1945.

Contributions to Pediatric Surgery

I should like to illustrate Dr. Ladd's thorough and consistent approach to clinical research through his contributions to the treatment of two well-known conditions, intussusception and pyloric stenosis, early in his career. In neither one were the methods of treatment original with him, yet the way in which the treatments were improved, organized, and delivered were typical of many other problems of clinical care which he studied and taught.

His first published paper was entitled "Treatment of Intussusception in Children." It appeared in 1911. In this paper he demonstrated (a) the fatal outcome of intussusception if left untreated; (b) the fact that 70% of the patients treated by enemas died; and (c) that mortality after surgical operation was 50%. He concluded by recommending that surgery be done early, without wasting precious time and the limited stamina of the patient in use of irrigations.

His next paper on this subject was published two years later in 1913 with J. Stone, the chief of the surgical service at Children's Hospital [2]. In this publication they reported a mortality of 45% in 20 cases treated surgically in the preceding 2 years. They also found that all the patients operated on less than 48 h after the onset of symptoms survived, while only one patient did so after a longer interval. They concluded by recommending that all cases be diagnosed and treated within 36 h of the onset of the typical symptoms.

In 1915, in a third paper [3], he reviewed their total of 63 cases, again comparing survival to the interval between the onset of symptoms and surgery. For those cases with less than 36 h from onset, there was 20% mortality; between 36 and 48 h, 55%; and between 48 and 60 h, 90%.

In his final study in 1934 [4], Robert Gross and he demonstrated a continuous improvement in the rapidity of referral and a continuous reduction in mortality in 372 cases. In their first 5 years, the mortality was 59%, while their most recent 5 years, it had come down to 14%.

Thus, Ladd collected the facts and established a policy, and at the same time he successfully publicized his recommendations to the medical community.

As he started working with infants and children, another common condition in need of attention was pyloric stenosis. Rammstedt's operation was described in 1912. As with any innovation, it had been received slowly. In 1918 he described the poor results prior to the use of the Rammstedt operation [5]. He then described the results of its use in 26 cases, allowing but 15% mortality. He emphasized the importance of a suitable diagnosis, early operation, carefully given anesthetic, and gentle supportive care both before and after surgery. He developed and taught a system for this which was gradually modified and improved over the years. His second report, in 1927 [6], reviewed the methods used in 197 cases and demonstrated 4.5% mortality. His third and final study was published in 1941 in the book *Abdominal Surgery of Infancy and Childhood* [7], which was written with R. E. Gross. In this study he described their current methods, which of course included the use of IV fluids. The mortality in 177 cases from 1935 to 1939 was 0.56%.

Each of these two examples demonstrate his thorough and consistent care for patients and his never-ending attention to details.

Since I knew him starting in 1938, he made teaching ward visits to every patient daily including Sunday. He stopped in the X-ray department to see all the films from the previous day. If there had been a death, he went to pathology to look at the autopsy findings. He stored away in his mind the observations made at the pathology laboratory, always with an eye as to how things could be improved with a new or better surgical approach or a change in the ward care. I recall sitting with him for 40 minutes while he investigated the mesentery and intestine of an infant who had died with intestinal nonrotation.

In addition to intussusception and pyloric stenosis, he left his mark on the methods of treatment for many other types of pediatric surgical ailments. In his early years there was no established group of surgeons to care for babies with cleft lip and cleft palate. To fill the void, Ladd taught himself to become an expert in this field. He wrote a number of papers on the subject and helped rehabilitate hundreds of these children. He accomplished a great deal of other necessary surgery which would now be cared for by plastic surgeons, including free-hand split thickness grafting for burns, and the care of such things as web fingers, birthmarks, and angiomas.

He developed ways to drain pneumococcal empyema from the chest; this was a frequent and serious complication of pneumonia. Later he became heavily involved in the problems of atresia of the esophagus. His closest associate, Thomas Lanman, wrote what was regarded as the basic study leading up to the cure of these infants. This study examined the damage caused by the presence of tracheoesophageal fistulas and the various possible surgical approaches for division of the fistula and anastomosis of the esophagus. The surgeons were then hampered by the lack of intratracheal tubes and positive pressure anesthesia.

In 1939 Ladd saved the life of a newborn infant named Millicent Collins by bringing out the upper esophageal pouch at the neck, by closing the lower tracheoesophageal fistula, and by establishing a feeding gastrostomy. This operation took place just 24 h after a successful similar operation performed by Logan Levin in Minneapolis. Ladd's little patient then had an antethoracic tube constructed from pedicle skin grafts from her neck to her gastrostomy. Partly due to the splendid and loving care given her in the hospital for the first 2 years of her life, and then the warmth of her parents when she finally went home, she has grown up to be a well-adjusted woman with a family of her own.

A wide range of conditions attracted his systematic and thorough attention. Biliary atresia was one, and in 1928 he reported twelve cases of which six (50%) were believed to have been helped. This hopeful report was tempered in 1935 when he and Robert Gross described 40 cases of which nine (22%) were thought to have improved.

In retrospect it may be that the type of cases he saw before 1928 may have been localized atresias of the common duct, a condition which is now less commonly encountered than a type of sclerosis of the entire lower duct system.

Abnormalities of the anus and rectum were studied in a paper written with Gross in 1934 [8]. In this article they considered the embryology, the associated anomalies, and the methods of treatment in 162 cases. Similar studies were made for other intestinal obstructions including atresias of the duodenum, malrotation with volvulus, and duplications.

Ladd and his associates did all of the urological surgery in the hospital. They pioneered much of this. Two particular lesions bear his stamp. One is Wilms' tumor, which he discussed in a paper in 1938 [9]. In this paper he recommended the abdominal approach for removal of the tumor rather than the classical flank incision usually used for nephrectomy. He described 45 cases of which 11 were believed cured using this approach. Up until that time there had been but eight other cures reported in the literature. Three years later he reported a further group, with Robert White, in which the mortality dropped from 92% in 1923 to 60% in 1941 [10].

Another difficult urological problem was that presented by children with exstrophy of the bladder. He and Lanman discussed their methods of excision of the bladder with reconstruction of the penis in males and with ureterosigmoid anastomosis in all patients [11]. This offered early hopes for rehabilitation.

In 1941 the concise, clear, and beautifully illustrated *Abdominal Surgery of Infancy and Childhood* appeared, which he wrote together with Robert Gross. This book stands as a model of surgical exposition, and was widely acclaimed in its time. It covered a wide variety of common conditions plus many of the more unusual ones. Each section gave an analysis of the results of the large number of cases seen at the Boston Children's Hospital, together with the author's most recent recommendations for treatment.

Organizations

Ladd was first and foremost a member of the old-style New England merchant class and a leader in the Harvard surgical community. This image was reinforced by the fact that he was brought to and from the hospital by his family chauffeur. In spite of this, he was highly approachable and had an excellent sense of humor. He also was always considerate of everyone with whom he came in contact. In 1940, after 13 years as head of the surgical services at Children's Hospital, he was honored by the Medical School, the hospital, and his colleagues and friends by the creation of the Ladd Professorship of Child Surgery. He held this chair until his retirement in 1945. Not only was he recognized as the authority in pediatric surgery at Harvard, but he became the acknowledged leader throughout North America. In the United States he was honored by membership in the highest surgical groups, including the New England Surgical Society, the American College of Surgeons, and the American Surgical Association. He was a founding member of the American Board of Surgery and of the Surgical Section of the American Academy of Pediatrics. The latter was brought into being by his contemporary and fellow pioneer pediatric surgeon H. E. Coe. He also helped found and was President of the American Association of Plastic Surgeons. Within these organizations he spoke up for the importance of the studies of pediatric surgery and yet he recognized that everything could not be done by pediatric surgeons. He hoped to keep the specialty under the umbrella of general surgery. In this, his wishes and pronouncements have been successful in that the accrediting body for pediatric surgeons was developed as part of the American Board of Surgery. He also favored the establishment of the American Pediatric Surgical Association, which has grown and flourished under the auspices of his trainees and now of their successors.

Ladd's Influence

Ladd had an almost unique group of qualities in that he developed new and sound methods of surgical treatment, he was a skillful practitioner of these same methods, and finally he was a superb teacher at all levels, from medical students to residents as well as to the practicing medical and surgical community. His teaching ability equalled the rest of his accomplishments. He had teaching rounds on Saturday mornings which were aimed at the medical students and the other hospital staff. His daily rounds were directed at the students and other surgical staff and would have made Socrates proud. We have seen how he developed understanding of children's surgical problems and their methods of treatment. As a surgeon he had a delicate and capable technique in which he utilized a surgical knife as an extension of unusally large hands, often within a miniature chest or abdomen. His writing was simple, clear, and well illustrated, thanks to a resident medical artist, Miss Etta Piotti, and an excellent hospital photographer, Mr. Harding.

The result of all these attributes was to attract an enthusiastic group of trainees. At first his residency was free standing. In 1939 he and Elliott Cutler at the Peter Bent Brigham joined their training programs into a combined training unit which achieved great popularity, offering as it did a combination of adult and pediatric surgical experience in varying mixtures.

Of his trainees, by far the greatest is his former resident and immediate successor, Robert E. Gross. Gross followed directly in Ladd's footsteps, although more as a great innovator of surgery and teacher. He continued the same system of using standardized methods and record keeping, with a continuous update of methods as improvements appeared, either within the hospital or at another institution. The teaching methods and schedules remained the same, and the number and caliber of the residency applicants remained high.

For any group of professionals, be it farmers or surgeons, the success of that group must rest on the individual strenght and wisdom of the members of the group, and then on their collective strength through their organizations. As a role model and leader, one could hardly have found a better man than W. E. Ladd. This extended to his personal life as well as his professional one. As far as I can see, his example has been carried along among his professional descendants to a remarkable degree. Almost all of the present pediatric surgeons in North America have been influenced in one way or another by the examples which he set. His trainees have included such men as Gross, Swenson, Clatworthy, and Koop. With the notable addition of Willis Potts in Chicago, these men have produced most of the teachers and practitioners who are the leaders of the present generation.

Ladd continued with his usual activities until his retirement after the end of World War II, at the age of 65. Following this he lived mainly at his estate outside of Boston, active in hunting and other outdoor activities and with his married children and his grandchildren nearby. He remained available to all of his students for his always carefully thought out counsel. He died in 1967. He was an ornament to his profession.

Summary

William E. Ladd (1880–1967) was the great pioneer pediatric surgeon of North America. His family had been New England merchants. He was educated at Harvard and worked within the Harvard Medical School during his entire surgical career. He began to limit his surgical practice to the care of infants and children at the Boston Children's Hospital soon after World War I.

One basis for his great contributions lay in the establishment of an accurate medical records system with a thorough follow-up of the patients. Another basic factor was the development of uniform policies and methods for each type of surgical disease. These policies and methods then underwent evolution as potential improvements appeared.

Using this general approach, Ladd influenced the improvement in care of almost all of the common types of pediatric disease treatable by surgery. Among the earliest were intussusception and pyloric stenosis. Later, among many other things, he developed useful systems for the treatment of hernias, rectal bleeding, biliary atresia, failure of rotation of the G.I. tract, rectal anomalies, and exstrophy of the bladder. He made unusual contributions to the care of Wilms' tumor and atresia of the esophagus.

He was a great teacher. His pupils have become the teachers of many other pediatric surgeons throughout the world.

Résumé

William E. Ladd (1880–1967) fut le grand pionnier de la chirurgie des enfants en Amérique du Nord. Il descendait d'une famille de négociants de la Nouvelle Angleterre. Il fit ses études à Havard et ne cessa jamais de coopérer avec la "Havard Medical School". Peu après la première guerre mondiale, au "Children's Hospital" de Boston, il commença à se consacrer entièrement à la chirurgie des enfants.

C'est à lui que revient le mérite d'avoir établi des dossiers très complets sur ses patients qu'il ne perdait pas de vue et qu'il faisait bénéficier de contrôles postopératoires très minutieux. Il s'est aussi employé à uniformiser les techniques et méthodes des diverses interventions chirurgicales.

Sur la base de ces principes, le Dr. Ladd a grandement amélioré et fait avancer les techniques chirurgicales. Au début de sa carrière, il s'est beaucoup occupé du pylore. Plus tard, il se consacra au traitement des hernies, hémorragies du colon, occlusions de la vésicule biliaire, anomalies intestinales, entre autres.

On lui doit aussi beaucoup en ce qui concerne le traitement de la tumeur de Wilms et de l'occlusion de l'œsophage.

Il fut aussi un grand enseignant et ses élèves, à leur tour, furent les maîtres de beaucoup de grands chirurgiens dans le monde entier.

Zusammenfassung

William E. Ladd (1880–1967) war der große Pionier der Kinderchirurgie in Nordamerika. Er stammte aus einer Familie von Kaufleuten aus Neuengland. Er studierte in Harvard, und als Chirurg setzte er die Zusammenarbeit mit der Harvard

Medical School fort. Kurz nach dem 1. Weltkrieg begann er am Children's Hospital in Boston sich ganz der Kinderchirurgie zu widmen.

Eines seiner Verdienste – ein Grundprinzip seiner Tätigkeit – war das Anlegen von genauen Patientenakten und die Einführung einer gründlichen Nachsorge. Ein weiteres Grundprinzip war für ihn die Vereinheitlichung von Vorgehen und Methoden für die einzelnen Arten von chirurgischen Fällen. Dieses Vorgehen und diese Methoden wurden ständig überprüft und dem jeweiligen Fortschritt angepaßt.

Von diesen Prinzipien ausgehend konnte Ladd die Behandlung der meisten chirurgischen Fälle verbessern und vorantreiben. Sehr früh widmete er sich der Intussuszeption und der Pylorusstenose. Später galt seine Aufmerksamkeit dem Fortschritt in der Behandlung von Hernien, Darmblutungen, Gallenblasenverschluß, Fehlrotationssyndrom, Darmanomalien u. a.

Er leistete einen großen Beitrag im Hinblick auf die Behandlung des Wilms-Tumors und des Speiseröhrenverschlusses.

Er war ein großer Lehrer. Seine Schüler wiederum wurden die Lehrer vieler großer Chirurgen in der ganzen Welt.

References

1. Ladd WE (1911) Treatment of intussusception in children. Bost Med Surg J 164 (20 May 1911)
2. Ladd WE, Stone J (1913) Progress and treatment of intussusception. Bost Med Surg J 168 (15 April 1913)
3. Ladd WE (1915) Intussusception. Bost Med Surg J (Dec 8, 1915)
4. Ladd WE, Gross RE (1934) Intussusception in infancy and childhood. Arch Surg 29:365–384
5. Ladd WE (1918) Congenital pyloric stenosis. Bost Med Surg J (June 6, 1918)
6. Ladd WE (1927) Congenital hypertrophic pyloric stenosis. Bost Med Surg J (Feb 10, 1927)
7. Ladd WE, Gross RE (1941) Abdominal surgery of infancy and childhood. Saunders, Philadelphia
8. Ladd WE, Gross RE (1934) Congenital malformations of the anus and rectum. Am J Surg 23 (1 Jan 1934)
9. Ladd WE (1938) Embryoma of the kidney (Wilms' tumor). Ann Surg 108:5 (Nov 1938)
10. Ladd WE, White RC (1941) Embryoma of the kidney (Wilms' tumor). JAMA 117 (Nov 29, 1941)
11. Ladd WE, Lanman TH (1940) Exstrophy of the bladder and epispedias. N Engl J Med 222: 130–134

Denis Browne: Colleague (1892–1967)*

J. Crooks[1] †

Denis Browne (Fig. 1) was an extraordinary man in whom strength of character and convictions stuck out like rugged and dangerous rocks upon which the unwary might easily founder. Those who understood him – or, perhaps it would be better to say, partially understood him – admired him almost to the point of idolatry, although they must have been aware of the thrust of purpose which would never leave time to admit them to closer friendship. He was an intellectual adventurer, a rebel and a cynic, and he made up his mind from a very early age to take nothing at its face value. It was easy to believe, when he expounded on the many and var-

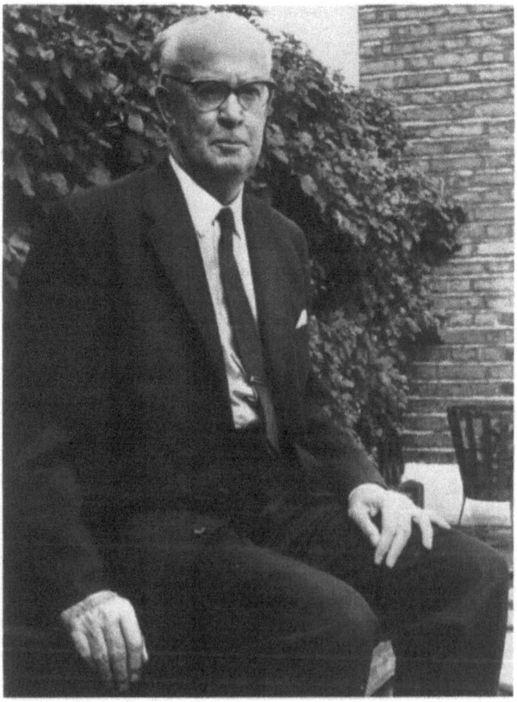

Fig. 1. Sir Denis Browne

* Reprinted from the *Selected Writings of Sir Denis Browne,* edited by H. H. Nixon, D. Waterston and C. A. S. Wink, by permission of the trustees of the Sir Denis Browne Memorial Fund

[1] Formerly Consultant Surgeon, The Hospital for Sick Children, Great Ormond Street, London, United Kingdom

Progress in Pediatric Surgery, Vol. 20
Ed. by P. P. Rickham

ious surgical procedures which attracted his special interest, that he had started from scratch and worked out all the logical solutions, and that he was ignorant of what others had written about that particular subject. This was not at all so; he was a voracious reader and had read almost everything about the subject, and then rejected it as based on erroneous assumptions or false reasoning. This was especially true of his conception of the fundamental part played by intrauterine position and pressure in the production of congenital deformities, starting with the various talipes and going on to curvature of the spine and dislocation of the hips. Of course, there are deformities which are due to lack of the proper and orderly cell multiplication and fusion which occur in a normal pregnancy where the foetus is free and easy. But in his last work, published soon after his death in *Advances in Teratology,* Volume 2, edited by D.H. Woollam and published by The Logos Press in 1967, and entitled "A Mechanistic Interpretation of Certain Malformations", one is convinced of the essential truth of his deductions by looking at the photographs, almost as surely as one was convinced by his demonstrations when he arranged the body of the newborn baby to show how it had lain in the uterus and how the deformities had arisen mechanically. He was working on this even during the few days in bed which preceded his death, and when I saw him then I thought what a wonderful life force and conviction were in this man, driving him on and on even when he was gravely ill. He was then still the supreme egotist, as the last sentences in this last published work show:

> In consequence I am reduced to giving a list of my own publications on the subject. As my thesis in this article is to suggest how the obvious has been overlooked or accepted teaching has been wrong, it is perhaps natural that this work has been ignored in other literature.

He quite rightly deemed himself greatly wronged by lack of recognition of the work which he knew to be true and of fundamental importance, and it was probably an essential character defect of someone like him that he gave not an inch in discussion, and overrode many of his colleagues, making enemies of them as he went. With a more gentle manner and modest approach he might have had an easy life with his genius acclaimed by everyone, rather than a life of struggle against ignorance and prejudice which, all the same, be greatly enjoyed.

It was a few years after the end of World War I, and Denis Browne was about 30 years of age, when I met him at Great Ormond Street Hospital for Sick Children. One of his duties then was to deal with the enormous tonsil and adenoid waiting list which that hospital had acquired as a legacy of the work of George Waugh in propounding the need for the operation to be done by careful dissection rather than by the generally accepted guillotine method. Browne was a demon for work and organised an operation session of 25 tonsils and adenoids a day from Monday to Friday, and 10 on Saturdays; on Sundays I suppose he thought about tonsils and adenoids and was engaged in his first clinical anatomical research. In this he showed the cause of bleeding after the tonsil operation and first described the large and tortuous vein which lies between the tonsil and the posterior pillar of the fauces. At Great Ormond Street, and, I hope, elsewhere, it is called "Browne's vein". He was at this time also engaged in developing suitable instruments to facilitate the operation, and these are to be found in all the main catalogues of instruments today. He had the habit and the art of attaching his name to them and went on doing this all his life, so using one of the few advertising channels open to the profession. Later on, of course, the various instruments, splints and operations he devised were gladly acknowledged as "Browne's", so that his name grew from being a household word at his hospital to an international name in the field of paediatric surgery. It is not the purpose of this character study to assess the inventions and achievements of this great paediatric surgeon, for they are referenced in the bibliography, but mention has to be made of the way the name of Denis Browne was first billed in lights on the medical hoardings, and of course it was kept lit and intensified over the years, not only by the published accounts of his major surgical thoughts and procedures, but by the continuous barrage of controversial, unforgiving and witty correspondence he contributed to medical journals.

In those early days when he was engaged in coping with these tonsil and adenoid lists he was casualty officer and lived out of hospital. The junior casualty officer dealt with the ordinary casualty work until Denis Browne arrived at a time which, no doubt, seemed to him suitable for starting his enormous operation sessions, but that time varied considerably and was confusing, if not irritating, to his juniors and the nursing staff. One day when I was awaiting his arrival a house surgeon told me not to be impatient, because Browne (we did not call him "D. B." in those days) would not be in for some time. He had just come from Regent Street on a bus and had seen Browne walking down Regent Street practising golf strokes with his umbrella. On an other occasion he would arrive on a foggy London day and announce that "the climatic conditions were unsuitable for surgery". He was right and had the courage of his convictions, and acted upon them. The mothers and children went home, and so did Browne. One day a friend of mine came to watch Denis Browne operating. He was thinking about tennis racquets that day as well as tonsils and adenoids, and made practice back-hand shots between cases with tonsil-holding forceps. "Very strange", my friend said. "He'll never make a surgeon." I wish I could meet that friend again and say in Cromwell's words: "I beseech you in the bowels of Christ think it possible you may be mistaken!"

After a year or two he became resident medical superintendent of the hospital, and the whole field of children's surgery was open to him. In those happy days nearly all the surgical chiefs disappeared in August and September, and it was then that the RMS. was able to extend his practical operative experience. At this time Denis was chiefly interested in harelip and palate operations, but also in the Ramstedt operation for pyloric stenosis. The supply of skilled anaesthetists then was not so abundant as it is today, and he developed a technique of doing this operation under local anaesthesia with remarkable improvement in the survival rate. It was at about this time, too, that the idea of the mechanistic cause of congenital deformities germinated in his mind. He made his first instrument for the non-operative treatment of talipes equino varus, which we used to call "Browne's beetle crusher".

Denis Browne was a strangely aloof RMS. At breakfast in the doctors' mess he sat, as was his right, at the top of the table, and propped *The Times* in front of him to exclude the rabble of the lesser house staff. He cooked his own lunch, which was always a three-egg omelette, and did not deign to dine in. He had an invaluable gift, a sort of instinct, which told him when he could be safely out of the hospital or when he had to be prepared to work there twenty-four hours at a stretch. He fostered this instinct so that, years later during World War II when he was largely responsible for air raid casualties, he seemed to know when a lull in the raids was due and would disappear, only to return as the first bombs fell. During his residency at the hospital as a young man this instinct served him so well that he was able to spend quite a bit of time with his wife, Helen Simpson, a successful writer who lived in a flat at the top of Sloane Street. It was against the rules in those days for men holding resident appointments to be married but Denis was always a rebel, and a successful one, and nobody found out.

Denis Browne was always interested in his cloths and appearance. He would arrive for the residents' Christmas dinner (I suppose from the comforts of his connubial flat) dressed in a full opera cloak and opera hat, and he was an impressive sight with all the grandeur of his 6 feet 4 inches, slight figure and vital face. When he became a consultant he wore a morning coat and sponge-bag trousers, and when he went shooting he had a real knickerbocker suit with capacious game pockets. We juniors envied him his flair for clothes and the means he had for satisfying it.

In those young days Denis Browne was a tennis player of Wimbledon standard, and on the residents' court at the hospital it was painfully obvious to us all that we could not give him a game. It is doubtful if he ever had time or inclination to be a frequenter of billiard saloons, but on the mess billiard table he was disposed to practice what looked like professional shots whenever there was a gap between his operating lists, and again none of us could give him a game. He was also a good shot, and interested in guns. I remember meeting him in Regent Street not so many years ago, carrying a gun in his hand. He explained that he was on the way from his gunsmith, who had been making a Browne modification. With his nature he could not leave the tennis racquet as it had so foolishly been made ever since tennis was played, with an oval face. He said one was as likely to miss the ball laterally as vertically, and so the face should be circular. The universal golf club he made, on which the angle of lift was altered by a butterfly nut and screw, also had a lot to be said for it. He demonstrated it in the residents' mess room so effectually that the ball entered the ward of the homeopathic hospital next door; fortunately, the broken panes of glass did not injure anyone. The Good Lord looks after His own. Denis Browne practised his tennis shots against a wall in his rather large bedroom, where he had painted a line at net level. The noise drove away his next-door neighbour, and the maid kept putting the bedroom chair in the middle of the wall. He therefore moved it to the end of the room and nailed it there. So on and on it went. He was adventurous, rebellious and difficult, but had an intellectual curiosity and an intense interest in technical problems.

Denis Browne had an extraordinary ability to shut himself off from the rest of the world when he was brooding on one of his theories. Those who did not know him well enough to admire and understand this were often offended because they seemed not to exist for him. But he was away in another world at these times, and when he came back his shy and sensitive nature made it difficult for him to re-establish ordinary human relationships. He nevertheless brought back from these voyages of thought treasures of surgical truths and practical remedies which are fundamental. These characteristics carried him on so that he made great contributions to children's surgery and in the end became recognised as its doyen.

His intolerance of ignorance, illogicality and conformity was equalled only by his dislike of committee procedure and compromise. He used to sit through medical committee usually without saying a word, but if he did it was to throw a practical spanner in the involved gear box, which was by no means synchromeshed, of medical politics. If the chairman asked for his opinion on the subject under discussion he would reply that he had given the matter no thought. During the meeting he was usually playing with a piece of metal or string, or working away with one of those wonderful all-purpose pocket knives, perfecting or inventing some mechanical device or surgical procedure. He had always been given to making things himself; at his first professional house in Queen Anne Street, the first door on the left led into a completely equipped workshop where he made the prototypes of his own splints, and later on he had a similar room in Wilton Street.

Before Helen Simpson died in the middle of the World War II, Denis Browne had been deeply involved in the world of letters and books. She wrote several successful novels and a few recondite history books, and her friends included Clemence Dane and Margaret Kennedy. Helen and Denis Browne wrote some most amusing letters to the medical press in the Sherlock Holmes style, which were signed by Denis Browne; I am told he wrote some of the chapters in Helen's books. He was interested in the use of words and as he wrote a considerable amount of surgical literature he became expert in concise description. Could anything be more briefly explicit than "My Gawd" or "C.B.I." written obliquely across the notes in his large hand? The C.B.I. (congenital bloody idiot) referred to the mother or grandmother – for children he had a loving tolerance! After Helen died he went through a very lonely period of his life when he was still living at Great Ormond Street to look after air raid casualties. He would often have his daughter to stay with him in the hospital, and when things were quiet they would go for long walks in the country. She says that what they talked about was the universe and Denis Browne and Denis Browne and the universe. They used also to go for runs through London at night in the blackout to keep fit. A policeman found it difficult to accept the innocent explanation of this tall, handsome man who was running after a good-looking blonde girl with long legs.

A few years later Denis Browne married Lady Moyra Ponsonby and they lived in Wilton Street until his death. He shared a professional house with Sir Wilfrid Sheldon and myself in Harley Street. There came a settled span of life when he went from strength to strength in his professional work, and his reputation spread throughout the world. His new work was on hypospadias, and he continued with the development of his theories on the mechanistic causation of congenital deformities. This is a very big and profound conception and an area of medical thought of enormous potential and importance. It was his main intellectual occupation until, and indeed during, his last brief illness.

Denis Browne was one of the founder members of the British Association of Paediatric Surgeons and its first and most illustrious president. The growth of this Association has been phenomenal and it has collected into its membership nearly all the paediatric surgeons in Europe, so that it is in fact much more an international than a national body. But it must give us all pride and satisfaction that its British origin is still enshrined in its name, and it is in part a monument to the genius of Denis Browne, who was the first surgeon in this country to devote himself entirely to children.

Such international fame led naturally to many invitations to lecture and give operating demonstrations in various parts of the world, and during the last few years of his life, when he had not so many fixed commitments in London, he was able to accept them. Such visits were very carefully planned and scheduled by Lady Moyra Browne, who was a trained nurse. There is a very satisfying recollection of this well-ordered and productive household in Belgravia, with Denis pursuing and initiating surgical truth, Moyra using her talent for organisation and administration to benefit the St. John's Ambulance Brigade (of which she is now Superintendent-in-Chief), and both of them enjoying the intellectual achievement of their son and the fortunate inheritance by their daughter of their combined physical endowments.

Denis Browne was of Irish descent, and his paternal grandfather, Captain Sylvester Browne, was a master-mariner who married an English girl and sailed his own ship, the Proteus, to Sydney with her in 1831. He lived in Sydney for a time and then in Melbourne, where he acquired several properties which proved a bad speculation, and in 1842 he moved to a sheep station.

Denis Browne's maternal grandfather was William Foster Stawell, who also sailed from Ireland to Melbourne in the ship of his distant cousin, whose daughter, Mary Greene, he married in 1856. He was a lawyer and was to become Attorney General, later Chief Justice, and, finally, Lieutenant Governor, of Victoria. Captain Sylvester Browne had two sons and seven daughters; the second of his two sons, Sylvester, married the elder of Sir William Stawell's daughters, and they were the parents of Denis. They were married in London in 1890 and on April 2, 1892, Denis was born to them in Melbourne. In 1901 when Denis was 9 years old they moved to a sheep station in New South Wales, where he had wonderful opportunities for riding and shooting and developing his skill at other country pursuits. The family remained there until 1914. Denis went as a boarder to Kings School, where he was a brilliant but difficult pupil. He did not like the orthodox games, and although he won the main school essay prize for divinity this did not indicate piety or saintliness, but just that he was much better than anyone else in the school at writing. His headmaster told his father that he was head and shoulders above all the other pupils mentally, and I think he might have added, physically. He got a scholarship to St. Paul's College, Sydney University, where he studied medicine. He won Blues for tennis and shooting and was nicknamed "Splinter Browne", because he was so tall and slim.

Denis was allowed to take his final medical examinations a year earlier than usual so that he could go off to the war, and he was drafted to Gallipoli. There he was seriously ill with typhoid when a ship arrived to take off "walking cases" only. Denis summoned bis batman and another man and they supported him until he got on board. The officer demanded to know who he was, and Denis, not liking silly questions even at the best of times, fainted on top of the officer and the ship sailed before things could be sorted out. After convalescing in Australia he returned to the war in France and became a Major in the Field Ambulance. At the end of the war he came to England, and did not return to Australia until he went in 1965 as Sir Denis Browne, KCVO, chevalier de la Légion d'honneur, emeritus surgeon to the Great Ormond Street Hospital for Sick Children, and the acknowledged leader of paediatric surgery. He was given an honorary fellowship of the Royal Australasian College of Surgeons.

In England, when he returned after World War I, he had no difficulty in becoming a Fellow of the Royal College of Surgeons of England, and soon found his way to Great Ormond Street. He did all the usual junior jobs in an unusual way; at the election for the key post of resident medical superintendent he was not successful and was passed over for a man whom the Medical Committee felt would not be so disturbing and would not upset their orthodox views. But soon after this the post fell vacant again; the surgeons had begun to see the light which was later to shine so brightly, and he was appointed resident medical superintendent, I should hazard with a good deal of trepidation. Later, when the next honorary consulting surgical vacancy on the staff occurred, Denis was appointed.

He was the first surgeon in England to devote himself entirely to children. The surgeons in London at that time regarded children's surgery as an interesting subbranch of surgery with a capital *S*. They typically had three or four hospitals where they spent a few hours each week, and the children's hospital was just one of them. It was for Denis to show by his great gifts and devotion to one children's hospital how much paediatric surgery could be advanced. He led the revolution, and now there are paediatric surgeons in all countries which can lay any claim to progress in medical science.

Can one trace the influences which were at work to produce Denis Browne? First of all his intelligence; he had intelligent forebears on both sides. Then adventurousness; could that be from his Irish descent? And then his bluntness of manner to some of his colleagues and his feeling that his work was ignored, or at least not accepted at its true worth by his fellow surgeons; could this be anything to do with being an Australian? And lastly his cynicism; this one can readily understand in anyone of intelligence who as a young man spent 4 years at war in Gallipoli and France.

Summary

The purpose of this character study is not to assess the achievements of this great paediatric surgeon but to describe this extraordinary, adventurous, rebellious and difficult man, his intelligence, intellectual curiosity and intense interest in technical problems, as well as his bluntness of manner which was confusing and irritating to some of his colleagues.

Denis Browne is described as a shy and sensitive nature, which made it difficult for him to establish ordinary human relationships, but also as a strangely aloof colleague with a flair for clothes, remarkable skills at riding, shooting, tennis, billiard and golf, and much admired by his juniors.

Denis Browne is also described as a demon for work, a man who had the courage of his convictions and acted upon them. Those who understood him admired him to the point of idolatry but he was also considered as the supreme egotist not giving an inch in discussions and overriding many of his colleagues, making enemies of them as he went and then deeming himself greatly wronged by lack of recognition. With a more modest approach he might have had an easy life with his genius acclaimed by everyone, rather than a life of struggle against ignorance and prejudice which, all at the same, he greatly enjoyed.

Résumé

Il n'est pas question ici de rappeler les mérites de ce grand chirurgien mais de faire le portrait d'un homme tout à fait extraordinaire, audacieux, rébarbatif et de caractère difficile, de décrire son intelligence, sa curiosité intellectuelle et sa passion pour la solution des problèmes techniques ainsi que son manque total de complaisance qui mettait très mal à l'aise beaucoup de ses collègues et les irritait.

L'auteur décrit Denis Browne comme un timide, un être d'une grande sensibilité qui avait grand mal à établir des relations normales et aussi comme un collègue bizarre et hautain qui appréciait l'élégance vestimentaire et le sport: bon cavalier, bon fusil, jouant remarquablement au tennis, au billard et au golf et faisant ainsi l'admiration de ses jeunes collègues.

Denis Browne est aussi présenté comme un acharné au travail, un homme qui agissait toujours en fonction de ses convictions. Ceux qui le comprenaient l'idolâtraient mais l'auteur le décrit aussi comme un homme ayant toujours besoin d'être admiré, ne cédant jamais un pouce de terrain dans une discussion, refusant tous les compromis et ignorant l'opinion de ses collègues dont il se faisait régulièrement des ennemis et qui par la suite se plaignait qu'on ne lui rendait pas justice et qu'on ne le comprenait pas. Il semble qu'avec un peu plus de modestie, il aurait mené une vie plus calme. Son génie se serait imposé plus facilement et il n'aurait pas été contraint de lutter sans cesse contre l'ignorance et les préjugés, ce que, par ailleurs, il adorait faire.

Zusammenfassung

In diesem Beitrag geht es nicht darum, die Verdienste dieses großen Kinderchirurgen aufzuzeigen, sondern darum, diesen ganz und gar ungewöhnlichen, kühnen, widerspenstigen und schwierigen Menschen sowie seine Intelligenz, seine intellektuelle Neugier und sein leidenschaftliches Interesse für technische Fragen, aber auch sein barsches Benehmen, das viele seiner Kollegen verunsicherte und verärgerte, zu beschreiben.

Denis Browne wird als schüchterner und empfindlicher Mensch beschrieben, dem es schwer fiel, normale menschliche Beziehungen aufzubauen, und gleichzeitig als merkwürdig unnahbarer Kollege, der Sinn für elegante Kleidung hatte und eine bemerkenswerte Fertigkeit im Reiten, Schießen, Tennis, Billard und Golf besaß, die ihm die Bewunderung seiner jüngeren Kollegen einbrachte.

Denis Browne wird auch als auf Arbeit versessen beschrieben und als ein Mann, der zu seinen Überzeugungen stand und danach handelte. Diejenigen, die ihn verstanden, vergötterten ihn geradezu, aber er wurde auch als in höchstem Maße geltungsbedürftig beschrieben, als ein Mann, der in Diskussionen nie einlenkte, sich über seine Kollegen hinwegsetzte und sich aus ihnen unweigerlich Feinde machte, um sich danach bitter über Ungerechtigkeit und mangelnde Anerkennung zu beschweren. Mit etwas mehr Bescheidenheit wäre sein Leben vermutlich ruhiger verlaufen. Jeder hätte ihn als Genie gepriesen, und er hätte nicht sein Leben lang gegen Unwissenheit und Vorurteile ankämpfen müssen, was ihm andererseits jedoch sehr viel Freude bereitete.

Denis Browne: Surgeon*

P. P. Rickham[1]

He was a man, take him for all in all, I shall not look upon his like again.

Shakespeare, *Hamlet*

Introduction

Denis Browne's appearance on the British surgical scene shortly after World War I was in many ways a unique occasion. As an outsider coming from far away he was appointed to the staff of one of the most exclusive hospitals in the British Isles and, casting financial considerations to the wind, he then proceeded to become the first surgeon in England to confine his practice entirely to children. His views on the pathology and anatomy of many paediatric surgical conditions differed widely from those of his elders. The methods of treatment devised by him were new and often revolutionary and were frequently attacked and criticized, but they worked. For the first time he was able to produce consistently satsifactory results in a branch of surgery which had hitherto had hardly anything but disasters to record.

His disregard for conventions, as well as his pungent wit, made him many enemies among the senior members of his profession. As he grew older, the attitude towards him slowly changed. He was still the outsider who wanted to teach orthopaedics to the orthopaedic surgeons, plastic surgery to the plastic surgeons, ear, nose and throat surgery to the otorhinolaryngologists, and most of all the general surgery of childhood to the general surgeons, and this was resented. Gradually, however, the brilliance of his teaching and the excellence of his surgery came to be appreciated by a new generation of surgeons, whose imagination he stimulated and to whom he showed a new and hardly explored field. It is little wonder that he won the admiration and loyalty of all the men whom he trained and who came into contact with him and his work.

Denis Browne was the father of modern British paediatric surgery, but his influence goes further than that. He was a truly original thinker. Some of his ideas may in the light of subsequent discoveries have been proved incorrect or only partially correct, but they were always new and exciting and at the same time based on fundamental facts. He was a very great surgeon, the nearest approach to a genius one is likely to encounter in surgery.

---

* Reprinted from Selected Writings of Sir Denis Browne, edited by H. H. Nixon, D. Waterston and C. A. S. Wink, by permission of the trustees of the Sir Denis Browne Memorial Fund

[1] Universitäts-Kinderklinik, Chirurgische Abteilung, Steinwiesstr. 75, CH-8032 Zürich, Switzerland

Progress in Pediatric Surgery, Vol. 20
Ed. by P. P. Rickham

Orthopaedics and the Aetiology of Congenital Deformities

> Children have become crippled in the following way. If the womb is narrow at that part in which the crippling is produced, it is inevitable that the body moving in a narrow space should become crippled in that part.
>
> *Hippocrates*

There is little doubt than Denis Browne regarded his research into the aetiology of congenital deformities as his most important single scientific contribution. His work on this subject spanned the whole of his long and active life, and he published more papers on this subject than on any other. As his theory on the causation of deformities was largely based on his observations of children with orthopaedic malformations, the subjects are best discussed together.

As early as 1931, in his first article on talipes equinovarus, he discussed the nature of the deformity and pointed out that this type of malformation could be explained by assuming that the foetus had suffered from continuous external pressure while pinioned in a cross-legged position against the concave walls of the uterus. The theory of the mechanical origin of congenital deformities was further evolved and enlarged in a study published in 1936, when talipes, torticollis, displaced ears, congenital facial paralysis, acrocephalosyndactyly, congenital dislocation of the hip, pressure dimples, arthrogryposis and a number of other conditions were postulated to be caused by selective or generalized intra-uterine pressure.

This theory was not new; it dated back to antiquity, but never before had it been put forward on the basis of such a wealth of clinical data. Browne's great powers of clinical observation were shown by his discovery of mutual deformities of different parts of the body, which further supported his views. He defended his opinions in numerous further articles, lectures and often highly sarcastic letters to medical journals. He also collected a large volume of clinical material in support of his theories. He was never a lover of experimental studies, especially not of animal experiments. He recognised that they were necessary for the progress of surgery, but thought that their importance had been overrated and analytical reasoning from careful clinical observations neglected. His views received scant recognition and often open hostility from embryologists, pathologists and orthopaedic surgeons. This only strengthened his belief that progress in modern medicine and surgery was too one-sided.

The mechanical theory of the causation of deformities led him to search for methods of treatment which would correct orthopaedic deformities by the use of selectively applied pressures and controlled movements. By the use of his splints permitting controlled movements he thus revolutionised the treatment of such conditions as talipes, congenital dislocation of the hip and scoliosis. He used his great ingenuity in the design of these splints and all his great technical skull in devising the correct methods of their application. He was at pains to point out that unless surgeons had personally watched him applying these splints they would not be successful in using his methods, and he deplored the numerous modifications of his appliances devised by men who had never taken the trouble to watch him applying them.

Denis Browne did not like open corrections of orthopaedic deformities, and repeatedly demonstrated the brilliant results achieved by his "conservative" methods when compared with operative corrections. During the later years of his life he came more and more to recognise the importance of active exercise for the strengthening of muscles as a necessary adjunct to splinting.

Anatomical Studies and their Clinical Applications

> How long will it take for this piece of knowledge to get into the anatomy books?
>
> *Denis Browne*

Anyone who knew Denis Browne could not help admiring his faculty for quickly getting down to the roots of any problem. When confronted by a surgical problem he would invariably start by studying the anatomy of the region involved, and he was not willing to accept the teaching of anatomists, however hallowed by time. For this reason he spent much of his time during the early years of his surgical career in London in the anatomy department of the London Hospital. He clearly saw the limitations of anatomical studies on "pickled" cadavers, where conditions were so very different from those found in the living body. He deplored the fact that it seemed to be impossible to get the professor of anatomy into the operating theatre to verify in the living what they believed to have discovered in the dead. He did not, of course, deny the value of anatomical dissections of cadavers per se; he himself used them, but only as an adjunct to his findings in the operating theatre.

He used his anatomical studies to elucidate problems which had puzzled him in surgical practice, such as incomplete descent of the then current teaching that in childhood the testicles could be pulled up by the cremasteric muscle into the inguinal canal. He was the first to describe the superficial inguinal pouch, but although he was ceaselessly demonstrating the presence of this obvious anatomical structure, and although he published several papers on this subject explaining among other things why hormone treatment for "undescended testicles" could not possibly work, his findings were not generally accepted by the anatomists. The same anatomical studies eventually enabled him to perfect the operation for inguinal hernia in infancy and childhood.

Denis Browne had similar experiences with other anatomical investigations, such as his studies of the anatomy and physiology of the pharynx which came to form the basis of his operation for cleft palate, and also his work on the surgical anatomy of the tonsil. He described the arterial supply and venous drainage of the tonsil for the first time in accurate detail. When one considers the tens of thousands of tonsillectomies carried out each year, it is surprising that the importance of this work was not immediately grasped. It is difficult to understand why Browne's anatomical approach was at first so widely ignored. In his opinion the main reason was probably that he was an amateur and not a professional, and professionals do not like outsiders to teach them their business. There is, however, a little truth in Browne's bitter comment that anatomists were reminiscent of medieval theologians in refusing to examine the truth of statements which conflicted with their own opinions.

Surgical Management and Techniques

> A surgeon specially skilled and interested in such cases is the final and not unimportant requirement.
>
> *Denis Browne*

It was in his development of the general surgery of infancy and childhood that Denis Browne made his greatest impact on paediatric surgery. With characteristic breadth of vision he studied most aspects of paediatric abdominal surgery, pre- and postoperative management, anaesthesia, operative techniques and instruments. He made advances in all of them and although today some of his views (for instance, those on anaesthesia) may have been superseded, others are still as pertinent as they were when they were first propounded.

Browne was the first surgeon to routinely employ transverse abdominal incisions in childhood, pointing out the shortcomings of the conventional median and paramedian incisions. Contrary to the teachings of the Boston school, he preferred immediate anastomosis following the resection of necrosed bowel to the temporary enterostomies practised on the other side of the Atlantic. He improved neonatal intestinal surgery by introducing his end-to-back anastomosis. His original studies on the pathological anatomy of pyloric stenosis led to a rationalisation and perfection of the operative technique.

Malformations of the perineum were the subject of many of Denis Browne's studies. Imperforate anus (a term he abhorred) was of special interest to him. His was one of the first comprehensive classifications of the many malformations collected under this heading, and he greatly advanced our knowledge of the embryological and pathological anatomy of the various "low" variations of this malformation. His ingenious and characteristically simple back-out operation solved many of the problems associated with the therapy of this condition.

Of his advances in the treatment of malformations of the external genitalia, his operation for hypospadias is probably the best known. In Dickson Wright's words, he created a fistula to end all fistulae, and his brilliant idea still forms the basis of most modern methods of treating this condition.

Many of Denis Browne's other advances in paediatric surgery were at the time as original and important as those which have already been mentioned, but have for one reason or other lost in importance owing to subsequent developments. He greatly improved the treatment of various infective conditions such as tuberculous glands, empyema and osteomyelitis, but today, when such infections have become less common because of vaccination and chemotherapy, this tends to be forgotten. It is also often forgotten that he was a pioneer of paediatric cardiovascular surgery in this country, because the great subsequent advances in cardiac surgery have overshadowed his original work.

Denis Browne's inventive genius was best seen in his development of numerous special surgical instruments and appliances. Their simplicity of design was matched only by the ease with which they could be used.

Personal Relations and Teaching

Denis Browne's imposing presence and strength of character impressed all who worked with him. He was a magnificent surgical technician, a perfectionist who constantly improved his techniques and insisted that his juniors should follow his guiding instructions in detail. Those who did not know him well often wondered how such a very tall man could manage to handle and operate on babies with such consummate skill. His gentleness was wholly remarkable, whether he was putting a small child at his ease when examining him or whether he was performing a difficult operation on the delicate tissues of a newborn infant.

He was an outstanding teacher, and infected his juniors with his own enthusiasm. He took a great personal interest in each of his pupils, watched over them and was as delighted about their successes as if they had been his own. Today his pupils can be found all over the globe, and during his later years he travelled widely and visited many of them.

Denis Browne has always kind and considerate to the parents of his patients, and it is little wonder that after his death so many of them showed their gratitude and appreciation of his devotion and skill by contributing to his memorial fund.

> The wounded surgeon plies the steel
> That questions the distempered part;
> Beneath the bleeding hands we feel
> The sharp compassion of the healer's art.
>
> *T. S. Eliot*

Summary

Denis Browne was the first surgeon in England to confine his practice entirely to children. The methods of treatment devised by him were new and often revolutionary and were frequently attacked and criticized, but they worked.

He regarded his research into the aetiology of congenital deformities as his most important single scientific contribution. In 1931, he published his first article on talipes equinovarus. He further enlarged his theory of the mechanical origin of congenital deformities in a study published in 1936. The mechanical theory led him to search for treatment by use of selectively applied pressures and controlled movements. He did not like open corrections. When confronted by a surgical problem he would invariably start by studying the anatomy of the region involved. He was the first to describe the superficial inguinal pouch. His anatomical studies eventually enabled him to perfect the operation for inguinal hernia in infancy and childhood and formed the basis of his operation for cleft palate and of his work on the surgical anatomy of the tonsil.

He was the first pediatric surgeon to routinely employ transverse abdominal incisions. He preferred immediate anastomosis to the temporary enterostomies. He introduced the end-to-back anastomosis. He helped rationalizing and perfecting the operative technique for pyloric stenosis. Malformations of the perineum were the subject of many studies. His operation for hypospadias is also well known.

His other advances in paediatric surgery, such as treatment of various infective conditions and cardiovascular surgery, were at the time original and important. His inventive genius was best seen in his development of numerous instruments and appliances. He was a magnificent surgical technician and constantly improved his techniques.

Résumé

Denis Browne fut le premier chirurgien en Angleterre à se consacrer entièrement à la chirurgie infantile. Ses méthodes étaient nouvelles et souvent révolutionnaires. Elles firent l'objet de fréquentes critiques mais les résultats obtenus témoignaient en leur faveur.

Sa contribution scientifique la plus importante, à ses yeux, est dans le domaine de l'étiologie des malformations. En 1931 parut sa première publication sur le pied-bot varus équin. En 1936, il publia les résultats d'observations renforçant sa théorie d'une cause mécanique. Se fondant sur cette théorie, il mit au point des méthodes de traitement par pression et mouvements. Il était contre les opérations de correction. Chaque fois qu'il était confronté à un problème chirurgical, il commençait par reprendre l'étude de l'anatomie de la région en question. Il décrivit pour la première fois la hernie congénitale. Ses connaissances en anatomie étaient telles qu'elles lui permirent de faire avancer considérablement la chirurgie abdominale des nouveaux-nés et des jeunes et de mettre au point sa méthode pour l'opération de la fente palatine. Elles lui furent aussi très utiles pour l'ablation des amygdales palatines.

Il fut le premier chirurgien à utiliser les incisions abdominales transversales. Il préférait l'anastomose directe à une entérostomie temporaire. Il introduisit l'anastomose entre l'extrémité et le dos. Il continua à rationaliser et perfectionner la technique d'opération de la sténose du pylore. Il publia plusieurs articles sur les malformations du périnée. Son opération de l'hypospadias est aussi très célèbre.

A l'époque, ses autres résultats dans le domaine de la chirurgie infantile, le traitement des maladies infectieuses et la chirurgie cardiovasculaire ouvraient tous une nouvelle voie et étaient d'une importance considérable. Son esprit d'invention lui permit de mettre au point de nombreux instruments et appareils. C'était un brillant opérateur qui ne cessa jamais de perfectionner sa technique.

Zusammenfassung

Denis Browne war der erste Chirurg in England, der sich ganz der Kinderchirurgie widmete. Seine Behandlungsmethoden waren neu und oft revolutionär. Sie wurden vielfach angegriffen und kritisiert, aber die Ergebnisse sprachen für sie.

Sein größter wissenschaftlicher Beitrag war – in seinen Augen – die Ätiologie der angeborenen Mißbildungen, 1931 veröffentlichte er seine erste Arbeit über den Talipes equinovarus. In einer 1936 erschienenen Untersuchung bekräftigte er seine Theorie einer mechanischen Ursache. Von dieser Theorie ausgehend suchte er nach Behandlungsmethoden auf der Basis von selektiver Druckeinwirkung und kontrollierter Bewegung. Er mochte operative Korrekturen nicht. Jedesmal, wenn er mit einem chirurgischen Problem konfrontiert wurde, beschäftigte er sich zu allererst mit der Anatomie der betroffenen Region. Er beschrieb als erster den angeborenen Leistenbruch. Aufgrund seiner anatomischen Studien war er dann in der Lage, die Bauchoperation bei Säuglingen und Kleinkindern zu verbessern sowie seine Methode für die Operation der Gaumenspalte zu entwickeln. Ferner waren sie ihm von großem Nutzen bei der Gaumenmandelchirurgie.

Er war der erste Chirurg, der grundsätzlich Bauchquerschnitte verwendete. Er zog die direkte Anastomose der Übergangsenterostomie vor. Er führte die End-zu-End-Anastomose ein. Er trug dazu bei, daß die Operationstechnik der Pylorusstenose rationalisiert und vervollkommnet wurde. Er schrieb mehrfach über die Perineummißbildungen. Sehr bekannt ist auch seine Hypospadieoperation.

Damals waren auch seine anderen Leistungen auf dem Gebiet der Kinderchirurgie, wie die Behandlung von Infektionskrankheiten und die kardiovaskuläre Chirurgie, bahnbrechend und von großer Bedeutung. Seine Erfindungsgabe ermöglichte es ihm, viele Instrumente und Geräte zu entwickeln. Er war ein glänzender Chirurg, der ständig seine Techniken verbesserte.

Robert E. Gross

H. W. Clatworthy[1]

Robert E. Gross devoted his lifetime to pediatric surgery. He was born in Baltimore, Maryland, on July 2, 1905, the son of Charles Jacob and Emma Houch. His father was the manager of the Stief Piano Company, and young Bob grew up in Baltimore, together with five sisters and two brothers.

As a boy, Gross was described as a sensitive, somewhat shy tinkerer, an avid reader, a keen observer, and a great lover of the outdoors. During high school summer holidays, he journeyed, first by train and later by "jalopy" to a central Minnesota farm to work, thereby deepening his instinctive concern for living things and nature's ways. These intensively rewarding summertime experiences led to his choice of Carleton College, located in a small central Minnesota town, for his early collegiate education. At that time, Gross had yet to establish any firm career plans, although he favored majoring in chemistry and initially embarked on such a course of studies. However, a Christmas gift from a friend was to change all of that. When Harvey Cushing's bulky biography of Sir William Osler arrived, he nearly dropped out of college to find the time to devour those two volumes. By the spring of his first year of college, he had decided to study medicine – and to attend Harvard Medical School because his newly found author-idol, Harvey Cushing, was teaching there. This he did in 1927 after graduating with Phi Beta Kappa honors from Carleton.

At Harvard, he was a top student whose enthusiasm for children's surgery, a then almost unknown and certainly officially unrecognized field of endeavor, was kindled during his 4th year by a 1-month elective rotation on the service of William E. Ladd. In 1931, he received his M.D. degree, was made a member of Alpha Omega Alpha for scholastic excellence, and selected a postgraduate training program with Burt Wolbach, then chairman of the department of pathology at Harvard Medical School and chief of the departments at the Peter Bent Brigham, Boston Children's, and Lying-In Hospitals. Wolbach was to become Gross's great friend and confidant, with whom he subsequently enjoyed a very productive professional relationship. For many years, they also shared Gross's only regular relaxation – early morning and occasional weekend horseback rides along the trails and through the woodlands of Framingham, Massachusetts, where these loyal friends chose to live with their families in delightful rural settings.

After completing the 2-year program in pathology with Wolbach and Sidney Farber at the Children's Hospital, Gross entered training as an assistant resident

[1] Children's Hospital, 700 Children's Drive, Columbus, OH 43205, USA

Progress in Pediatric Surgery, Vol. 20
Ed. by P. P. Rickham

in surgery with Elliott Cutler, who had succeeded Cushing as the Moseley Professor of Surgery at the Peter Bent Brigham Hospital and with Ladd, who then occupied the first chair of pediatric surgery to be established in the United States. This combined program provided an incredibly broad exposure to surgical discipline. The initial responsibility for all surgical patients was shouldered by the house officers and included cases involving most the currently recognized surgical specialties. During these formative years as a resident, Gross also began his writing career, publishing alone or with his mentors a total of ten papers on diverse subjects.

At the Children's Hospital, Gross was uniquely prepared through his knowledge of developmental anatomy and pathology to study the major congenital malformations afflicting his young patients. These early fundamental observations were to guide him in his future studies. He found particular inspiration in the collected papers of William Halsted of the Johns Hopkins Medical School, and Alexis Carrell, a vascular experimentalist working at the Rockefeller Institute, as well as in the history of Elliott Cutler's own vigorous efforts to devise a cure for mitral stenosis in the laboratories and operating theater of Brigham Hospital. Therefore, it was not surprising that after these 3 years of basic training in a wide variety of surgical problems, Gross should decide to devote his considerable talents and energy towards solving problems relating to congenital malformations in children, particularly those involving the circulatory system.

However, in 1937, before beginning his final chief residency years, he had an opportunity to travel abroad as Harvard's George Gorham Peters Traveling Fellow, which took him on a 9-month tour of the most active surgical centers of Britain and the Continent. His stay in London and at the Royal Hospital for Sick Children in Edinburgh was particularly memorable. There, he spent several of his fellowship months in the laboratories observing the experimental approach to surgical problems.

Upon his return to Harvard in 1938, he assumed his chief residency at the Boston Children's Hospital (Fig. 1). There, while serving under Ladd and enjoying the stimulation and encouragement of another pediatric medical colleague, John Hubbard, he worked out the surgical approach to the ligation of the ductus arteriosus in the laboratory and autopsy rooms. In August 1938, during Ladd's holiday from the hospital and with the approval of the acting chief, Thomas Lanman, he performed the first successful ligation of a patent ductus. This initial success involved a 7-year-old girl who had been examined by Paul Dudley White, the esteemed cardiologist of the Massachusetts General Hospital. White described Gross's accomplishment as "a brave procedure and obviously one that has been carefully considered" [1]. This hallmark operation introduced the era of modern cardiovascular surgery and was the first of a long series of major contributions by Gross and his colleagues to this field of surgery.

In the ensuing years in which his referred practice was developing, and only 2 years after the completion of his chief residency in pediatric surgery, he coauthored *Abdominal Surgery of Infancy and Childhood* with Ladd [2], which quickly became the standard textbook in this field. In addition, he contributed a

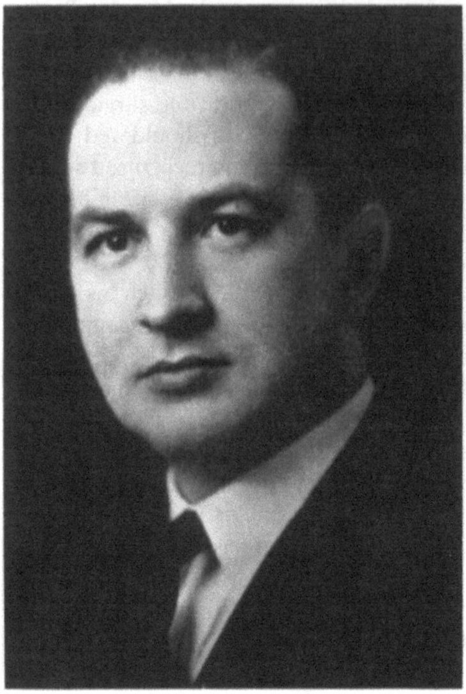

Fig. 1. Robert E. Gross, circa 1938, after gaining fame for performing first operation to close a patent ductus arteriosus in a 7-year-old girl

wide variety of articles dealing with biliary atresia, anorectal malformations, intussusception, aberrant pancreas, tumors of the peripheral nerves, brancheogenic anomalies, vinyl ether (Vinethene) anesthesia, as well as articles dealing with a number of improvements on the original ductus ligation, including the division of the patent ductus arteriosus. In the laboratory, he actively pursued means of treating other, aortic anomalies that might lend themselves to some form of correction. In 1945, he was able to report the first successful treatment of coarctation of the aorta performed in the United States. In the same year, he effectively treated an infant with a "vascular ring" by dividing an abnormally aberrant retroesophageal right subclavian artery that had compressed and thus partially obstructed the airway and the esophagus.

During this period, Gross collaborated with Charles Hufnagel to bring about an achievement of major import. The successful reconstruction of long strictures and the repair of aneurysms associated with coarctation of the aorta required bridging a gap with some type of graft. Lucite tubes had been studied but never used. Instead, the first practical means of preserving and sterilizing aortic arterial homografts was developed for use in this type of surgical repair – an advance which laid the foundation for modern reconstructive vascular surgery.

In 1946, Ladd retired, and Frank Ingraham, pioneer pediatric neurosurgeon, served as the interim chief of surgery at the Children's Hospital until 1947, when Gross was named the William E. Ladd Professor of Children's Surgery at Harvard Medical School and became surgeon-in chief of the Children's Hospital.

The next two decades were indeed golden years for this innovative, perfectionist, pragmatic, and incredibly skilled surgical leader. Now he was free to address a broad range of surgical problems of infancy and childhood and to expand his research laboratories and surgical training program. Through personal example, he demonstrated practical applications of research at the bedside, setting proficiency standards and improving the survival rate for an increasingly wide variety of congenital malformations and neoplasms peculiar to the young. His contributions to the literature, which eventually exceeded 250 publications, exerted a powerful influence on the treatment and care of children all over the world and culminated in the publication of a classic textbook, *The Surgery of Infancy and Childhood* [3]. This book, published in four languages and multiple editions, found its way into the offices and operating rooms of physicians and surgeons treating children in every civilized country.

Dr. Gross had an enormous influence on pediatric surgical training through the development of a 3-year program in children's surgery, which included rotations on all the then existing surgical specialty services at the Boston Children's Hospital. This program was particularly effective because it afforded a broad exposure to a wide variety of cases and to Gross's insistence on the surgeon's responsibility of *taking care of his or her own patients.* Not surprisingly, 12 of the currently approved 21 pediatric surgical training programs in the United States and Canada are now directed by former residents of Gross. Seventy-four surgeons who had their primary training in pediatric surgery with him are currently practicing this specialty. Nearly half of the total membership of the American Pediatric Surgical Association, of which he served as the first President, trace their educational roots back to this "golden era", which started in 1947 and ended with his retirement in 1970. In addition, countless colleagues in thoracic, cardiovascular, and general surgery throughout the world journeyed to his wards and operating rooms to hone their knowledge of child care and surgical techniques and to participate in the investigative efforts so enthusiastically pursued in the laboratories created and fostered by Gross personally.

During this Gross era, it was not surprising that new developments tumbled like snowflakes into the patient care programs. Some survived, some did not. The successful closure of a pulmonary aortic window and the staged skin flap closure of huge omphaloceles worked very well. A few, such as the atrial well permitting the leisurely, careful, and unhurried repair of primary intra-auricular septal defects, represented a relative miracle at the time. However, this technique was soon to be discarded in favor of deep hypothermia; later, together with Savage, a skilled technician in the laboratory, a miniaturized extracorporeal pump system capable of maintaining the circulation and oxygenation of small patients during the correction of major intracardiac anomalies was developed. Unfortunately, the Savage pump could not cope with the tiniest infants suffering from cyanotic heart disease. A hyperbaric chamber capable of accommodating the patient, the staff, and the oxygen supply was thus used to provide an environment in which such operative procedures could be carried out successfully, as reported with William F. Bernhard in 1963. Although inconvenient for personnel, the chamber was indeed effective for certain otherwise insoluble intracardiac anomalies, and its use continued for approximately 10 years.

During this era, the honors bestowed on this man of achievement were many indeed. Gross was elected to the presidency of the American Association of Thoracic Surgeons and the American Pediatric Surgical Association. He was the recipient of five honorary degrees, including a doctorate of science from his alma mater, Carleton College, as well as three from foreign institutions. A total of 26 medals were bestowed on him in recognition of his pioneering efforts in pediatric and cardiovascular surgery. A few highlights of this list were enumerated by William Scott, himself a Gross trainee, when, as president of the American Surgical Association, he was privileged to award Gross the third gold medal given by that association in the 93 years of its history. Included were honorary degrees from Louvain University, Turin University, and the University of Sheffield, and medals and awards such as the William E. Ladd Medal from the American Academy of Pediatrics, the first Denis Browne Gold Medal given by the British Association of Paediatric Surgeons, the Albert Lasker Award in both public health and in the treatment of heart disease, the Rodman E. and Thomas G. Sheen Award from the American Medical Association as the nation's outstanding physician in 1969 (see Appendix A).

To his students, Gross was a gentle, perhaps even shy man. In the operating room, he was a master surgeon, working swiftly and quietly. Watching him, one always had the impression of being in the presence of greatness. On the rare occasion in which an operation did not go well, Gross accepted all the blame himself. For years, he had a large sign hanging in the operating room: "If an operation is difficult, you are not doing it well."

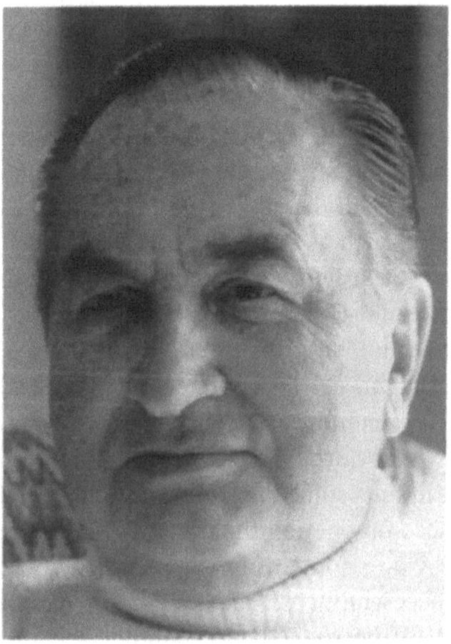

Fig. 2. A relaxed Dr. Gross, age 75, at the time Harvard Medical School initiated the Robert E. Gross Professorship Fund in honor of his many accomplishments in pediatric and cardiovascular surgery

Shortly after completing his last book, *An Atlas of Children's Surgery* [4], Gross, who had suffered from lumbar and sciatic ailments for some time, underwent a laminectomy at the Peter Bent Brigham Hospital. The first operation went poorly, and a second was eventually necessary. During the next few years, he was plagued by incapacitating pain that practically immobilized him. He retired to a cheery New England farmer's cottage high on a hillside overlooking the Connecticut River near Brattelboro, Vermont. There, mercifully, he gradually improved and once again became mobile and intellectually active, as he remains today.

During this prolonged recovery period, further heartwarming accolades came from those who knew him best. In 1979, when the Boston Children's Hospital completed its new multidisciplinary intensive care units, the fifth floor, which was to serve the cardiovascular and general surgical patients, was dedicated to Gross. The following year, on the occasion of Gross's 75th birthday, the dean of the Harvard University Medical School hosted a dinner in recognition of Gross's accomplishments during the past 40 years and formally announced plans for developing a Robert E. Gross Fund to provide a million dollars or more to establish a Robert E. Gross Professorship in perpetuity. Insofar as feasible, the post is to be occupied by a pioneering teacher-surgeon who is primarily involved in the primary care of patients and in the investigation and dissemination of knowledge concerning congenital and acquired surgical conditions afflicting infants and children. Nearly 400 donors, including friends, associates, trainees, and grateful patients, have responded so that the success of this effort is now assured.

In his 1980 American Pediatric Surgical Association presidential address, the late Robert Allen provided us with a warm and realistic look at Bob Gross, the chief [5]. This thoughtful resumé culled from the memories of his colleagues and students is delightful reading. Allen summarized with a paragraph that is worth repeating:

> "Genius is a gift. Dr. Gross was given that gift. Greatness, however, had to be achieved by hard work. Through his surgical-technical advancements, his publications, his residency training program, the genius and greatness of Dr. Robert E. Gross contributed more to pediatric surgery than any other surgeon in this century."

Need anyone say more!

Appendix

Honors and Appointments of Robert E. Gross

Phi Beta Kappa, Carleton College	
Alpha Omega Alpha, Harvard University Medical School	
F. Mead-Johnson Award, American Academy of Pediatrics	
Rudolf Matas Vascular Surgery Award, Tulane University	
Children's Service Award, Toy Manufacturers of America, New York	1954
Albert Lasker Award, American Public Health Association	1954

The Roswell Park Gold Medal of the Buffalo Surgical Society	1956
The Gold Medal of the Louisville Surgical Society	1957
Officer of the Order of Leopold, Belgium	1959
Albert Lasker Award of the American Heart Association	1959
The Laeken Award, Brussels, Belgium	1959
Gold Medal of the Detroit Surgical Association	1959
The Billroth Medal, New York Academy of Medicine	1959
Gold Medal Award, The Golden Slipper Square Club of Philadelphia	1961
President, American Association for Thoracic Surgery	1963–64
William E. Ladd Medal Award, Surgical Section, American Academy of Pediatrics	1965
The Gold Cross of the Royal Order of Phoenix of the Greek Government	1965
The Denis Browne Gold Medal of the British Association of Paediatric Surgeons	1968
Dr. Rodman E. Sheen and Thomas G. Sheen Award, American Medical Association	1969
The Alfred Jurzykowski Medalist, New York Academy of Medicine citation with Dr. Farber and Dr. Neuhauser and the Children's Hospital Medical Center	1970
The Henry Jacob Bigelow Memorial Medal	1970
First President, American Pediatric Surgical Association	1970–71
Tina Award, Foundation for Children, Houston, Texas	1971
Distinguished Service Medal, American Surgical Association, Chicago, Illinois	1973

D. Sc. (hon.) Carleton College, Northfield, Minnesota	1951
M.D. (Hon. Causa) University of Louvain, Louvain, Belgium	1959
M.D. (Hon. Causa) Turin, Italy	1961
D. Sc. (hon.) Suffolk University, Boston, Massachusetts	1962
D. Sc. (hon.) University of Sheffield, Sheffield, England	1963
Honorary Fellow, Royal College of Surgeons of England	1973
D. Sc. (hon.) Harvard University, Boston, Massachusetts	1984

Summary

Born in 1905, Gross graduated with honors from Carleton College and the Harvard Medical School. After spending 2 years in pathology, he entered his surgical training at the Peter Brent Brigham Hospital and at the Boston Children's Hospital with Dr. William E. Ladd, who occupied the first Chair of Pediatric Surgery in the United States.

After 3 years of basic training with a wide variety of surgical problems in both adults and children, he decided to devote his considerable talents toward solving some of the problems of children with congenital malformations. After having returned to Harvard to assume the Chief Residency in Surgery at the Boston Children's Hospital, he worked out a surgical approach to the closure of the patent ductus arteriosus, and he performed the first successful ligation of this structure. Two years later, Gross co-authored with Dr. Ladd *Abdominal Surgery of Infancy and Childhood.*

In the laboratory Gross was actively pursuing the treatment of anomalies of the heart and great vessels. With Dr. Charles Hufnagel, he developed a practical method of preserving, sterilizing, and using aortic homografts to bridge damaged aortic areas, and thus introduced modern reconstructive vascular surgery.

In 1947 Gross was named Professor of Children's Surgery at Harvard Medical School and Surgeon-in-Chief of the Boston Children's Hospital. His contributions to the literature included the classic textbook *Surgery of Infancy and Childhood.* Gross was elected President of the American Association for Thoracic Surgery in 1964, and served as the first President of the newly formed American Pediatric Surgical Association in 1970. New ideas and techniques tumbled like snowflakes from his laboratory into the patient care program.

After completing his last book, *An Atlas of Children's Surgery,* he retired to a New England farmer's cottage to recover from incapacitating pain following laminectomy.

Résumé

Gross est né en 1905, a été étudiant du "Carleton College" et de la "Harvard Medical School" où il a été reçu à l'examen avec mention. Après 2 ans de pathologie, il se spécialisa en chirurgie au "Peter Brent Brigham Hospital" et au "Children's Hospital de Boston" où exerçait alors le Dr. William E. Ladd qui occupait la toute première chaire de chirurgie infantile aux Etats-Unis.

Après 3 ans de chirurgie générale et après avoir été mis en présence de toutes sortes d'affections des adultes et des enfants il décida de se consacrer entièrement aux enfants souffrant de malformations. Il retourna à Harvard où il avait été nommé "chief resident" à l'Hôpital des Enfants de Boston. Il trouva une solution chirurgicale au problème du canal de Botal ouvert et réussit la première ligature. Deux ans plus tard, il publia, en coopération avec le Dr. Ladd *Abdominal Surgery of Infancy and Childhood.*

Il consacra ses travaux de recherche au traitement des malformations cardiagues et vasculocardiaques. En coopération avec le Dr. Charles Hufnagel il mit au point une méthode pratique pour conserver les allogreffes de l'aorte, les stériliser et les utiliser pour des pontages. Ce fut le début de la chirurgie vasculaire reconstructive moderne.

En 1947, il fut nommé à la chaire de chirurgie infantile de la "Harvard Medical School" et en même temps directeur du service de chirurgie infantile de l'Hôpital des Enfants de Boston. Il publia le manuel *Surgery of Infancy and Childhood.* En 1964, il fut nommé Président de l'Association Américaine de Chirurgie du Thorax et en 1970, il était le premier Président de l'Association Américaine de Chirurgie Infantile qui venait d'être fondée. Son laboratoire était une mine d'idées et de conseils pratiques pour le plus grand bien des patients.

Après avoir terminé son dernier ouvrage *An Atlas of Children's Surgery* il fut obligé de se retirer en Nouvelle Angleterre, car il souffrait de douleurs intolérables après avoir subi une laminectomie.

Zusammenfassung

Robert E. Gross wurde 1905 geboren, besuchte das Carleton College und die Harvard Medical School, wo er die Abschlußprüfung mit Prädikat bestand. Er blieb zunächst 2 Jahre in der Pathologie und begann danach seine Fachausbildung als Chirurg am Peter Brent Brigham Hospital und am Children's Hospital in Boston bei William E. Ladd, der den ersten Lehrstuhl für Kinderchirurgie in den USA innehatte.

Nach einer 3jährigen Ausbildung in der allgemeinen Chirurgie, während der er mit den verschiedensten chirurgischen Fällen bei Erwachsenen und Kindern konfrontiert wurde, beschloß er, seine überragende Begabung der Behandlung von Kindern mit angeborenen Mißbildungen zu widmen. Er ging zurück nach Harvard, wo er als Chief Resident am Boston Children's Hospital berufen worden war. Dort entwickelte er eine chirurgische Lösung für die Schließung des offenen Ductus Botalli, und ihm gelang die erste Ligatur. Zwei Jahre später schrieb er in Zusammenarbeit mit Ladd *Abdominal Surgery of Infancy and Childhood.*

Seine Forschungsarbeit galt der Behandlung der Herzfehler und der Mißbildungen der großen Herzgefäße. Mit Hufnagel entwickelte er eine praktische Methode, um Homotransplantate der Aorta haltbar zu machen, sie zu sterilisieren und sie zur Überbrückung von geschädigten Aortabereichen zu verwenden. Dies war der erste Schritt zur modernen rekonstruktiven Gefäßchirurgie.

1947 wurde Gross als Ordinarius für Kinderchirurgie an die Harvard Medical School berufen und wurde gleichzeitig ärztlicher Direktor der chirurgischen Klinik des Children's Hospital in Boston. Er verfaßte das Standardlehrbuch *Surgery of Infancy and Childhood.* 1964 wurde er Vorsitzender der Amerikanischen Gesellschaft für Thoraxchirurgie und 1970 der erste Vorsitzende der neugegründeten Amerikanischen Gesellschaft für Kinderchirurgie. Aus seinem Labor kamen unzählige Anregungen für die Patientenversorgung.

Nach Beendigung seines letzten Werkes *An Atlas of Children's Surgery* mußte er sich nach Neuengland zurückziehen, da er infolge einer Laminektomie unter so großen Schmerzen litt, daß er nicht mehr tätig sein konnte.

References

1. Warren R (1984) Patent ductus arteriosus. JAMA 251:1203–1207
2. Ladd WE, Gross RE (1941) Abdominal surgery of infancy and childhood. WB Saunders, Philadelphia
3. Gross RE (1953) The surgery of infancy and childhood. WB Saunders Company, Philadelphia
4. Gross RE (1970) An atlas of children's surgery. WB Saunders Company, Philadelphia
5. Allen RG (Dec 1980) Presidential address: the evolution of pediatric surgery. J Pediatr Surg 15(6):711–718

Max Grob (1901–1976)

U. G. Stauffer[1]

Introduction

On December 21, 1976, paediatric surgeons throughout Europe learned of the death of Max Grob (Fig. 1). The news came as a surprise; he had died quite unexpectedly, without having been ill, during the work he loved so well, on the way to a consultation. Thus the father of paediatric surgery in Switzerland, one of the founders of the specialty of paediatric surgery in the German-speaking countries and one of the great pioneers of paediatric surgery with a worldwide reputation, had departed from us. I have had the oppurtunity and the privilege of spending the last 5 years of Grob's period as director of the surgical clinic at the University

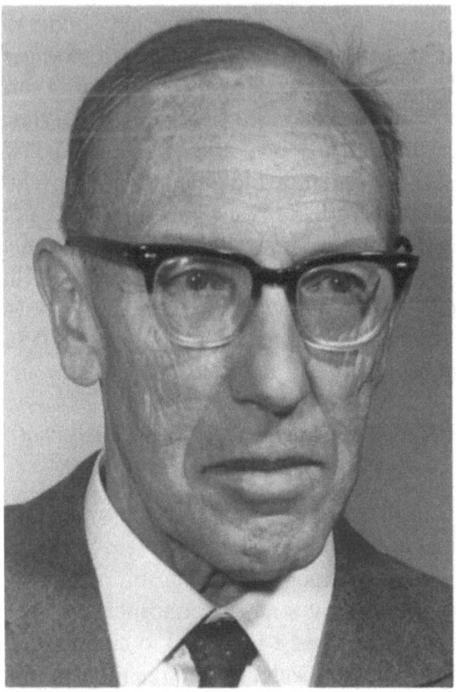

Fig. 1. Prof. Max Grob

[1] University Children's Hospital Zurich, Professor of Paediatric Surgery, University of Zurich, Switzerland

Progress in Pediatric Surgery, Vol. 20
Ed. by P. P. Rickham

Children's Hospital in Zurich with him as his senior resident. This article is an attempt to highlight some of the life and work of Max Grob, which cannot be separated from the development of paediatric surgery as a specialty.

The Beginnings

Max Grob was born in Hottingen, Zurich, the son of a primary school teacher. He attended primary school and grammar school in Zurich, and after his matriculation in 1921 he proceeded to study medicine at the University of Zurich. After his final examinations in 1928 his first appointment was as first-year resident to Professor Bernheim at the cantonal infants' hospital in Zurich, where he worked until 1930. He initially wanted to become a paediatrician. The director of the University Children's Hospital at that time, Guido Fanconi, was, however, able to offer him only an unpaid assistant's post in 1930. For financial reasons Grob could not afford to accept this. Fanconi advised him to apply to E. Monnier, who was in charge of the surgical department at the same hospital. The position of the only surgical house officer had just become vacant. Monnier (1877–1940) was an excellent surgeon and generally highly esteemed, but he was mainly engaged in the treatment of adults, and his work at the department of paediatric surgery at the children's hospital was only a sideline, and merely an honorary appointment. Grob was so fascinated by this task that instead of staying one year with Monnier he remained for five, and decided to devote himself exclusively to paediatric surgery. He was the first surgeon in Switzerland to make this decision. At the time the professional prospects did not seem particularly favourable for a paediatric surgeon. When Max Grob told his chief that he intended to devote himself exclusively to paediatric surgery, Monnier said anxiously: "You know, one just can't make a living practising paediatric surgery". In those days this attitude was only too easy to understand, but Max Grob did not left himself be discouraged. He completed his surgical training with Paul Clairmont (1875–1942), the professor of surgery at the University Hospital of Zurich, with whom he worked from 1935 to 1936. In his usual blunt way, Clairmont told Grob emphatically: "Paediatric surgery is not a specialty!"

Max Grob had other ideas. In the *Neujahrsblatt der Gelehrten-Gesellschaft,* 1976, he described the surgical treatment of children at that time as follows:

> In fact, in those days children were almost everywhere operated on by general surgeons. Apart from a few exceptions, which included my own teacher Monnier, they simply did not have the necessary experience. I can still remember quite well how there was always a particularly strained atmosphere in the operating theatre at the University Hospital when a baby had to be operated on, even if it was only an inguinal hernia. As a rule, an intervention of this type took a disproportionately long time because the same complicated procedures were applied as in adult patients, although this was not at all necessary.
>
> The lack of experience, often linked with inadequate diagnostic skill and inadequate operating technique, increased the operative risk. Long, complicated interventions in neonates and babies in particular were associated with a

high mortality. This was true mainly for those cases in which severe congenital malformations had to be corrected and which were thus exceptionally demanding for the surgeon. Either the surgeon had to take the plunge and commit himself to a desperate venture or – not uncommonly – he abandoned any thought of operation and left the child to its fate. In addition, he was often unable to manage any severe inflammatory conditions, such as suppurative osteomyelitis, pleurisy and peritonitis. All these conditions were associated with a mortality amounting, for instance, to 16% in the case of a perforated appendix. These rather depressing circumstances were not exactly propitious, when it came to the recognition of paediatric surgery as a specialty and to the awakening of interest in the specialty, nor could one hope to reap any laurels in this field.

In the same New Year pamphlet, Max Grob summarized the situation in Europe and the United States at that time as follows:

In Europe there were few centres at that time dealing exclusively with paediatric surgery. At the Hôpital des Enfants Malades in Paris such men as E. Kirmisson, A. Broca and L. Ombrédanne rendered outstanding services in the development of paediatric surgery even as early as the end of the last century and at the beginning of the present one. They were later followed by R. Drachter at the University Children's Hospital in Munich and Denis Browne at Great Ormond Street Hospital for Sick Children in London.

There was only one centre of this sort in the USA at this time, at the children's hospital in Boston, directed by W. E. Ladd, who worked there from 1910 to 1945 as a paediatric surgeon. It was he who founded paediatric surgery as a discipline in its own right in the United States. Thanks to his pioneering work in this field he was offered a chair of paediatric surgery at the Harvard Medical School – but this was not until 1940. It was the first and at that time the only chair in the USA.

In these pioneering days of paediatric surgery Max Grob went unerringly on his way, though reservations were expressed from many quarters. The time with Clairmont was followed by a 6-month course of study in Paris at the Hôpital des Enfants Malades, where the surgical department was then directed by L. Ombrédanne. In this department Grob made a study of the techniques used in paediatric surgery, in particular in paediatric urology. With Veau, he also familiarized himself with the treatment of cleft lip, jaw and palate. Thus trained, Grob opened a private practice in Zurich in late 1936. Despite his 8-year training, however, he was not allowed to use the title of specialist in paediatric surgery. He therefore established himself as a specialist in paediatrics and surgery. In Switzerland the title "surgeon" could not be supplemented by the qualifying phrase "specializing in paediatric surgery" until 1952. It was another 22 years after that, in 1974, that a proper specialist degree in paediatric surgery was established in Switzerland.

At the same time as Grob started his private practice he was nominated deputy head of the surgical department of the children's hospital in Zurich. After 2 years of private practice as a paediatric surgeon he was unanimously elected by the committee of the children's hospital in 1939 to be Monnier's successor.

The Development of the Specialty at the Clinic in Zurich

On becoming the director of the surgical department, Max Grob gave up his private practice and devoted himself entirely to his duties at the children's hospital. It was wartime and the national borders were closed, so that any exchange of experience in this new specialty on an international level was out of the question. Thus, years of extremely intensive research work began for Grob, most of which he had to develop entirely on his own. Under his direction Zurich soon became the centre of modern paediatric surgery throughout the German-speaking world. Grob's main interest was in surgical correction of congenital malformations, and in addition he was a general surgeon in the truest sense of the word, who applied himself to problems of urological, neurological, thoracic, orthopaedic, plastic and traumatological surgery, and devised brilliant methods of treatment. All those who were abel to work with him during this period admired his composure and control throughout even the most complicated operations. In addition, he was interested in the field of cardiac surgery, which was evolving at the time. After detailed theoretical studies and careful preparation, the limitations of the modest premises in which the surgical department of the children's hospital was housed did not prevent him from carrying out the first heart operation in Switzerland: a Blalock-Taussig operation in a child with Fallot's tetralogy. He was successful.

In subsequent years he operated on numerous children suffering from a very wide variety of congenital heart defects and in this way he was able to preserve many a young human life for the future. In the winter of 1957–58 he introduced artificial hypothermia (hibernation) for the first time, which permitted him to undertake intracardial interventions without blood flow for a short period, whether for closure of a septal defect or for dilatation of a stenosed exist of the pulmonary artery. In 1959, Grob also carried out the first operation in Switzerland using a heart-lung machine. In those days heart operations of this kind could be successfully performed only after detailed examination and preliminary work in countries outside Switzerland and a critical evaluation of the material available. Grob was also exceptionally well informed on the pathophysiology of the heart, and a splendid operator. In addition, he was confident and determined and had enormous personal courage. Especially in the field of cardiac surgery that he loved so well, Max Grob displayed later his outstanding qualitites both as a person and as a master of his subject when he handed the department of cardiac surgery in Zurich over to the next generation of surgeons on the appointment of the Swedish cardiac surgeon, Ake Senning.

Max Grob also did pioneering work in the field of surgical treatment of cleft lip, jaw and palate. In these subjects Zurich soon occupied a leading position. In abdominal surgery, Grob was the first surgeon in Switzerland to perform a pull-through operation for Hirschsprung's disease (congenital megacolon), and he was also the first to undertake surgical correction of a "short oesophagus", as hiatus hernia was called in those days.

Recognition of the Specialty at University Level

In 1952 Max Grob received a higher degree from the University of Zurich for his monograph on anomalies of the gastrointestinal tract, which is still the definite work on the various forms of intestinal malpositions. His great didactic skill and comprehensive overall knowledge were shown in his brilliant textbook of paediatric surgery, which appeared in 1957 and became a classic, making the name of Grob famous in all parts of the world. He also published innumerable other contributions in Swiss and foreign specialist journals, which were often of historic significance. In 1957, Grob was offered the chair of paediatric surgery at the University of Munich. After due consideration, however, her declined this honour and thus his own city and the University of Zurich were able to keep him. In the same year the administrative council of the canton of Zurich made him the first associate professor of paediatric surgery in Switzerland, following the recommendation of the faculty of medicine. This was a milestone in the development of paediatric surgery which, for the first time, was recognized as a new academic subject. Grob's predecessor, Monnier, had already given one weekly lecture on problems concerned with paediatric surgery, but as a rule only two or three students had attended. Nonetheless, on the principle of *tres faciunt collegium* the lecture was held regularly. Soon after Grob's appointment as associate professor, teaching in paediatric surgery was incorporated into the mandatory main course in paediatrics. This special subject is now taught in all five faculties of medicine in Switzerland by full professors, following the first step made in this direction by the University of Zurich in 1970, a year before Grob's retirement, as a mark of esteem for his life's work.

International Contacts

Numerous guests from Switzerland, all the European countries and the United States came to Max Grob at the children's hospital in Zurich to spend various periods of time as observers and pupils. In 1950, on the occasion of the International Congress of Paediatricians in Zurich convened by Fanconi, Grob and his team had their first opportunity of making close contact with a number of leading paediatric surgeons working abroad, especially those working in England. Three years later (1953), the first society for paediatric surgery, the British Association of Paediatric Surgeons (BAPS) was founded in London under Denis Browne, and it had an international character from the start. In addition to 40 British surgeons, 19 surgeons from the remainder of Europe and from further afield were accepted for membership. Grob was one of these. One of the 40 founder members of the BAPS, P.P. Rickham of Liverpool, later became Grob's successor as director of the Children's Surgical Clinic in Zurich. Following the example of the BAPS, the Swiss paediatric surgeons started to organize annual meetings from 1963 onwards, and in 1969 finally founded the Swiss Society for Paediatric Surgery, of which Grob was the first president. The constant increase in the number of scientific articles written by the members of the rapidly growing sector of paediatric surgery, which had formerly been disseminated among many different journals and were therefore difficult to find, provided the stimulus for the founding of journals for paediatric surgery, in which all the relevant papers could appear together. Thus, the *Annales de Chirurgie Infantile* started to appear in France in 1959, and the *Rivista di Chirurgia Pediatrica* started in Italy in the same year. They were followed in 1964 by the *Zeitschrift für Kinderchirurgie und Grenzgebiete* in Germany, Austria, Holland and Switzerland, which was founded by Fritz Rehbein of Bremen; Grob often worked with him and the two men were close friends. The *Journal of Pediatric Surgery* followed in the United States in 1966 for the English-speaking world. The breakthrough of paediatric surgery as a specialty, to which Grob had made such an essential contribution as a pioneer, had thus been achieved.

The Last Years in Zurich; the Swiss School of Paediatric Surgery; Tributes

Max Grob was still in Zurich in 1969 when the surgical department moved into the new building that he had helped to plan. Thus, in the last 2 years he was in office Grob was in charge of one of the most modern and best-equipped paediatric surgery units in the whole of continental Europe. During his period of office from 1939 to 1971 the yearly numbers of surgical patients had risen three times, and the number of operations four times. When he retired in 1971 there were about 20 paediatric surgeons working in Switzerland, two-thirds of whom had emanated from the Zurich school either directly or indirectly. There are also numerous foreign paediatric surgeons, who, after training in Zurich, carried Max Grob's name into all parts of the world. Thus it is no wonder that honours were lavished upon this brilliant surgeon, including, for example, the award of an honorary readership at the University of Madrid and honorary memberships of the American Academy of Pediatrics and of the British, German, Austrian and Swiss societies of paediatric surgery. In 1969, he was awarded probably the greatest honour of all, the Denis Browne Memorial Medal of the British Association of Paediatric Surgeons. On his retirement as director of the Children's Surgical Clinic in Zurich, Max Grob was able to hand over a modern 110-bed clinic in a new building with three assistant medical directors and ten assistants to his successor, P.P. Rickham of Liverpool. Thanks to his tireless application, his immense ability and his tremendous perseverance linked with brilliance, he had made Zurich into one of the great centres of paediatric surgery in Europe.

Private Life

Anyone who had the good fortune to have a close personal relationship with Max Grob or to work with him was able to find out what a humane person was behind this man who had always remained reticent and modest despite all his outward success. He was hardly ever to be seen in the front row at a congress. He would sit beside one of his trusted colleagues in the auditorium holding a notepad, only speaking if he was asked to describe his own relevant experience, and then his concise and lucid answer often became the central point of the whole debate.

Max Grob's love of tradition and history manifested itself in his loyal membership of the "Gesellschaft zur Konstaffel", an association that is over 600 years old and which used to rule Zurich in collaboration with the guilds in the early Middle Ages. It is still in existence today, most visible in the traditional spring fair in Zurich, the "Sechseläuten". He loved his country home in Gerra on Lake Maggiore in Ticino. There Grob was seen as a lovable and humorous host, and occasionally also as a highly skilled cook. Those of his friends who have watched night falling over the lake while sitting with the Grobs at the open fire will never forget the experience. In Ticino Grob also found enough leisure to indulge in his love of music and poetry and to enjoy painting. In view of the professional and scientific workload, there was otherwise not a great deal of time for social or political commitments. This intensified Grob's need for the comfort of family life. Fate was, however, not kind to him. In 1963 he and his five children lost wife and mother. In 1965 he married his second wife, his assistant medical director, who later became director of the surgical children's department at Triemli Hospital. She also succumbed to an insidious illness in 1973, after which he took over her job as a temporary arrangement 2 years after his retirement from the directorship of the Zurich University Hospital. In this position he then met his third wife, who was with him until the end of his life.

For his colleagues of the first generation of paediatric surgeons and for his many pupils, Max Grob remains the good friend and great teacher whose charisma will live on beyond his death. For our younger colleagues he is the great Swiss pioneer of paediatric surgery whom the Swiss Society of Paediatric Surgery honoured by founding the Max Grob Lecture in 1971, given annually as part of the meeting of the Society. His name will remain immortalized in gold letters on the roll of honour of pioneering research workers and scientists.

Summary

Max Grob's first appointment in 1928 was as a first-year resident at the cantonal infants' hospital of his native town, Zurich. He then worked with Monnier in the surgical department of the same hospital and was so fascinated by his task that he decided to devote himself exclusively to paediatric surgery and completed his training with P. Clairmont at the University Hospital of Zurich in 1936. This was followed by a 6-month course in the surgical department directed by L. Ombredanne at the Hôpital des Enfants Malades, Paris, where he studied the techniques used in paediatric surgery and in particular in paediatric urology. With Veau, he familiarized himself with the treatment of cleft lip, jaw and palate. Back in Zurich in late 1936, he opened a private practice as a specialist in paediatrics and surgery. Two years later he was elected to be Monnier's successor at the children's hospital. It was wartime, and there was no exchange of experience on an international level. His main interest was in surgical correction of congenital malformations and cardiac surgery. He carried out the first heart operation in a child in Switzerland and was successful. He operated on a wide variety of congenital heart defects and introduced artificial hypothermia. He was the first to use a heart-lung machine and also did pioneering work in the field of surgical treatment of cleft lip, jaw and palate. He was the first surgeon in Switzerland to perform a pull-through operation for Hirschsprung's disease and to undertake correction of a "short oesophagus".

In 1957 he was made the first associate professor of paediatric surgery in Switzerland, and teaching in paediatric surgery was incorporated into the mandatory main course in paediatrics. When he retired in 1971, there were about 20 paediatric surgeons working in Switzerland. The last part of the chapter deals with the international contacts and the private life of M. Grob.

Résumé

Max Grob commença à exercer la médecine à l'Hôpital Cantonal de sa ville natale Zürich. Il y resta de 1928 à 1930. Il fit ensuite partie de l'équipe du chirurgien Monnier et décida de se consacrer entièrement à la chirurgie des enfants. Il finit de se spécialiser à l'Hôpital Universitaire de Zürich où exerçait P. Clairmont. Il fit ensuite un stage de 6 mois à Paris, à l'Hôpital des enfants malades dont Ombredanne était alors directeur. Là, il se familiarisa avec les techniques d'interventions dans le domaine de la chirurgie et de l'urologie des enfants. Veau lui enseigna le traitement chirurgical des fentes labiopalatines. De retour à Zürich, il ouvrit un cabinet de pédiatrie et chirurgie. Deux ans plus tard, il succédait à Monnier à l'Hôpital des Enfants. C'était alors la guerre et tous les contacts internationaux avaient cessé. Max Grob se consacra à l'époque au traitement chirurgical des malformations et des affections du coeur. Il fut le premier à opérer un enfant atteint d'une affection cardiaque en Suisse. Il opéra ensuite diverses malformations cardiaques et introduisit l'hypothermie artificielle ainsi que le coeur-poumon artificiel. Il fut aussi un pionnier dans le domaine des opérations des fentes labiopalatines, et de la maladie de Hirschsprung.

En 1957, il fut nommé professeur sans chaire de chirurgie des enfants. Quand il se retira en 1971, il y avait déjà 20 chirurgiens des enfants en Suisse. La dernière partie du chapitre traite des contacts internationaux et de la vie privée de M. Grob.

Zusammenfassung

1928–1930 hatte Max Grob seine erste Stelle am Kantonshospital seiner Heimatstadt Zürich. Er arbeitete dann mit Monnier in der chirurgischen Abteilung desselben Krankenhauses und war von dieser Aufgabe so begeistert, daß er beschloß, sich ausschließlich der Kinderchirurgie zu widmen. Bei P. Clairmont am Universitätskrankenhaus Zürich beendete er seine Facharztausbildung. Dann folgte ein 6monatiges Praktikum in der chirurgischen Abteilung des Hôpital des enfants malades, Paris, die von Ombrédanne geleitet wurde. Dort hatte er Gelegenheit, die Operationstechniken der Kinderchirurgie und Kinderurologie zu erlernen. Veau machte ihn mit der Behandlung der Lippenspalte sowie der Kiefer- und Gaumenspalte vertraut. Er kehrte dann nach Zürich zurück und eröffnete eine Privatpraxis als Facharzt für Kinderheilkunde und Chirurgie; 2 Jahre später wurde er zum Nachfolger von Monnier am Kinderspital gewählt. Es war Krieg, und internationaler Erfahrungsaustausch fand nicht statt. Er war auf sich gestellt und interessierte sich in erster Linie für die chirurgische Behandlung von angeborenen Mißbildungen und für die Herzchirurgie. Er unternahm die erste Herzoperation bei einem Kind in der Schweiz. Er operierte zahlreiche verschiedene Herzfehler und führte die künstliche Hypothermie ein. Er benutzte als erster eine Herz-Lungen-Maschine, und seine Arbeit auf dem Gebiet der Lippen-, Kiefer- und Gaumenspalte war bahnbrechend. Als erster Chirurg in der Schweiz führte er eine Durchzugsoperation bei der Hirschsprung-Krankheit durch und korrigierte als erster den „kurzen Ösophagus".

1957 wurde er zum ersten außerordentlichen Professor für Kinderchirurgie in der Schweiz berufen, und Kinderchirurgie wurde zum Hauptfach in der Kinderheilkunde. Als er 1971 emeritiert wurde, gab es in der Schweiz schon 20 Kinderchirurgen. Der letzte Abschnitt dieses Beitrags behandelt Grobs internationale Kontakte und sein Privatleben.

The Dawn of Paediatric Surgery: Johannes Fatio (1649–1691) –
His Life, His Work and His Horrible End*

P. P. RICKHAM[1]

Introduction

Isolated operative procedures on children have been performed since antiquity, but there is no general agreement as to who was the first surgeon to operate systematically on congenital deformities of neonates and infants. Felix Würtz, who lived in Basel from 1518 until 1576 or 1578 and practised surgery in his home town, is thought by many to be the father of paediatric surgery [1]. Würtz wrote a book on wound surgery in four parts [2]. It was allright as far as it went, but it cannot be compared with the masterpiece written by his contemporary, Ambroise Paré, in Paris. Added to Würtz's surgical textbook was *The Children's Book,* which forms the basis for the claim that he was the first paediatric surgeon. Würtz was a friend and pupil of the great Paracelsus, or, to give him his full name, Theophratus Bombast Paracelsus von Hohenheim, who dominated the European medicine of his time [3]. His medicine was, however, deeply rooted in the scholastics of the Middle Ages. He rejected anatomical dissections and the use of operations [4], and this view is faithfully reflected in *The Children's Book.* Würtz did not describe one single operation, and the only descriptions of surgical therapy are concerned with the splinting and bandaging of deformed limbs; in other words, he did not practice paediatric surgery at all.

In my opinion, the honour of being the first paediatric surgeon belongs undoubtedly to that remarkable man Johannes Fatio (Fig. 1), who lived in Basel a century after Würtz.

His Life

Johannes Fatio was born in Basel in 1649, the son of a well-to-do merchant of Italian descent. The family, Italian Protestants, had taken refuge in Switzerland like so many of their fellow believers, and came to Basel in 1620 [5]. Fatio's father married into one of the best-known Basel families. His mother was the daughter of the lawyer Henric Petri. As we shall see, the relationship with the Petri family, and especially Fatio's friendship with his cousin, Dr. Jacob Henric Petri, did cast

* Based on a lecture given at the Greek Paediatric Surgical Association, Chios, 1983

[1] Universitäts-Kinderklinik, Chirurgische Abteilung, Steinwiesstr. 75, CH-8032 Zürich, Switzerland

Progress in Pediatric Surgery, Vol. 20
Ed. by P. P. Rickham

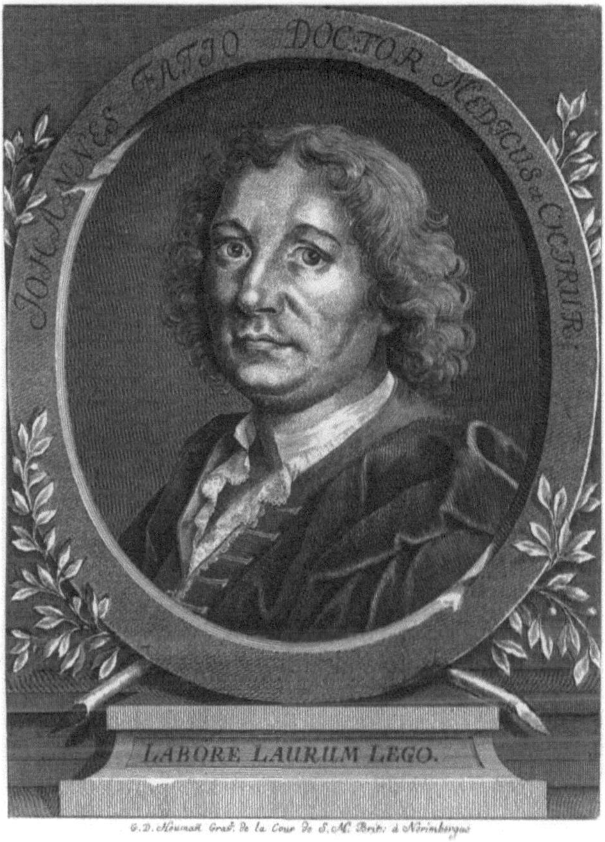

Fig. 1. Johannes Fatio: engraving by Daniel Heumann. (From University Library, Basel)

a shadow on his whole life. Very early on in his life, Fatio decided to become a surgeon. In those days there were two ways to take up surgery. One could study at university to become a doctor of medicine and, by paying an extra 5 guilders, it was possible to become a doctor of surgery as well, at least from 1604 onwards. In 1647 the University of Basel may have introduced an examination in surgery, but it is not certain whether this examination was ever held. Qualified doctors never operated themselves; operations were carried out by barber surgeons, the second way to take up surgery. Fatio must have been an apprentice to a barber surgeon and passed his master degree in 1672, when he became a member of the barber surgeons' guild at the age of 23. However, in 1662 at the age of 13 years, he had already immatriculated in medicine at the University of Basel. For reasons which are unknown, he never studied there [6, 7].

In order to understand some of Fatio's difficulties, we have briefly to examine the state of the University of Basel during the seventeenth century. This university, the oldest in Switzerland, was founded in 1460 by Pope Pius II, when Basel was still a free city of the Holy Roman Empire (Fig. 2). In 1501 Basel was one of the last cantons to join the Swiss federation. The population was converted to the

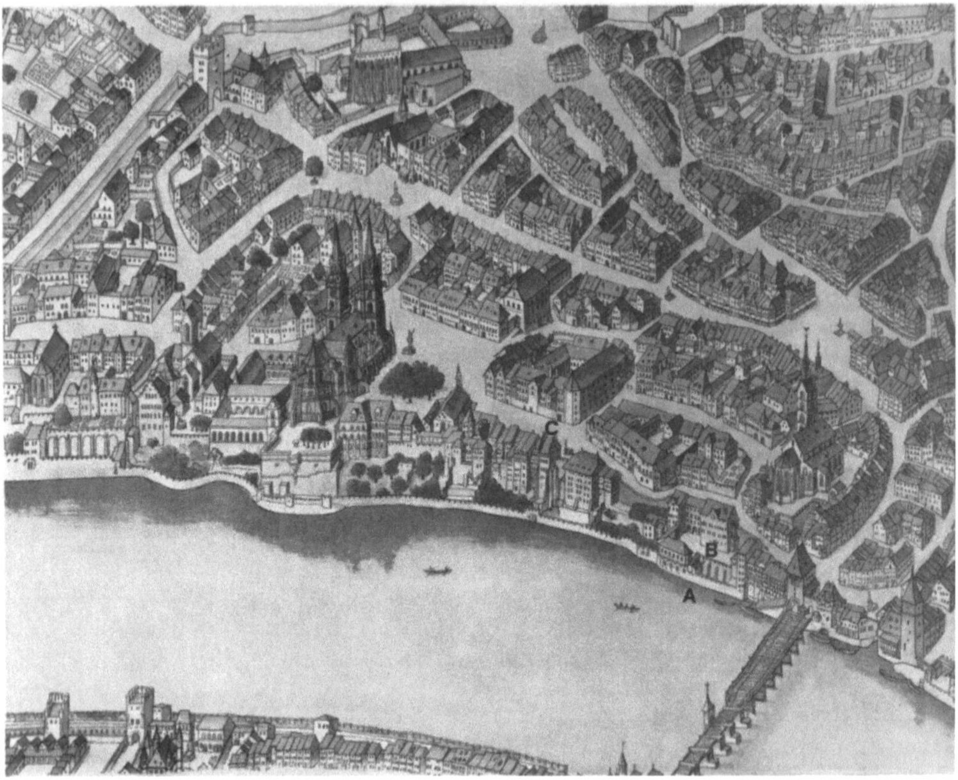

Fig. 2. Basel in 1615; part of the town plan drawn by Merian. *A*, Lower university college; *B*, university library; and *C*, upper university college in former Augustinian monastery. (From University Library, Basel)

Protestant faith by Ocolampadius in 1528, and the Catholic bishop was evicted. During the sixteenth century, Basel became one of the foremost centres of learning and art. Names like Erasmus and Hans Holbein the Younger only highlight the galaxy of talents working and living in the city. In the faculty of medicine brilliant men abounded – Paracelsus, Caspar Bauhin and Samuel Plattner, to mention but a few who taught there. Vasalius carried out public anatomical dissections, and virtually every scientific European book was published in the city [8].

The seventeenth century showed, however, a steady decline. The republic's strength depended on the importance of its craftsmen, who were joined together in guilds. Their importance gradually diminished as big merchants and industrialists took over the running of the canton [9]. The Protestant and free Basel acted like a magnet for Protestant refugees from the surrounding countries, especially Germany, France and Italy. There were many Italian Protestants, like the Fatio family, the most famous among them being the Socins, who nearly continu-

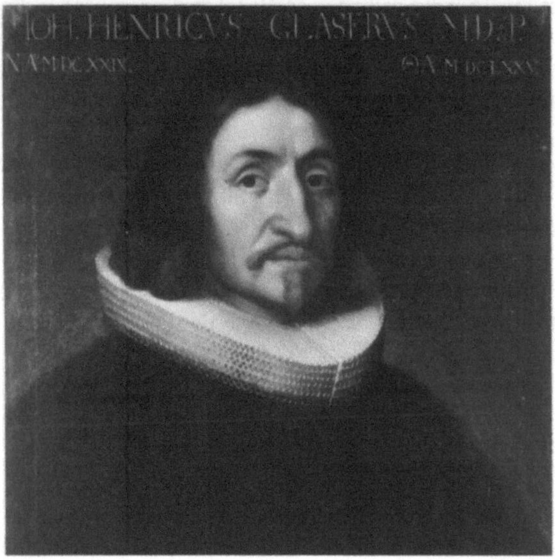

Fig. 3. Johannes Heinrich Glaser (1629–1675)

ously provided one of the two lord mayors throughout the second half of the century. The most powerful family were the Burkhardts, Protestants who originally came from the Black Forest. They were not only always lord mayors, but members of the family held almost every important office, including chairs of medicine at the university. Both families fought each other in government, parliament and town. Bribery and corruption prevailed and when trying to obtain a position it became much more important to know the right people or to bribe one's way in than to be capable of doing the job. Not surprisingly, the standard of the university and its medical faculty deteriorated, although it retained its pomposity and decorum.

Fatio seems to have had few friends amongst the medical hierarchy. Of the three professors of medicine, only one, Johan Henricus Glaser (Fig. 3), was a progressive and active medical teacher [6]. He reintroduced dissection of bodies, which had not been practised for half a century. Like John Hunter 100 years later, he had difficulties in procuring bodies for dissection; in 6 years he was able to produce a total of only seven bodies. The dissections were in public, as had been the dissections carried out by Nicolaus Tulp in Leyden which were depicted by Rembrandt [10], but Glaser dissected only half of the body. Then the auditorium was cleared of all but medical students, and Fatio demonstrated the common surgical procedures on the other side of the body. Although he had no official standing in the university, his friendship with Glaser seems to have given him a certain status. Unfortunately Glaser died in 1675 after only 7 years as professor, and Fatio was left without a friend in the university, although by that time he already had an extensive surgical practice in the city.

Fatio now decided to take a medical degree, and as it seemed to be impossible in Basel, he went to the Protestant University of Valence in the Dauphiné and took his doctor's degree there. In 1678 he returned to Basel and presented a dissertation (no unfortunately lost), in order to be recognized as a qualified physician in his home town. His application was rudely rejected, not because of the quality of his work, but because Basel had not recognized a foreign degree for over 100 years [6].

During the following 13 years, Fatio had an enormously successful surgical and obstetrical practice in Basel. Although officially a quack, all the important physicians, including the professors, asked for his help and consulted him. We know this because of his case histories, where he always mentioned the name of the doctor who referred the patient to him and the names of the physicians who watched him doing a particular operation. We can only surmise what he thought of them.

His Work

He seems to have been a prolific writer, but unfortunately none of his works, including his textbook of surgery, was ever published, for reasons which we shall discuss later on. Only his book on obstetrics written primarily for midwives, *The Helvetic Reasonable Midwife,* has survived [11], a remarkable book (Fig. 4). It is in four main sections, of which the first three are devoted to obstetrics, full of common sense and far ahead of his time, but do not concern us here. It is the last section on the affection of neonates and infants which will be discussed here.

The first chapter deals with the general management of healthy neonates. In the second chapter he describes special affections of neonates, and already in the first paragraph dealing with infants who will not breath after delivery, he astonishes the reader by describing mouth-to-mouth respiration as the most efficient method of resuscitation. He advises the midwife to take a few drops of wine into her mouth and then to blow them the infant's mouth repeatedly, while pinching the infant's nostrils. He warns of the danger of bleeding from cutting the lingual frenulum, an operation which he thought hardly ever necessary. He operated for urethral meatal stenosis and atresia, inserting a thin leaden tube postoperatively, if necessary. At least twice, in the presence of many witnesses, he carried out a successful operation for peno-scrotal hypospadias in boys of 2 years of age, passing a trocar from the glans along the shaft of the penis, mobilizing the abnormal urethral opening, and passing a leaden tube along the newly made channel into the bladder, where it was left for 16 days while the hypospadias opening was closed by strapping. In a 3-year-old girl he operated on a hydrometrocolpos causing urinary obstruction, incising the imperforated hymen and being surprised that it was not urine but a milky fluid that exuded. Low anal atresia with perineal or vulval fistula was treated by dilatation with or without a backcut. In high rectal atresia he warned against injuring the anal sphincter, made a cruciate incision at the site of the anal dimple, and passed a triangular trocar upwards until meconium exuded. He then kept a metal tube in place for some time, lubricating it with honey. He clearly distinguished between pigmented naevi and haemangiomas;

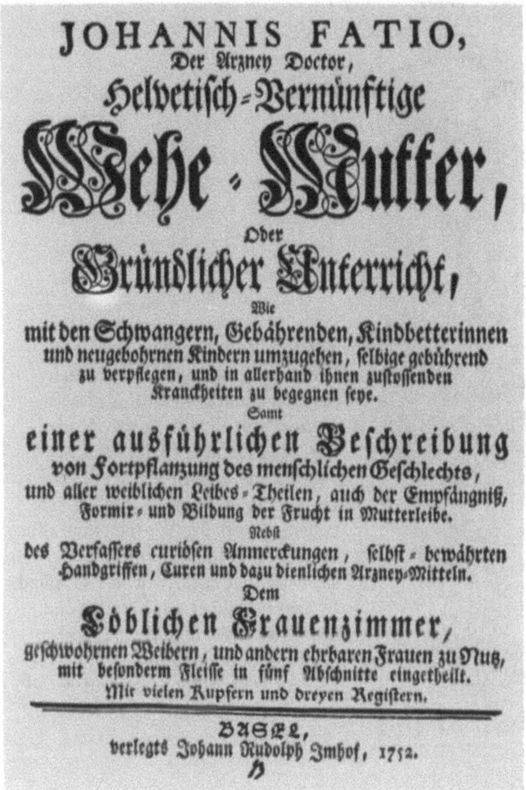
JOHANNIS FATIO,
Der Arzney Doctor,
Helvetisch-Vernünftige
Wehe-Mutter,
Oder
Gründlicher Unterricht,
Wie
mit den Schwangern, Gebährenden, Kindbetterinnen
und neugebohrnen Kindern umzugehen, selbige gebührend
zu verpflegen, und in allerhand ihnen zustossenden
Kranckheiten zu begegnen seye.
Samt
einer ausführlichen Beschreibung
von Fortpflanzung des menschlichen Geschlechts,
und aller weiblichen Leibes-Theilen, auch der Empfängniß,
Formir- und Bildung der Frucht in Mutterleibe.
Nebst
des Verfassers curiösen Anmerckungen, selbst-bewährten
Handgriffen, Curen und dazu dienlichen Arzney-Mitteln.
Dem
Löblichen Frauenzimmer,
geschwohrnen Weibern, und andern ehrbaren Frauen zu Nutz,
mit besonderm Fleisse in fünf Abschnitte eingetheilt.
Mit vielen Kupfern und dreyen Registern.
BASEL,
verlegts Johann Rudolph Imhof, 1752.

Fig. 4. Title page of Fatio's *Helvetic Reasonable Midwife:* first edition printed 60 years after his death in 1752. (From University Library, Basel)

warned against treating haemangiomas, as they often disappear; and, if necessary, treated them by applying ammonium chloride.

In Chap. 3, infant feeding was discussed; in Chap. 4, constipation; in Chap. 5, vomiting; in Chap. 6, fits; in Chap. 7, disturbances of sleep; and in Chap. 8, neurological disorders. Here he described hydrocephalus in great detail, including the setting-sun sign. Skin diseases were described in Chap. 9, eye diseases in Chap. 10, and diseases of the nose in Chap. 11. In Chap. 12 diseases of the mouth were reported, and here he described how he successfully treated a ranula by uncapping it. The next chapters on teeth, cough, worms and dehydration are of secondary surgical interest. Chap. 17 on diseases of the umbilicus is perhaps the most brilliant one. He clearly distinguished between umbilical hernia (which rarely needed any treatment) and exomphalos, which had to be reduced and the defect strapped together. In those days many children with exomphalos were born with rupture of the membranes and prolapse of coils of the intestine. He returned the gut carefully into the abdomen and closed the defect by continuous strapping.

His star case was that of the conjoined twins, Elizabeth and Catharine Meyerin, born on November 24, 1689, the mother being 42 years old. Fatio was called on the following day, and in the presence of both lord mayors and a galaxy of medical

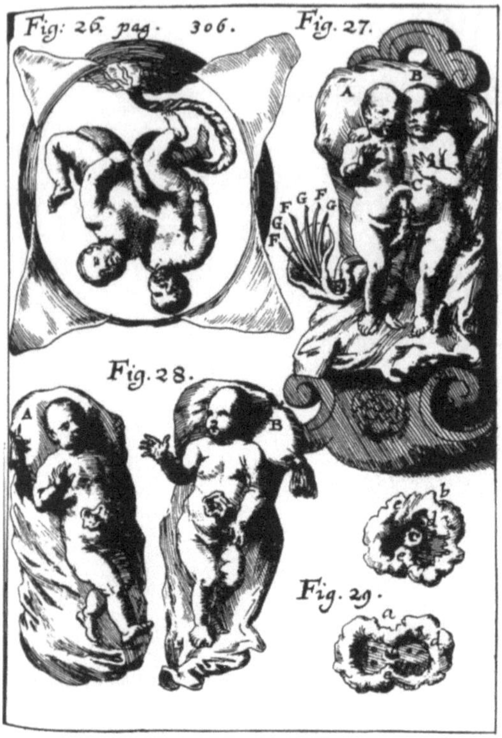

Fig. 5. Fatio's conjoined twins, published by E. König in *Miscellanes curiosa physico-medica academise naturae curiosorum lipsise,* Norimbergae, Fracofort (from the Josephin Library Institute of Medical History, University of Vienna). *Fig. 26,* The twins in utero; *Fig. 27,* the twins after delivery and ligation of the cord, showing that each twin was supplied by two umbilical arteries and one umbilical vein; *Fig. 28,* the twins after ligation and division of the isthmus connecting them; and *Fig. 29,* the structures in the isthmus in twin *A* and twin *B*

men he proceeded to separate the xypho-omphalopagus twin. They were joined from the xyphoid processes down to the single umbilicus (Fig. 5). Fortunately, the midwife had tied the cord at a distance from the infants. Fatio was thus able to isolate the umbilical vessels and follow them to the navel, where he tied them separately (Fig. 5). He then transfixed and tied the bridge between the two infants with a silken cord, and cut the isthmus (Fig. 5). It has been said that he was lucky that there was no liver in the isthmus, but this is by no means certain, and it would hardly have made any difference. The ligature fell off on the 9th postoperative day and both children recovered. This was the first successful separation of conjoined twins and it remained the only successful one until the second quarter of this century. A young physician, Emmanuel Koenig, was present as a spectator during this operation. One year later he published the case history of the twins in Nuremberg, using Fatio's illustrations but never even mentioning his name [12]. The twins are, therefore, always referred to as the Koenig case in the medical literature. Sic transit gloria!

His Horrible End

The intolerance political situation of the canton of Basel rapidly deteriorated, ending in what Swiss historians like to belittle as the "91 Happenings", which were in fact a fully fledged revolution. The developments leading to the revolution are too complex to relate here in detail, nor were they confined to the year 1691. A few explanatory words must, however, be added in order to aid understanding of the complicated events.

The republic of Basel was in theory ruled by the guilds, each of which elected six representatives to the "great council", parliament of 200, every year. "The little council" or government should have been elected by the great council, and was composed of the two lord mayors and the masters of the guilds. In the seventeenth century, the citizens were practically powerless and public elections became a farce. Members of little and great council stayed in office until they died, and when a vacancy occurred the councils decided the successor, usually giving the post to the highest bidder. As has already been mentioned, the big families dominated politics; the big merchants, factory owners, lawyers and retired senior officers filled the parliamentary ranks; and craftsmen were in a small minority. To the evil of bribery and corruption further misdeeds were added. The coinage was several times debased, the expropriated lands of the monasteries were given away as presents, duties were arbitrarily raised, and payment to the Protestant clergy was insultingly and drastically cut [7]. Already in 1688, these malpractices infuriated the population to such an extent that they forced the members of the government and parliament to kneel and take a public oath that they had never paid or received bribes. They all did do so, although it was common knowledge that hardly one of them had not sinned in this respect. Every Sunday the clergy vituperated from the pulpits against a government of perjurers. In 1690 a secret committee of discontented citizens formed under the leadership of Fatio's cousin, the lawyer Dr. Jacob Henric Petri. Fatio was persuaded to become a member of this committee and was soon one of its leading exponents, thanks to his brilliant oratory and the great popularity he had among his many patients, especially the women whom he had so frequently and unselfishly helped. In November 1690 the great council still felt strong enough to cite Fatio to appear before the council and told him rudely "to shut up once and for all", but the revolution could not be postponed any longer [9].

On January 25, 1691, the guilds elected a committee of citizens and asked Henric Petri to become protector general. This general rebellion did not please the Swiss federation at all, as they were at this time in great difficulties with Louis XIV of France, who had built an enormous fortress at Hüningen near the border of the canton of Basel. Disunity within their ranks was the last thing the Swiss could then afford. Zürich, Berne and Lucerne sent representatives to Basel in order to mediate, but this was of no avail. After the wife of one of the lord mayors and the wife of the chief guild master, as well as several members of parliament, were shown to have blatantly tried to bribe their fellow citizens, the people took up arms and imprisoned government and parliament in the town hall. They were not allowed to leave until the chief guild master and 29 members of parliament had resigned, and further parliamentary members were forced to resign the following week [7].

Meanwhile, Fatio had worked out a new constitution consisting of 178 articles; on May 29 all members of parliament and government had to accept this constitution and the great city seal was affixed to it. The new constitution was extraordinarily progressive. There was universal franchise, including the farmers living outside Greater and Lesser Basel, and periodic elections of the parliament, which would in its turn elect the government. Important decisions like foreign treaties, the value of the coinage and custom duties could be passed only by referendum. In fact, the 1691 Basle constitution worked out by Fatio largely foreshadowed that of France of 1789. This was Fatio's hour of triumph, but the reaction set in fast. The members of parliament who had been ousted formed a secret club of "Malcontentes". Both the disposed lord mayors, Socin and Burckhardt, found that now the time for family squabbles had passed and the common enemy had to be got rid of. They allied themselves with the citizens of Lesser Basel, the part of the city on the other side of the Rhine. Fatio realized the coming danger and proposed an amnesty for all acts committed during the rising. However, only a minority of government and parliament confirmed the amnesty by oath [7].

On September 21 armed citizens of Lesser Basel invaded the city. The town hall into which Fatio had retreated was surrounded, he was chased from room to room, and was finally taken prisoner at the point of the sword and committed to one of the city towers. His rescue was twice attempted by an armed up rising of Basel's population under the leadership of his brother-in-law, the barber surgeon Mosis, but the up risings were a lamentable failure and the ringleaders, including Mosis, were imprisoned.

Government and parliament now acted with indecent haste. The fact that the amnesty was law and that they were about to commit a judicial murder made them rightly fear grave repercussions from the Swiss federation. Fatio was tortured twice. His arms were tied to a rope and he was pulled up with the aid of a pulley and suddenly dropped several metres, so that the arms came out of their sockets. As this did not have the desired effect, the procedure was repeated with weights tied to his feet. There was in fact nothing for Fatio to confess. All the other revolutionary leaders had been caught with the exception of his cousin, Petri, who had escaped into Germany, where he continued to live in constant fear of being murdered by agents from Basel. Fatio quite correctly stated that he thought that the constitution he had given Basel was the best and most just any city had ever had. In fact, there was no reason for this torture other than that of cruelty.

On Sunday, September 28, Fatio was brought before his judges. In order to spread the guilt of judicial murder as widely as possible, the whole of the Greater and Lesser Council had to appear as judges, a procedure similar to that practised 40 years earlier in the trial of Charles I. Fatio was accused of having ruled without the consensus of the people and of having behaved like a Roman dictator [7]. There was a grain of truth in this accusation: Fatio would have never achieved what he did in so short a time had he proceeded with scrupulous concern for the law.

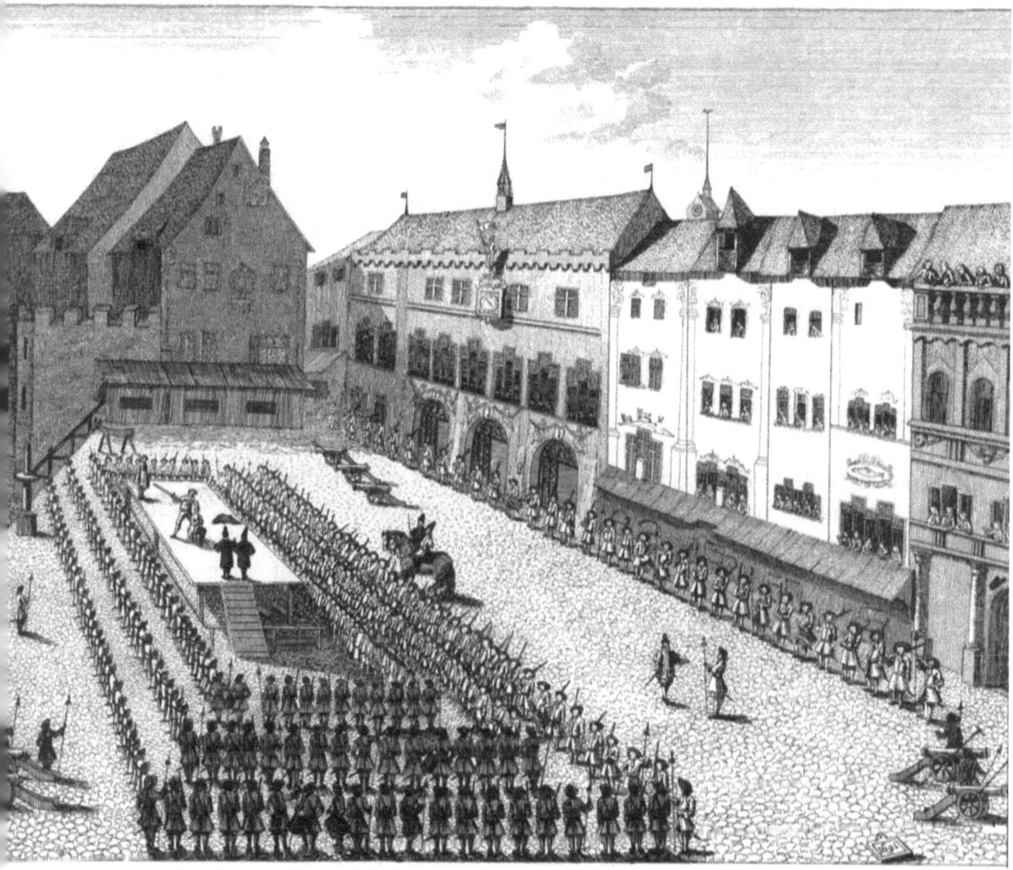

Fig. 6. Fatio's death: drawing 1691. (From the State Archives of Basel and the University Library, Basel)

He was condemned to death and on the following Monday, September 28, was conducted by a company of soldiers with drums and pipes to the market place, where a special platform had been erected (Fig. 6). The place was crammed with people and the soldiers had difficulty keeping them back. Many of the men and a multitude of women were in tears because he was a well-loved man. Fatio, always a dandy, had arrived in a black velvet coat and a white silken scarf. The hangman wanted to remove it, but Fatio asked him for patience. He prayed aloud: "Oh Lord, in my need I turn to Thee. Lead me to eternal salvation". He then turned to the member of the two councils who filled the windows of the town hall and asked their forgiveness for any inconvenience he might have caused them, and to the people, exhorting them to work diligently and not to get involved in matters that were not their concern, as he had done. He removed and folded his coat, bound his hair up with the scarf, and was beheaded at five minutes to five in the afternoon.

So greatly was he hated that the ousted members of parliament played football with his head on the Rhine bridge joining the two Basels. His head was then put on a pike and stuck on the roof of the Rhine Gate, where it was still to be seen 60 years later.

The complete disappearance of his works except for one of them, *The Helvetic Reasonable Midwife,* published anonymously 70 years after his death, shows that resentment and fear of him lingered on in the government for a long time. He was a man so far ahead of his time, both as a surgical and a political thinker, that one can understand that his political contemporaries feared him just as we today can have nothing but admiration for him.

Summary

Johannes Fatio was probably the first surgeon who systematically studied and treated surgical condition of children. Born in Basle in 1649, he never studied medicine at the university there but became a member of the barber's guild. Later he studied medicine and became a doctor of the University of Valence. He returned to Basle to practice surgery, midwifery and paediatric surgery. He wrote a number of medical books, but only one, *The Helvetic Reasonable Midwife,* still exists. In it he devotes a whole section to surgical afflictions of children. He describes ingenuous operations for such conditions as hypospadias, hydrocolpos, imperforate anus and many more. He was the first surgeon successfully to separate conjoined twins.

He became involved in the turbulent politics of the city of Basle and was largely responsible for the overthrow and modern ratio of the Basle parliament and government. In the following counter-revolution he was captured, imprisoned, tortured and executed. All his written works were destroyed by the authorities; The Helvetic Reasonable Midwife was published 70 years after his death.

Résumé

Johannes Fatio fut probablement le premier chirurgien à se consacrer entièrement à l'étude et au traitement des cas de chirurgie des enfants. Il est né à Bâle en 1649. Il n'avait pas fait d'études de médecine à l'université mais était membre de la corporation des barbiers. Plus tard, à Valence il fit des études de médecine et obtint le titre de docteur en médecine de l'Université de Valence. De retour à Bâle, il exerça la chirurgie, l'obstétrique et la chirurgie des enfants. Il écrivit plusieurs livres dont un seul "Helvetic Reasonable Midwife" nous est resté. Dans cet ouvrage, un chapirtre entier est consacré à des cas de chirurgie des enfants. Il décrit des méthodes d'intervention très au point en cas d'anomalies morphologiques telles qu'hypospadias, hydrocolpos, imperforation et autres. Il fut le premier chirurgien à réussir à séparer des siamois.

Il prit part à la vie politique très mouvementée de la ville de Bâle et continua à renverser le parlement et le gouvernement. Pendant la contre-rérvolution qui suivit, il fut arrêté, emprisonné et torturé jusqu'à ce que mort s'ensuive. Tous ses écrits furent brûlés ou détruits par les hommes alors au pouvoir, à l'exception de l'ouvrage mentionné plus haut qui fut publié 70 ans après sa mort.

Zusammenfassung

Johannes Fatio war vermutlich der erste Chirurg, der sich systematisch dem Studium und der Behandlung von kinderchirurgischen Fällen widmete. Er wurde 1649 in Basel geboren, studierte nie Medizin an der Universität, aber er gehörte der Zunft der Barbiere an. Später studierte er Medizin, und es wurde ihm der Doktortitel an der Universität von Valence verliehen. Er ging dann zurück nach Basel, wo er Chirurgie, Geburtshilfe und Kinderchirurgie praktizierte. Er schrieb mehrere Bücher, aber nur das eine: *Helvetic Reasonable Midwife* ist noch erhalten. In diesem Werk widmet er einen ganzen Abschnitt den kinderchirurgischen Fällen. Er beschreibt wohldurchdachte Operationsmethoden bei Hypospadie, Hydrokolpos, Imperforation und vielen anderen Mißbildungen. Ihm gelang zum ersten Mal die Trennung von siamesischen Zwillingen.

Er nahm Anteil am bewegten politischen Geschehen der Stadt Basel und war maßgeblich beteiligt am Sturz des Parlaments und der Regierung in Basel. In der darauffolgenden Gegenrevolution wurde er festgenommen, eingekerkert und zu Tode gequält. Alle seine Schriften wurden von den Machthabern vernichtet, nur die oben erwähnte wurde 70 Jahre nach seinem Tod veröffentlicht.

Acknowledgment. I should like to thank Dr. Marie-Louise Portmann, Director of the Medical History Library of Basel, for her help with the literature and illustrations. Without her profound and expert knowledge, this paper could not have been written. Professor W. Zenker kindly arranged for the supply of Fig. 5 from the Medical History Library of Vienna.

References

1. Ruhrah J (1925) Pediatrics of the past. Hoebar, New York
2. Würtz F (1563) Practica der Wundartzney. Basel
3. Karcher J (1944) Paracelsus. Nova Acta Paracelsica 1:82
4. Nigst H (1949) Die chirurgischen Vorlesungen von Paracelsus in Basel 1527/1528. Helvetica Chirurgica Acta 16:157
5. Huber-Burckhardt A (1913) Die Basler Familie Fatio. Sonntagsblatt der Basler Nachrichten 28/29:121
6. Burckhardt A (1917) Geschichte der medizinischen Fakultät zu Basel 1460–1900. Reinhardt, Basel
7. Gerster J (1917) Johannes Fatio. Inaugural Dissertation. Schwabe, Basel
8. Bonjour E (1971) Die Universität Basel. Helbing and Lichtenhahn, Basel
9. Ochs P (1822) Geschichte der Stadt und Landschaft Basel, Vol 7. Schweighäuser, Basel
10. Rickham PP (1963) Nicolaas Tulp and Spina Bifida. Clin Pediat 2:40
11. Fatio J (1752) Helvetisch-Vernünftige Wehe-Mutter. Johann Rudolph Imhof, Basel
12. Koenig E (1690) In: Miscellanea Curiosa Academiae Imperialis Leopoldinae. Wolfgang Manrith Endteri, Nuremberg

The History of Oesophageal Atresia and Tracheo-Oesophageal Fistula – 1670–1984

N. A. Myers[1]

As this is the history of oesophageal atresia, it is appropriate and virtually obligatory to commence with reference to two classical contributions – that of Durston [31] in 1670 and that of Gibson [46] in 1697. However, at the outset it is equally appropriate to give credit to those who have previously researched the history, none more thoroughly than Ashcraft and Holder [7] and, in more recent times, Chang [24]. With many of the contributions in the literature, introductory and later paragraphs frequently describe events of historical significance, and these contributions are also acknowledged.

In addition, by way of a prologue, history is always in the making, and although no one would deny the excitement of the past, present-day history is equally important with its changing emphasis and with new developments concerned with neonatal support, tracheal stabilisation and methods of improving the outlook for the "high risk" group of patients. Large series are now frequently reported from many centres, and comparison of such series has enabled the results of treatment to be assessed. Nevertheless, when today's history is reviewed in the decades ahead it will become clear that there are still many contentious areas and that there is lack of uniformity of opinion regarding many aspects of management.

The recorded history of oesophageal atresia commenced in 1670, when Charles II was on the throne of England. In that year William Durston [31], Doctor in Physick, described oesophageal atresia in a conjoined twin. His description is to be found in the *Philosophical Transactions of the Royal Society* under the heading "A Narrative of a Monstrous Birth in Plymouth, October 22, 1670: Together with the Anatomical Observations Taken Thereupon. ..." The description commences as follows: "One Grace Battered the wife of a shoemaker of honest repute and mother of five children, now come to the full time to be delivered of a sixth birth, about twelve o'clock at night began to have travelling pains." Later in the description, it becomes clear that Durston delivered a thoracopagus monster and when he performed a necropsy, having with some difficulty "obtained the father's leave to dissect it", he found "one navil-vein, and one liver ... and one stomach with the oesophagus or gullet perforate and open from the mouth of the left head; but the oesophagus from the mouth of the right head descended no lower than a little above half an inch off the midriff, and there it ended".

In their erudite essay entitled "The Story of Esophageal Atresia and Tracheoesophageal Fistula", Ashcraft and Holder [7] mention Durston's description, but

[1] Royal Children's Hospital, Flemington Road, Parkville, Victoria 3052, Australia

Progress in Pediatric Surgery, Vol. 20
Ed. by P. P. Rickham

prefer to give pride of place to Thomas Gibson, commenting that in Durston's monster "there is little to link this unique anomaly with the one which we know now as so characteristic an entity".

Ashcraft and Holder were, of course, referring to the most commonly encountered anomaly, and certainly credit for the first description of this must go to Thomas Gibson. (History relates that Gibson's wife Anne was the granddaughter of Oliver Cromwell, Lord Protector of England.) In 1697 Gibson wrote the following in his *Anatomy of Human Bodies Epitomized:*

> About November 1696 I was sent for to an infant that would not swallow. The child seem'd very desirous of food, and took what was offer'd it in a spoon with greediness; but when it went to swallow it, it was like to be choked, and what should have gone down returned by the mouth and nose, and it fell into a struggling convulsive sort of fit upon it. It was very fleshy and large, and was two days old when I came to it; but the next day died. The parents being willing to have it opened, I took two physicians and a surgeon with me. ... We blew a pipe down the gullet, but found no passage for the wind into the stomach. Then we made a slit in the stomach, and put a pipe into its upper orifice, and blowing, we found the wind had a vent, but not by the top of the gullet. Then we carefully slit open the back side of the gullet from the stomach upwards, and when we were gone a little above half way towards the pharynx, we found it hollow no further. Then we begun to slit it open from the pharynx downward, and it was hollow till within an inch of the other slit, and in the imperforated part of was narrower than in the hollowed. This isthmus (as it were) did not seem ever to have been hollow, for in the bottom of the upper, and the top of the lower cavity, there was not the least print of any such thing, but the parts were here as smooth as the bottom of an acorn-cup. Then searching what way the wind had passed when we blow from the stomach upwards, we found an oval hole (half an inch long) on the fore-side of the gullet opening into the aspera arteria a little above its first division, just under the lower part of the isthmus above mentioned.

These contributions of Durston [31] and Gibson [46] may be regarded as the two classic contributions in the history of oesophageal atresia, but many further contributions were to follow. In order to appreciate the significance of latter, it is helpful to recognise the several phases in the history of oesophageal atresia, namely:

The First Phase – Before 1670. This is the pre-recognition phase; as far as can be ascertained, the condition had not been recognised or described before 1670.

The Second Phase – Commencing in 1670. This year marked the first documented report. For over 250 years, although there are an increasing number of references in the literature, the year 1670 is the year in which the *pre-survival era* commenced. When did this era end? It is usually stated that it came to an end in 1939 when Ladd [88] and Leven [95] independently operated on two babies who survived. Both babies had the commonly encountered anomaly, namely, proximal oesophageal atresia with distal tracheo-oesophageal fistula, and in both survival with alimentary continuity was achieved utilizing a multi-staged approach. Further reference to the details of the management of these babies will be made later. Others, however, would state that for all practical purposes the pre-survival era gave way to the survival era in 1941, when Cameron Haight [53] first achieved success by means of end-to-end oesophageal anastomosis. Certainly this technique has become the corner stone of treatment during the past 25 years, but by the time Haight achieved survival, Ladd's and Leven's patients were both in their 2nd year of life, although still awaiting oesophageal replacement.

If we are to be "purists", however, we must refer to the year 1935 as the year when the pre-surival era came to an end and the survival era commenced, because on February 16, 1935, a patient with an isolated oesophageal atresia was born, investigations revealed "a blind proximal pouch", and gastrostomy was performed on the following day. Successful oesophageal replacement was not achieved until 1951, by which time the patient was aged 16 years! History records that the gastrostomy was performed by James Donovan, and that the alimentary continuity, using jejunal interposition, was effected in 1951 by George H. Humphreys II [76, 67].

Thus, the pre-survival era spanned nearly 300 years; during the latter years of this period, more and more surgical endeavours were made, and it is therefore possible to recognise a surgical era during the pre-survival era. This surgical era commenced in 1888, and thus spans both the pre-survival and survival eras.

The Third Phase. This is the survival era, which commenced with the early successes of Ladd, Leven and Haight. The first surviving patient with an "H"-fistula – tracheo-oesophageal fistula without oesophageal atresia – was born in 1931, but the fistula was not closed until 1938 [79]. Further reference will be made to this case later, when this type of anomaly is considered in more detail.

In summary, therefore, the pre-survival era ended in the 1930s, the original survivals being obtained in the following cases:

1931: H-fistula (reported by Imperatori [79] in 1939)
1935: Oesophageal atresia without tracheo-oesophageal fistula
1939: Proximal oesophageal atresia with distal tracheo-oesophageal fistula (Ladd and Leven [88, 89, 94–96])
1941: Proximal oesophageal atresia with distal tracheo-oesophageal fistula with successful oesophageal anastomosis (Haight and Towsley [53])

Many would also recognise a more recent phase – the era of salvage. To appreciate the significance of this concept, which is basically philosophical, it is necessary to foreshadow some later comments, because in the early years of survival mortality remained high when the baby was of low birth weight, when it had another life-threatening anomaly, or when the diagnosis was "late" and associated with established pneumonia. Today many such babies survive, hence the "era of salvage", but it is well to remember that common sense must prevail and early salvage of the oesophagus of a baby who has an additional condition incompatible with life, e.g., trisomy 18, is pointless. It is beyond the scope of this paper to analyse the ethical and philosophical concepts associated with such combinations as oesophageal atresia and mongolism or oesophageal atresia and severe hydrocephalus, but the practising paediatric surgeon must have a positive attitude to such matters. A balanced point of view has been put by Rickham [145] who in 1969 summarized the situation clearly and concisely:

> An attempt has been made to deal briefly with these difficult ethical problems in as practical a manner as possible. Strictly speaking this is not a matter of morality, but of deontology, the science of duty (after the Greek deon, or what must be done). Whilst moral standards are more or less consistent throughout the Western world, deontology differs from locality to locality ... as science and medicine progress and the community develops and becomes more and more complex, ethics will change as well. It is the duty of medical men to see that the development of the ethics of their profession keeps in step with the scientific development.

In another erudite and meaningful contribution entitled "Oesophageal Atresia: Triumph and Tragedy", Rickham [146] some years later stresses the long-term problems in babies of low birth weight with oesophageal atresia, particularly when associated anomalies were present. When Rickham stated:

> This is the tragedy of oesophageal atresia; we have become too good in getting these children to survive and we fear that ... the long term results of oesophageal atresia in these groups of children ... may present a very pessimistic report,

many in the audience that day did not agree. In the light of later experience (Myers [120]), there can be little doubt that Rickham's prediction was to prove correct.

The history of oesophageal atresia must therefore be considered against the background of recognition, the pre-survival era, surgical endeavours, surgical success and the era of salvage, and in addition of an increasing awareness of ethical and moral issues and responsibilities. That the community as a whole may be involved in such problems is indicated by reference to the lay press and in particular to an article entitled "The Hardest Choice", which appeared in a widely distributed lay periodical in 1974 [182].

Reference has already been made to the "team" approach and perhaps this, above all, has significantly improved the survival figures. To reduce the mortality from 100% to almost zero has required technical expertise, but in addition the surgeon has found it necessary to seek help from paediatricians, radiologists, pathologists, biochemists, haematologists, bacteriologists and, last but by no means least, anaesthetists. Skilled nursing – for 24 hours every day, and perhaps for weeks and months on end – has been required, and it is almost impossible to describe this aspect adequately. Certainly, experience has shown that there is frequently a narrow margin between medical care and nursing care, and the borderline is far from clearly defined. With increasing complexity of treatment and increasing size of the "team", it has been essential to adopt a system of mutual trust; only in this way have satisfactory results been achieved in the more seriously ill babies.

Cameron Haight achieved his first survival at a time when another great man, Winston Churchill, declared:

> This may not be the beginning of the end, but at least it is the end of the beginning.

It is with the beginning that this paper has concerned itself first, but one cannot but agree with the final comment made by Ashcraft and Holder [7] in their review of the story of oesophageal atresia and/or tracheo-oesophageal fistula:

> To those who are not satisfied with the present outlook there remains much of this sotry to be written.

To return to the early history: after the classic contributions of Durston and Gibson in the seventeenth century, the eighteenth century was singularly lacking in references to oesophageal atresia. However, despite this lack it is interesting to note that in 1793 John Hunter [77] drew attention to the possibility of providing a substitute for deglutition; describing the management of a patient with paralysis of the muscles of deglutition, he wrote:

"... This disease is only rendered dangerous from the want of a substitute for deglutition. It becomes our duty to adopt some artificial mode of conveying food into the stomach, by which the patient may be kept alive while the disease continues, and such medicines may be administered as are thought conducive to the cure." Although John Hunter was not referring specifically to oesophageal atresia, it is pertinent to note that the method he suggested and adopted was ultimately to become a very important part of the treatment for oesophageal atresia – viz. transoesophageal tube feeding.

Several interesting articles were written in the nineteenth century; the early references were mainly clinical, but as the century progressed, references were made to the possibility of operative treatment of the anomaly, the first such attempt being made by Charles Steele [167] in 1888.

Early in the nineteenth century, Martin [107] reported the second known case of oesophageal atresia with a distal tracheo-oesophageal fistula: this occurred in 1821 and was apparently comparable to the case reported by Gibson. Review of the writings of Morell Mackenzie [123, 124] (to whom further reference will be made shortly) and Plass [135] is thus inclined to be confusing, because Morell Mackenzie actually gives credit to Mondière [115] for describing a case "in which there is deficiency of the portion of the oesophagus with intercommunication between the alimentary and respiratory tract" which occurred in 1821, and states that "in 1825 a similar case was recorded by Martin". The important point is that early in the nineteenth century increasing attention was being paid to the type of anomaly under discussion, and there can be little doubt that various authorities were describing anomalies without knowledge of previous or simultaneous descriptions. In this connection, Thomas Hill [60] wrote an interesting account in the

Boston Medical and Surgical Journal in 1840, and it would appear most unlikely that Hill had ever heard of the condition, which adds even greater interest to his description. His patient – the newborn infant of Dr. and Mrs. Webster – also had rectal agenesis with a recto-urinary fistula. Hill must, therefore, be given credit for the first description of a combination of anomalies which has frequently been encountered since. Hill's clinical description warrants repetition: "The infant had been noted to salivate excessively since birth, and with each feeding it would cough, become cyanotic, and regurgitate all its food." His diagnosis was "spasmodic stricture" of the oesophagus, and he suggested a warm enema might relieve the spasm. When the nurse attempted to give the enema, she found not even a vestige of an anus. Autopsy subsequently revealed oesophageal atresia with a distal tracheo-oesophageal fistula and "an imperforate anus with a fistula to the bladder neck".

This description indicates that Hill was a very good observer; one only has to review case histories as recent as the past decade to find examples where identical symptoms were attributed to such conditions as prematurity, cerebral birth injury or pulmonary atelectasis, and no thought was given to the possibility of oesophageal obstruction.

In the same year, 1840, Thomas Mellor [111] of Charlton-upon-Medlock, near Manchester, England, wrote to the Editor of *The Medical Gazette* in the following manner:

Sir,

I am induced to transmit the accompanying case for insertion in your excellent journal, in consequence of its extreme rarity, and under the conviction it may prove interesting to your numerous readers, should you deem it worthy of publication.

In the month of August 1839, Mrs. P., the mother of four healthy children, was delivered of her fifth, a fine, well formed infant, after a perfectly natural labour of a few hours' duration. When in due time the infant was put to the breast, it was observed that the nipple was scarcely retained in the mouth beyond a minute, when the little creature became apparently convulsive, and almost instantly rejected the nutriment which it had taken. On my subsequent visit I was made acquainted with the above particulars, when I felt disposed to assent to the opinion expressed by the mother, that flatulency might be the cause of the symptoms, and accordingly prescribed a simple carminative. This was almost immediately rejected, as the milk had been, the infant notwithstanding manifesting the greatest eagerness to supply its instinctive wants. Inferring the existence of some obstruction in, or malformation of the oesophagus, I attempted to pass a common bougie, which however proceeded only for a very short distance, and then became curved upon itself, apparently not having arrived further than the commencement of the oesophagus. Matters went on in this way for six days, no other evacuation having taken place from the bowel than the meconium, and the infant continuing to apply its mouth to the breast with no other result than that of a slight convulsive paroxysm so soon as the pharynx became filled, and the immediate repulsion of its contents. Early on the morning of the seventh day it died, when a post-mortem examination disclosed the existence of little more than the membranous pouch of the pharynx, which terminated in a cul-de-sac a little below the cricoid cartilage, no trace of the oesophagus being visible beyond this part. The stomach presented no deviation from its ordinary form and dimensions, with the exception of its cardiac orifice, where there existed a slight bulging at the part corresponding with the termination of the gullet and which was firmly united to the diaphragm. Further, a probe, introduced at this aperture, could not be made to pass into the stomach. Between this point and the sternum not the slightest trace of oesophagus, or any bend of connections whatever with the pharyngeal portion, existed. The stomach contained nothing but air and a little mucus; the other viscera appeared perfectly normal.

In juxtaposition with the foregoing case of defective conformation, I may mention an instance lately communicated to me by Mr. Heath, a highly respectable practitioner of this town. In this, the infant, which was of ordinary size, presented symptoms very analogous to those above described, and survived until the eighth day. On inspection after death, the duodenum was found to be obliterated to the extent of an inch or more, no further malformation having ben observed.

I will close this communication with an extract from Meckel's *Manual of General, Descriptive, and Pathological Anatomy,* vol. iii, Page 375, to which I was induced to refer, thinking it not improbable that I might therein meet with examples corresponding with that first described. In place of this, however, I find only the following remarks bearing upon the point in question: – "It sometimes, though rarely happens, that the pharynx and oesophagus terminate in a cul-de-sac, the one at its lower part, the other superiorly, in consequence of a primitive defect of conformation. In the first case the cavity of the mouth at least is almost always developed in an imperfect manner, and the lower jaw is either entirely, or in a great measure wanting. The same thing occurs when the pharynx opens into the neck by too narrow an orifice".

Hoping that I shall not be considered as trespassing too far upon your columns, by requesting the insertion of the preceding,

I remain, sir,

Your very obedient servant,

THOMAS MELLOR.

In 1856 J. W. Ogle [126] described "Malformed Trachea and Oesophagus: Congenital Communication Between Them", and the report reads thus:

The specimen showed complete obliteration of a portion of the oesophagus, at about one inch from its pharyngeal opening, the upper part being very dilated. Below the obliterated part there was an opening at the anterior surface of the oesophagus, which directly communicated with the larynx, at a point about a quarter of an inch above the bifurcation of the latter into the bronchi, and hence the stomach and oesophagus were only continuous with the mouth by

> means of the glottis. This opening was valvular in form, the posterior part of the trachea above the opening being continuous with the posterior part of the oesophagus, which was patent below the communication; whilst the anterior part of the oesophagus was continuous with the lower, or crescentic lip of the opening. No other malformation was noticed.
>
> The preparation was removed from the body of an infant, who only lived to the fourth day. The child was of healthy appearance when born, and sucked at the breast vigorously; but it seemed that most, if not all the milk, returned through the nares. It became convulsed before death, and appeared to die without suffering pain.
>
> It is probable that some slight amount of milk found its way by the trachea, and thence into the oesophagus, as the child lived so long, but this was evidently only in spite of the laryngismus, which its passage through the glottis caused, and was totally insufficient to support life.

As one delves into the early literature concerned with oesophageal atresia, many famous names are to be found; one of these is Hirschsprung [62], who in 1861 was able to find ten cases in the literature, and who added four of his own.

Another very well-known medical figure in the nineteenth century, Morell Mackenzie (whose involvement with the ultimately fatal illness of the Crown Prince, subsequently Kaiser, of Germany was to lead to much vitriolic discussion), made a very substantial contribution to the literature in 1880 [123]. His review of previous contributions, his attention to detail, and the pertinence of his observations, many of which were frequently ahead of his time, prompt quotation of the following extracts from his article which appeared in the *Archives of Laryngology,* under the title of "Malformations of the Oesophagus", on December 30, 1880:

> Malformations of the oesophagus, in all probability, are of extremely rare occurrence. All the recorded cases which I have been able to collect do not number more than 56, and I am only able to add one from my own observation, making altogether 57 examples. These facts are especially significant when we remember that the presence of the affection, in viable infants at least, is attended by such striking symptoms, that it is hardly possible for it to escape notice, whilst its inevitably fatal result affords an invariable opportunity of investigating its cause. At the same time, it must not be forgotten that Hirschsprung himself personally observed four examples of the condition in less than seven months in a town of only 108,000 inhabitants, and that within three weeks Ilott met with two cases in a country district near London. It is, indeed, possible that if still-born infants, and especially monsters, were more uniformly submitted to careful dissection, malformations of the oesophagus would be found of more frequent occurrence than the small numbers of recorded cases would lead us to suppose. The earliest recorded examples of deformity of the oesophagus are two cases published by Blasius [15] in 1674: in one of these the tube bifurcated and again united, in the other there was saccular dilatation of the gullet at its lower end.

Morell Mackenzie then goes on to refer to the contributions made by Mondière and Martin, and again refers to Hirschsprung's "small work of considerable merit". He continued:

> Of complete deficiency there are 5 cases on record, viz., those of Sonderland, Lozach, Mellor, Heath and a specimen in the Museum of the Army Medical Department of Netley.
>
> Of blind determination there are 9 examples, viz., those of Reoderer, Marrigues, Lallemand, Van Cruyck, Brodie, Durston, Pagenstecher, Warner and Pinard.

Morell Mackenzie mentions names which rarely appear in the literature of oesophageal atresia; thus of his latter nine examples only Durston has been mentioned in this article and among the previous group, only Mellor. This epitomises the gaps in any historical record, and if there are omissions in the nineteenth and earlier centuries it is inevitable that there will be even more in the present century.

Mackenzie also wrote: "Of patients in which there was no intercommunication between the oesophagus and air-passages, with deficiency of a portion of the former, or, as they have been called, 'inosculating' cases, there are 37 examples, the communication being with the trachea in 34 and with one of the bronchi in 3." He also refers to "intercommunication between the oesophagus and trachea (the oesophagus being otherwise normal)", and specifically refers to Lamb; reference to Lamb's [91] classic contribution will also be made later.

So much has been written and so much discussion has taken place during recent years regarding the causation of congenital malformation that one cannot but admire and draw attention to Mackenzie's assessment of the situation:

> The essential cause of congenital malformation of the oesophagus is involved in the same obscurity that hangs over the whole subject of teratology. ... It is probable, however, that it is the third cause which is the most potent, and that by far the larger number of malformations of the oesophagus are due to disease of an embryo previously well formed, the main argument in support of this view being that even in cases where the oesophagus is partly absent, there are almost always traces of the obliterated portion. The most generally accepted view of the immediate cause of oesophageal malformations is that they depend on 'arrested development'. This view is probably correct, but it does not go far enough; it does not explain the cause of the arrested development. ... The frequent co-existence of other deformities with malformation of the oesophagus has been regarded as evidence that the latter depends on imperfect evolution, and not on disease. This is merely begging the question; the facts sustain well the theory that in such cases the embryo is extensively diseased. If a glance be taken at the normal development of the oesophagus and trachea as recently described by Kolliker, it will facilitate the comprehension of the mode in which the malformation may arise through some slight morbid deflection of the normal process. ... The symptoms of congenital malformation of the oesophagus are so characteristic, that when present they will at

once be recognized. The infant may appear healthy whilst at rest, but the moment it attempts to swallow, the most distressing attacks of suffocation supervene, and there is great danger of one of these proving fatal. ... In other cases, the use of a bougie will allow the condition of the canal to be made out, the instrument being arrested at the end of the oesophageal pouch.

The pathology varies according to the nature of the deformity. In those cases in which the oesophagus is absent, the pharynx ends in a cul-de-sac, and the stomach is generally adherent to the diaphragm. ... In cases of blind termination, the gullet may terminate quite high up ... or may reach nearly to the stomach. ... The cases, however, in which there is deficiency of a greater or less amount of the middle third of the oesophagus, with inosculation of the gullet and air-passages, are the most common, and the most interesting to the pathologist. Here the upper part of the oesophagus usually terminates in a dilated pouch about half an inch above the bifurcation of the trachea, whilst the lower portion generally originates from the trachea still closer to the bifurcation, and passing downwards enters the stomach in the usual way. The portion of the oesophagus immediately proceeding from the trachea is generally very narrow, but as it descends it acquires its normal size. The upper portion, or pouch, is always much dialted, and its walls considerably thickened. ... On dividing the trachea, the opening of the oesophagus may generally be seen as a small aperture situated in the posterior wall of the trachea and directed downwards. Sometimes the opening is described as oval and sometimes as round. ... As regards the associated deformities, in one instance there was spina bifida, absence of anus, and a single horse-shoe kidney placed over the spine. In two cases there was trifurcation of the trachea, and in two others there was atelectasis pulmonum.

... The diagnosis of this deformity is easy – in fact there is no disease for which it can be mistaken. The absolute inability to swallow, which cannot fail to be observed from the first time the infant attempts to suckle, is characteristic; whilst, if a measured quantity of milk be administered with a teaspoon and the ejected fluid collected, it will be found it is all returned. The diagnosis can be further verified by the passage of a catheter. ... If ... a catheter of suitable size cannot be passed the distance indicated, it may be presumed that there is a congenital obstruction.

Morell Mackenzie's observations of the pathology and symptomatology belong to the classical era; although quoted to enable one to appreciate something of the history of oesophageal atresia in the pre-survival era, it cannot be denied that his writings have something of value to teach us today – for all concerned with the early diagnosis and assessment of congenital anomalies of the oesophagus.

It was not surprising that an increasing number of reports appeared following Mackenzie's contribution and, as will later be shown, since the pre-survival era gave way to the survival era an increasing number of survivals have been reported from an increasing number of centres, but that aspect of the history will be dealt with later.

In 1919, Plass [135] surveyed the literature, and his comprehensive review contained 136 verified cases; by 1931, Rosenthal [149, 150] had collected 255 patients in his review, but even in 1944 recognition of the problem was still uncommon and the total number of patients reported in the literature was still of interest. Thus, Ladd [88] in that year mentioned Rosenthal's reported 255 cases and then wrote: "... in 1933 O'Hare reported 281 cases and by 1941 Ashley was able to collect 314 cases. From the records of the Children's Hospital in Boston, can be added 72 cases, which brings the total close to 400. These figures make it apparent that atresia of the oesophagus is a much more frequent anomaly than it has usually been considered to be."

It was previously suggested that there have been three phases in the history of oesophageal atresia, the first phase preceding recognition; the second phase being the pre-survival era which commenced in 1670; and the third phase, the survival era. From a therapeutic point of view, it is perhaps more convenient to look at this history in terms of the following eras:

1. Pre-surgical era
2. Surgical era, which can be subdivided into two eras:
   a) pre-survival
   b) survival
3. "Recent"

With this classification in mind, it is evident that there will be considerable overlap, but as far as surgical treatment is concerned credit for pride of place is given to Timothy Holmes [69], who suggested the possibility of operative treatment. Perhaps, however, the most significant comment he made – and this was in 1869 – was: "... and in any case the attempt ought not, I think, be made." Strangely enough, although perhaps it was not so strange, Holmes was more hopeful "in cases where no such communication can be made out...", referring, of course, to the anomaly where atresia exists without a distal tracheo-oesophageal fistula. Over the years it has become increasingly clear that although the presence of a tracheo-oesophageal fistula does lead to specific problems, absent in pure oesophageal atresia, from a surgical point of view it is preferable to be confronted with the type of patient Holmes was referring to when he wrote: "... and in any case the attempt ought not, I think, be made". Holmes has been accused of being "vague", but his suggestions regarding the possibility of surgery are of renewed interest today when miscellaneous attempts have been made to establish oesophageal continuity where a long gap exists and thereby to avoid oesophageal replacement using colon or some substitute.

In the same year (1869) Thomas Annandale [6], a lecturer on surgery in Edinburgh, wrote: "Examples of this form of congenital malformation cannot be considered to be of much practical importance to the surgeon owing to their extreme rarity and also to the fact that they do not admit of operative interference." Perhaps it is equally relevant to quote M. Sédillot [156], as did Annandale:

> In any case where the oesophagus is simply obliterated, withered or interrupted, gastrotomy would give the hope of saving the child without other acci-

dents, save those related to the operation itself. If there were a communication between the inferior tip of the oesophagus and the trachea, one could fear that the substances carried into the stomach would be regurgitated into the respiratory tract; but the narrowness of the abnormal orifice and its natural tendency to close because there is no reason for it to exist should reassure against the eventuality of this problem, which it is not possible a priori to suspect.

The true surgical era commenced in 1888 when Charles Steele [167] of London operated on a baby. His own description, entitled "Case of Deficient Oesophagus", is by far the best way to describe this experience, and he wrote in the following manner in the issue of *The Lancet* dated October 20, 1888:

The following case appears to be of interest from both a surgical and an anatomical point of view. I was lately asked to see in consultation an infant twenty-four hours old who, shortly after being given nourishment, a little of which was taken readily, became very livid, had difficulty in breathing, and then returned the food and appeared to worsen.

The gentleman in attendance wisely introduced a sound, and found that it passed about five inches and encountered an impassable obstruction. He then asked me to see the child, and I repeated the sounding with the same conclusion. We diagnosed that there was either a membrane across the oesophagus, or that it ended in blind terminations; and I advised that through the night enemata of dessertspoonfuls of peptonised milk should be given every two hours, and that by daylight the stomach should be opened and the oesophagus explored; if a membrane could be made out across a continous canal, that it should be perforated in order to give a hope of life; and that, if we found any distance existed between the extremities, we could do no more; the parents, however, might feel that every possible endeavour had been made to save their child's life. This was agreed upon, and the father willingly acceded. On the following afternoon I was asked to perform an operation. The infant took chloroform well. I openend the abdomen above the umbilicus in the middle line, exposed the stomach, and stitched it at four points to the skin, having some difficulty to keep the liver from protruding. The stomach was then opened, which was perfectly healthy, and of course empty. A bougie was passed down the oesophagus as before, and another upwards from the stomach for a short distance; but, they did not approach each other by what we judged to be an inch and a half. I then cut a gum-elastic catheter in half, and passed it from below, introducing up it a long slender steel probe, and pressed it upwards as much as was justifiable, in case the lower part of the tube might be twisted or narrowed, and capable of being rendered pervious. All was of no avail, however; so the stomach wound was closed with sutures, also the abdominal wound, and we felt sure that the oesophagus was deficient for about an inch and a half. The infant slept for some time, and died twenty-four hours afterwards. The next afternoon, we made an examination, and found the oesophagus terminated above and below in blind rounded ends an inch and a half apart, and there was no cord or connexion between the parts.

All the wounded portions were quite healthy, and the appearance led to the conclusion that had there been a membranous occlusion a happy result might well have been hoped for.

Steele has been credited by some writers with having been the first surgeon to perform gastrostomy for oesophageal atresia; in fact, it is obvious that he did not do this, but only a gastrotomy. En passant, it is to be noted that history records that the first gastrostomy for oesophageal atresia was performed by Hoffman [64] in 1898; initially he attempted a primary repair through the neck, but failing to achieve his purpose, he resorted to gastrostomy. Gastrostomy had been introduced for feeding purposes for a variety of conditions in the latter half of the nineteenth century; the first survival is credited to Verneuil [189].

However, another early report appeared in the *Guy's Hospital Reports* of 1858 [52], describing "a stableman of 47 years who was admitted to Guy's Hospital under the care of Dr. Habershon, complaining of severe dysphagia ... sanctioned by the presence of the medical and surgical staff, I performed the operation, there being no experience in British surgery to guide me ... the opening in the stomach was enlarged slightly ..." It would seem that this preceded Verneuil, and again emphasises difficulties in accurately tracing some aspects of the history.

Despite present-day variations from centre to centre, gastrostomy has proven to be of inestimable value in the management of oesophageal atresia. In the pre-survival era it was initially the sole form of treatment; when more definitive treatment was attempted, it became part of a staged plan. In the survival era there are many who have advocated that gastrostomy should always be performed; those who are not necessarily proponents of this view would agree that it is virtually obligatory for a wide variety of the problems which may be associated with oesophageal atresia, and certainly that it is obligatory for many specific pre- and post-operative complications.

The period following Hoffman contains a few surgical contributions in the early years and then an accelerating number of reports as the 1930s began, culminating in the classic contributions of Leven, Ladd and Haight.

In 1913 Brennemann [17] described three patients, two of whom were treated surgically; before looking more closely at the operations attempted, it is again interesting to read the clinical description, which so closely fits the description of so many patients in this and other series. Brennemann wrote:

> Congenital atresia of the oesophagus is everywhere considered one of the rare anomalies. ... Shukowsky, with a hospital experience of 50,000 new-born babies saw only one case. And yet within a period of one year three of these cases came under my observation. ... While many different kinds of congenital anomalies of the oesophagus are described, one type is the rule ... this is the so-called 'inosculating type', in which the upper end of the oesophagus ends in a free dilated pouch, while the lower end passes from the stomach into the trachea.

Brennemann's clinical description was indeed typical, and reference can be made to his first case, where he writes:

> Case 1. Baby O ... born at full term. Family history negative. Birth weight 5 pounds 9 ounces; ... Outside of the fact that it had a very low temperature (92 F) a few hours after birth the baby attracted no special attention until it began to expel mucus from the mouth. Four hours after birth the nurse recorded 'Spitting up mucus'; two hours later, 'Mucus almost continually coming from nose'; and following a teaspoon of water, 'Water coming back through the nose'. On the third day she recorded [baby taken] 'to mother; almost strangled; milk came back through nose'.

Brennemann then describes his finding:

> From the lower angle of the mouth there flowed a constant stream of stringy mucus and saliva, running over and excoriating the cheek and chin. In front of each nostril, there was a considerable quantity of white, frothy discharge that bubbled to and from with each respiration. When the child was nursed or given water from a bottle it swallowed greedily, but after one swallow the milk or water came back through the mouth, and in jets from both nostrils, synchronous with each act of swallowing. Then with the first breath it would suddenly stop nursing, would cough, become deeply cyanotic, and look as if it were choking to death. After expelling the water by coughing, and especially if the baby was inverted, it would gradually return to normal. ... A rubber catheter inserted through the mouth and always ending abruptly at distance of about 12 cm from the lips, clinched the diagnosis.

Jejunostomy was performed on this baby by L. L. McArthur; death occurred 5 days later.

Brennemann's second patient was admitted "when three days old, with a probable diagnosis, for obvious reasons, of broncho-pneumonia. There was some fever, the breathing was rapid, both lungs were covered with moist rales, and there were spells of alarming cyanosis. The baby had retained nothing since birth".

This description parallels so closely the description in the histories of many of the babies in whom there has been diagnostic delay that it warrants this re-statement.

This second baby had a gastrostomy performed by H. M. Richter on the 5th day of life "leaving a catheter in situ through which the baby was fed on breast milk", but "when the tube was clamped after food was introduced, the child would soon cough, breathe 100 to 150 times a minute, become deeply cyanosed, and would seem to be literally choking to death. If the tube was now open to prevent the child from dying, the milk would well out through it, often in spurts as the child coughed. ... So alarming were the symptoms of drowning in this instance that it was not repeated. When the stomach was empty and the tube open there was an audible to and from movement of air through the tube".

The third patient in Brennemann's series "... had all the essential symptoms and findings of the other two. ... The diagnosis was established on the third day by the inability to pass the catheter into the oesophagus more than about 12 cm from the lips". It was decided that an operation was not indicated. The baby died on the 8th day.

In his discussion, Brennemann comments on many factors which have continued to be significant to this day – birth weight, associated anomalies, cause of death, associated sclerema, symptomatology (particularly attacks of suffocation and cyanosis), the abdominal findings and the diagnosis. Then when he comes to discuss treatment, he comments thus:

> No treatment so far has been of any avail. To attempt to feed such an infant by mouth only hastens the fatal end. Rectal feeding in the new-born can be only a very temporary measure. A radical operation that would aim at a restitutio ad integrum is hardly to be considered in the new-born and not much more so in the older child if it should survive. Hoffmann attempted it, but abandoned it for a gastrostomy.
>
> Temporizing operations have accomplished nothing because of the practical impossibility of nourishing the child under the conditions imposed. Gastrostomy, recommended by Sédillot, has been performed a number of times (Steele, Hoffmann, Happich, Villemin [190], Kirmisson, Dickie, Demoulin, etc.). In every case, as in Case 2, the result has been the same, the fluid introduced into the stomach has flooded the lungs, and invited death by suffocation and bronchopneumonia. It is clearly contra-indicated in cases in which a communication between the stomach and trachea has been diagnosed, and these probably constitute 80 to 90 per cent of all cases of atresia. Surgical closure of the cardiac end of the esophagus, if possible, would make this operation more rational, but would make any later radical operation still more formidable. In cases in which there is a simple blind termination of the upper end, with no lower end communicating with the trachea, simple gastrostomy would be the operation of choice.
>
> Jejunostomy, recommended by Demoulin, and performed in Case 1, would seem sounder theoretically, but it is very doubtful if a new-born infant, thus handicapped, ever could be nourished sufficiently by jejunal feeding to more than simply prolong its life a few days, to say nothing of building it up for a future radical operation. These cases are unfortunately rarely diagnosed before so enormous a loss in weight has taken place that this alone jeopardizes the child's life. Even if a child could be fed in this manner it would be doomed to perpetual feeding through a tube, and to other embarrassments that would make life unbearable; or else it would have to submit later to a radical operation that would offer little if, indeed, any hope. While the utter hopelessness of these cases, if untreated, justifies surgical procedures that would otherwise seem too daring; nevertheless the physician who, after making his diagnosis of congenital atresia of the esophagus, decides to let his little patient die undisturbed, as in Case 3, can amply justify his course.

No one would deny that at that time this philosophy was basically correct; even today, it is essential to remember that we must not leave a child in a situation of "embarrassment that would make life unbearable".

In a second contribution from Chicago 5 years later, Brennemann [18] was to reiterate his clinical observations and his philosophy regarding surgical management, stating that "... pediatric limitations will form an insurmountable barrier"; however, a ray of light appeared in one of his comments that "in these otherwise hopeless cases, however, one gives the surgeon a full range with a clear conscience".

Brennemann mentioned Richter as the surgeon involved in the case of the second of his patients, and we now find a very famous and oft-quoted contribution from Richter himself. In the same year (1913), Richter [143] wrote an article entitled "Congenital Atresia of the Oesophagus; An Operation Designed for Its Cure – With a Report of Two Cases Operated upon by the Author". This contribution presented two particularly important aspects of the problem. Firstly, Richter drew attention to basic problems which seemed insurmountable at the time, but secondly, he was very near to finding a solution, and in addition attempted an operative technique which was 50 years later to become standard practice for the poor-risk baby in many centres. Further reference will be made to this when recent developments in the staged management of oesophageal atresia are considered.

With reference to the first of these points, Richter wrote: "The essentially fatal factor in the anatomy consists of a communication between the upper end of the distal segment and the trachea or bronchus, allowing of free communication between lungs, gullet, and stomach; forced respiration, as in crying etc., distends the stomach; attempts at vomiting fill the air passages with stomach contents (secretion), resulting in drowning (cyanosis)."

Considering treatment, Richter commented on Hoffman's attempt and dismissed his approach: "His attempt was by way of the neck, an obviously impossible route."

It should be noted that Richter also commented on Brennemann's first patient, strangely enough suggesting that the jejunostomy was performed by A.E. Halstead, and this highlights some of the difficulties in tracing the precise history of this and other conditions. Perhaps more important was the point made by Richter that "jejunostomy cannot, of course, obviate the fatal outcome of the tracheo-oesophageal fistula".

We now come to the classic paragraph which has been quoted and re-quoted, and which indicates Richter's clear thinking at a time when thoracic surgery had not really entered its infancy and neonatal surgery was even younger:

> Direct anastomosis of the ends, with closure of the trachea, in an infant less than a week old is certainly a hazardous proceeding. I am not certain however, that it may not prove impossible, and, if so, would be the ideal operation. I do not wish to dismiss the idea of immediate union of the two segments of the oesophagus. The technical difficulties would be rather greater than that of the operation here suggested. The greatest obstacle would be the danger of infection; however, I expect to attempt it at the first favourable opportunity. ... The present problem seems to be to close the communication with the trachea, do a gastrostomy, and so feed the child. The recent development of thoracic surgery justifies the hope that later in life a means of utilizing the gullet may be found.

Richter outlined his plan of operation as follows:

1. Closure of gullet at tracheal junction via trans-thoracic route
2. Gastrostomy

The description that follows is very clear and does not require to be quoted in its entirety; nevertheless, it is not without interest to note the following of Richter's comments: "Lack of familiarity with the surgical anatomy of the parts will obviously be a source of embarrassment to most general surgeons. The abdomen was first opened, a small opening made in the anterior wall of the stomach at the intended site of gastrostomy, and a pliable uterine sound introduced, passed up through the cardia into the gullet." (This too was to be introduced as a very helpful manoeuvre in enabling recognition of the lower end of the oesophagus in the type of oesophageal atresia where a long gap exists.)

Many years later Cameron Haight was to describe the situation very clearly, commenting that it was unfortunate that Richter had no further experience with the lesion: "This was unfortunate because had he had such experience a satisfactory solution to a difficult problem might well have been obtained much earlier than was the case."

Richter thus should be remembered in two ways – firstly, he accepted the possibility of restoration of alimentary continuity with preservation of the oesophagus, and secondly he actually adopted a technique which was to prove life-saving for many critically ill babies. At this point it is therefore not without interest to refer to many articles written during the past 15 years, e.g. the contribution by C. Everett Koop and James P. Hamilton [86] – "Atresia of the Esophagus: Increased Survival with Staged Procedure in the Poor Risk Infant." In a series of 41 patients, 13 were initially managed by the 'Richter technique', i.e. the upper oesophageal pouch was left intact, the tracheo-oesophageal fistula closed, and gastrostomy performed.

Although it is acknowledged that the surgical era commenced in 1888 and although as time passed there was to be more and more emphasis on operative correction, anecdotal experiences were still reported before and after the 1913 contributions of Brenneman and Richter. Of course, the following references are but a few, but they are representative and reflect thinking at the time. In 1899 Stewart and Thomson [169] "exhibited a 'congenital malformation of the oesophagus' – the baby was born on the evening of 28th December; the labour was tedious but easy; the mother had had a fall down stairs at the 4th month". Perhaps the most interesting part of their description is the following:

> On the following day the child was seen by Dr. John Thomson [no doubt not the same Dr. Thomson of Teviot Row referred to by Annandale 30 years earlier], who having passed a tube which was stopped at the same point, confirmed the diagnosis of malformed oesophagus, either atresia or a transverse septum. The child seemed then so weak, besides having crepitations over both lung fields, that it was thought better to leave him alone. However, on the morrow (1st Jan.) the child looking better and the lungs having to a great extent cleared up, it was thought advisable to give him a chance of operation. He

(Dr. Stewart) therefore with the assistance of Major Mitchell and Dr. Miles did a gastrostomy after the manner of Witzel.

Some years earlier, in 1890, the section entitled "Organs of Digestion" in the *Transactions of the Pathological Society of London* contains a presentation by Samuel G. Shattock [159] regarding a "dissection of a still-born child of about full term, with congenital atresia of the oesophagus". Shattock makes the pertinent comment that "congenital atresia of the oesophagus is indeed a malformation of remarkable uniformity", and he also comments that "the atresia as a matter of deduction, therefore must be regarded as secondary to its origin. ... The continuity frequently present between the two parts of the oesophagus points also strongly to this; the longitudinal fibres are sometimes readily tracible by dissection from one segment to the other. Nevertheless, the constancy of its situation points to its having a relation with some constant phase in the development process".

Was it only coincidence that over 30 years later C. E. Shattock [158] presented a six-line report under the heading "Specimen of Congenital Malformation of Oesophagus"? The report is short enough to quote in toto.

> ... The child was aged 10 days, had lost 2 lb. in weight since birth, and regurgitated all food immediately after swallowing. The stomach and intestines were much distended with air. Post-mortem – The patent lower portion of the oesophagus extended upwards from the cardiac orifice to open into the trachea about its bifurcation. The upper portion of the oesophagus ended blindly about this level.

It is interesting to note that the baby lived 10 days without treatment.

In 1914 Losee reported two cases of oesophago-tracheal fistula from the Lying-In Hospital, New York; in the first of these "a gastrostomy was performed and feeding was carried on through a tube". This baby died on the 10th day from "inanition and bronchopneumonia". Losee [104] also commented: "These infants all die from 2–12 days after birth regardless of any treatment. I think that such cases as these should be reported in order to keep ever-present in the eyes of the attending physician the occasional occurrence of these anomalies so that an early diagnosis and definite prognosis may be made."

Others who contributed to the literature during this relatively long period include Huntington, Young and Foote [78] in 1919 and Reynolds and Morrison [141] in 1921, and both of these contributions discuss cases, reports and theories regarding the aetiology of the anomaly. There are some extremely interesting references appended to the Reynolds/Morrison article, all of which would be worthy of review, and the depth of the early literature is indicated by referring to three of these: Dam – "Cas d'Imperforation de l'Oesophage", Policlinique, Bruxelles; Spicer – "A Case of Abnormal Development of the Oesophagus (1907)"; and Jackson – "A Case of Congenital Atresia of the Oesophagus (Michigan – 1915)". But even earlier than this, in England in November 1903, William Thomas [180] spoke on "Congenital Occlusion of the Oesophagus", describing a baby he had seen in October 1901. He quaintly refers to this experience thus: "Whilst looking over the stock of a Second Hand Book Seller, I came across a copy of Gibson's 'Anatomy'", and he also – and this is of even greater interest – refers to a baby operated on "by Mr. F. J. Stewart at the Hospital for Sick Children, Great Ormond Street, London". His final paragraph reads:

> I only know of one case which has been operated on – i.e., Mr. Stewart's, to whom I am indebted for particulars. The child did not recover but lived for 14 days, the longest time on record. Perhaps in the future, when these conditions are discovered early, greater success may be attained. Rectal feeding has prolonged life in at least one case and might with advantage accompany other treatment, and careful examination should be made to insure that there is no congenital deficiency of the rectum or other part of the alimentary canal.

From Philadelphia in 1909, Griffith and Lavenson [49] reported in the *Archives of Pediatrics* on "Congenital Malformation of the Esophagus with the Report of a Case", their article having previously been read before the 20th Annual Meeting of the American Pediatric Society in Delaware. One can only imagine the discussion which took place at such meetings and the anecdotal experiences shared. Griffith and Lavenson discussed treatment in the following manner: "This is entirely discouraging. Cases of stenosis have recovered, but all instances of complete obstruction have died. The weakness of the child and its early age makes operative interference a questionable procedure. Yet gastrostomy offers the only hope." Again reference should be made to Griffith and Lavenson's bibliography with its 76 references, some already familiar, others not. In the same year (1909) Cameron and Lightoller [22] contributed to the literature from Australia, describing "A Case of Congenital Malformation of the Oesophagus", their baby living 5 days. In 1920 Henry Shaw [160] of New York reported a case "typical of the great majority of these malformations", and stated: "The diagnosis is simple. An operation was not advised. Two days later the baby died." Shaw also drew attention to the passing report by Thomas Gibson in 1696, Shaw commenting that "this case ... is so quaintly described that it bears repetition" and also adding a little history regarding Dr. Thomas Gibson himself. In addition, Shaw epitomised the interest in isolated experiences, pointing out that "in a discussion of Griffith's paper read before the American Pediatric Society in 1908 Dr. Putnam [136] of Boston reported a case which has escaped notice".

Shaw's comments on Thomas Gibson were the following:

> Dr. Gibson was Physician General to the British Army in 1718–1719. An interesting side-line of his character is found in the diary of Thomas Hearne of Oxford under the date of September 8, 1717 and the extract reads thus: – 'Sept. 8. On Saturday (Sept. 5) came to Oxford two of the daughters of Richard Cromwell, son of Oliver Cromwell, protector, one of which is married to Dr. Gibson, the physician, who writ the Anatomy; the other is unmarried. They are both Presbyterians, as is also Dr. Gibson, who was with them. They were at the Presbyterian meeting-house in Oxford on Sunday morning and evening; and yesterday they, and all the gang with them dined at Dr. Gibson's, provost of Queen's College, Oxford, who is related to them, and made a great entertainment from them, expecting something from them, the physician being said to be worth 30,000 libs. They went from Oxford after dinner.'

In the same year (1920) Kastner [82] addressed the Milwaukee Medical Society, and he too quoted Thomas and Gibson – accurately! He concisely summarized prevailing attitudes: "Though congenital atresia of the esophagus receives an unwarranted neglect in most text books, many authors have, expecially in recent years enriched the literature with accounts of the condition", and: "The charitable view then would be that these cases fall not with impartiality, but that like the malicious paper snow storm of the melodrama, they pursue the unfortunate up and down stage and snow on him and him alone. None the less, it will be just as well to remember that it is a human fraility to recognize most readily what is familiar – so this subject, perhaps with profit, may be opened again."

It is not surprising that Kastner concluded: "So when we consider the peculiar anatomical conformation of the anomaly, the unfavourable field for successful surgery that the delicate economy of the new born offers plus the limitations of intrathoracic surgery, these cases may be called hopeless from the beginning."

Kastner warrants mention, if for no other reason, for his philosophy and phraseology.

In 1920 Reynolds and Morrison [141] of New York commenced their report in the following manner: "Cases of congenital malformations of the esophagus are extremely rare and many standard works on embryology, anatomy, pathology or pediatrics dismiss the subject with but a few words. In the large necropsy service of Bellevue Hospital only one case has been recorded in the last sixteen years. The etiology of the condition still remains in doubt although several theories to explain it have been brought forward." (This is still true 60 years later!). Interestingly, Reynolds and Morrison commented in the course of their article: "In the matter of treatment, the only hope of saving the child is to perform gastrostomy as soon as the condition is diagnosed. The technic may be difficult as the liver may be large and the stomach contracted, as in Case 1, in which there was no tracheo-esophageal fistula. On the other hand, where a tracheo-esophageal fistula is present, as in Case 2, the stomach may be ballooned out with gas."

It is therefore apparent that there were many who contributed to the literature, including Hirsch [61] in 1921, Willard [201] in 1922, Weiss [198] in 1923, and also in 1923 E. Dargan Smith [165], whose address was given as Kweilin, SI, China. Part of Smith's article warrants notice:

> It is evident that in the treatment of esophageal atresias, a distinction must be drawn between the minority of cases in wich there is an uncomplicated atresia, and those with an associated esophago-respiratory fistula. The logical procedure in cases of the first type is gastrostomy. Unfortunately, this relatively favourable group constitutes only about one-fifth of the cases encountered. A variety of methods has been used in an effort to relieve cases of the second type with uniform lack of success. Simple gastrostomy has been tried repeatedly but all the infants died from operative shock or were drowned in the milk which passed through the fistula. Jejunostomy suggested by Demoulin in 1904 has proven equally futile. Following jejunostomy, while the milk is introduced below the stomach, gastric secretions stimulated by the process of digestion may still enter the respiratory tract.

> ... Should one of these little patients live, then, several years later ... the fistula could be closed ... two portions of the esophagus united. ... The carrying through of one of these cases to a successful conclusion would require the solution of a series of problems in technic and the exercise of fine judgment, but the satisfaction of success would be immeasurable. Should the condition of the patient, or the judgment of the surgeon, decide against this rather formidable series of operations a continued gastrostomy life is conceivable.

In 1927, Holderman [67], who was surgeon-in-chief at the Locust Mountain Hospital in Shenandoah, Pennsylvania, reported the case of a patient on whom a Witzel gastrostomy was performed. Perhaps one of the more interesting comments in his report is: "Roentgen-ray Diagnosis: Congenital atresia of the esophagus with congenital diverticulum. This patient, it was noted, had thirteen ribs on each side".

In 1923 McClellan and Elterich [122] from Pittsburgh made their contribution; they had also clearly researched the literature, but had perpetuated an error previously made in citing "Thomas" rather than "Gibson". Reference can also be made to Flood [35] (1926) and his comment that "nothing unusual was noticed during the pregnancy except a moderate hydramnion", and to Mathieu and Goldsmith [109] from Portland, Oregon, who in 1933 summarized the symptomatology thus:

1. Absolute inability to retain fluids.
2. Regurgitation of fluid through the nose and mouth associated with attacks of dyspnea, cough and cyanosis when put to the breast or when gavaged. The attacks are constant and occur with each attempt to give fluids by mouth.
3. Frothy fluid at the nares and flow of saliva by mouth.
4. Failure to pass a catheter into the esophagus more than 10 to 12 cm from the lip margin.
5. Air in the stomach if a tracheal fistula is present.
6. Moist rales throughout both lung fields.
7. Gradually increasing temperature with development of bronchopneumonia.
8. Increasing dehydration, loss of weight and malnutrition.
9. Inevitable death within two weeks usually from bronchopneumonia.
10. Associated congenital anomalies.

In their discussion with reference to prognosis and treatment, they comment that "surgery must be held forth as the only optimistic procedure for lessening what is now an inevitable death". And, as with others, they draw attention to Brennemann's philosophy. Also in 1933, Reitter [140] described "A Case of Congenital Atresia of the Upper End of the Esophagus with Tracheo-Esophageal Fistula".

Many of these contributions drew attention to the duration of life of these babies, as did C. Kessick Bowes [16] as long ago as 1897 when, in his report in the *British Medical Journal,* he concluded: "The case is an extremely interesting one, not only on account of the rare malformations, but also on account of the length of time the child lived without any nourishment whatever."

When Brown Kelly [83] of Glasgow described "Congenital Abnormalities at or Near the Upper End of the Oesophagus", his description appeared in the *Journal of Laryngology and Otology,* reference being made to the interesting fact that this journal was founded in 1887 by Morell MacKenzie and Norris Wolfenden; there is little doubt that he was probably unaware of many of the surgical endeavours which had been made on these babies, but he was aware that "of all the maldevelopments of the gullet, atresia is the most serious as it invariably has a fatal issue". During this period, there was an increasing interest in the diagnostic aspects of atresia of the oesophagus as illustrated by Tucker and Pendergrass [186], whose contribution was entitled "Congenital Atresia of the Esophagus: A New Diagnostic Technic". It is interesting to note that in the patient they described "gastrostomy was done by Dr. I. S. Ravdin and the lower end of the esophagus was tied off". These references ranging from Bowes in 1897 to Brown Kelly and others in the 1930s encourage us to attempt to trace the pathways of treatment. In 1923, as has been mentioned, Smith made a contribution to the literature (let us bear in mind that throughout the literature there are references to the role of gastrostomy and jejunostomy as the sole procedures and their failures). Smith's philosophy, being very logical, was based on the fact that since gastrostomy feedings with a patent fistula were fatal and direct attempts to divide the fistula disastrous, an alternative was necessary; for this reason he suggested ligation of the oesophagus at the cardia combined with gastrostomy.

In 1925, in a textbook of thoracic surgery, Lilienthal [98] suggested that operative treatment could take the following form: "Division of the tracheoesophageal fistula and 'anastomosis' of the atretic oesophagus by tieing each pouch over a rubber tube stent." At this stage, thoracic surgery was in its infancy, and as Ashcraft and Holder state: "Few surgeons could be expected to be as agressive and direct as Richter."

The remaining years of the pre-survival era were to be marked by despair and hope, and isolated examples of babies living for varying periods – sometimes several months – following a variety of surgical measures. Although ultimately survival was to be the reward for surgical ingenuity, it is to be noted that advances in paediatric medicine, particularly in the care of the newborn, advances in anaesthesia, and, in due course, the introduction of chemotherapeutic agents and antibiotics, were all to parallel surgical advances and play their part in the success which would ultimately be achieved. Not the least of these parallel advances was the increasing knowledge of homeostatic factors in the new-born and its clinical application, with particular reference initially to water and electrolyte balance, but later to acid-base balance.

There were many workers in the field during the 14 years (1925–1939) which were to precede the first case of survival, and of these the following are definitely worthy of note: Mixter [114], Ravdin [138], Tucker and Pendergrass [186], Gage and Oschner [42], and Scott [155]. Rosenthal [149], Tucker, and Gage and Oschner followed Smith's approach, namely ligation of the oesophagus coupled with gastrostomy, whereas Mixter followed the original Richter plan. Scott (in 1928 and subsequently in 1934) divided the oesophagus at the cardia and, on at least one occasion, combined this with exteriorization of the distal oesophagus. The attempt to control the lethal factor of a patent tracheo-oesophageal fistula by an operation on the stomach foreshadowed later developments when gastric division was advocated as a form of staging; for example, by Meeker [110] and Randolph [137].

Other surgeons who addressed themselves to the problem included Gamble [43] and Leven [94]; Gamble's contribution in 1938 was entitled "Tracheo-Esophageal Fistula, Description of a New Operative Procedure and Case Report". He stressed that "the treatment was essentially a surgical problem", and that "there is gradually becoming evolved from the cumulative efforts of many operators a procedure which it is hoped will ultimately result in the saving of some of these children", stating that "we cannot subscribe to the philosophy of Brennemann"; previous reference has been made to this.

Gamble summarized the role of surgery thus: "The surgical approach to this problem is either by directly attacking the condition or by indirect methods. In the direct approach at least three stages are necessary to relieve this condition. The indications in the first stage are: 1) To provide a means for nourishing the child; 2) To prevent regurgitation of food; and 3) The prevention of pulmonary complications. The second stage is concerned with the reconstruction of the esophagus, and the third stage has to do with the re-establishment of the continuity of the gastro-intestinal tract. The operation performed upon our second case was designed to fulfill these requirements."

Clearly, Dr. Vilray P. Blair [14] of St. Louis, Missouri, was the discussant of Gamble's paper and in his discussion, Blair made some semi-philosophical observations:

> Doctor Gamble has presented a very intriguing surgical problem, and the ingenuity evidenced by him, and his comparatively large experience with this rare occurrence, leave little if anything to be added, especially by one who has never even seen any. However, based upon some experience with extensive operations on very young babies, I would corroborate the emphasis he has put upon the importance of early operation. ... I believe one would be more apt to succeed if this part of the operation were performed within the first 24 hours – better still within the first four hours after birth; conceivably this might save a gastrostomy. If done at all, I am inclined to believe that the baby's best chances for ultimate recovery with normal life will be inverse to the age at which both of these are accomplished. ... A day old baby normally withstands a tremendous amount of trauma such as being pulled by the neck through a tight parturient canal. The second possibly greater advantage is that in the event of death the loss of a day old baby is a minor tragedy compared with one a mother has fondled and suckled. I hope for the sake of both baby and parents that Doctor Gamble's next case will be turned over to him before it has had its first bath.

No comment is needed on Blair's philosophy.

Leven's initial approach was to transect the stomach and it was only later that he altered his plan to gastrostomy, fistula division and cervical oesophagostomy.

An excellent summary of these many events is to be found in the article written by Humphreys [74] in 1944, based upon the paper presented at the meeting of the Society of University of Surgeons, Nashville, Tennessee, earlier in that year. The article contains a summary of 153 operative cases, including 19 "reported here for the first time". For those interested in the history of the operative treatment of oesophageal atresia, Humphreys points out that the tracheo-oesophageal fistula, which "must be assumed to be present in all cases", must be eliminated before any procedure to provide for feeding is embarked upon. He summarized earlier attempts when he said: "A long and uniformly dismal record of fatalities following gastrostomy alone attests the fact that drowning by feeding always results unless the communication between the stomach and trachea is closed or unless the anomaly is one in which a fistula is not present." He also observed that "these basic principles have been slow to emerge". The obvious failure of gastrostomy led first to the hope that by jejunal feeding regurgitation could be avoided; it was, however, found that not only was jejunostomy an unsatisfactory method of feeding, but also that material soon found its way back into the stomach. His references to Richter, Lilienthal, Iglauer, Heatley and others lead up to an excellent summary of the original survivals achieved by the multi-stage approach reported by Leven and Ladd.

Later, in 1956, Humphreys [75] was to report experience with "136 cases of congenital esophageal atresia with or without fistula" seen at Babies Hospital or born in Sloane Hospital, both now units in the Columbia-Presbyterian Medical Center in New York, in the half-century between 1903 and 1953. It is extremely interesting to note that the discussants on this occasion included Shaw of Texas, Cameron Haight and Willis Potts.

In summary, therefore, the history before 1939 shows that one way or another every effort had been made to control the blind upper pouch and/or to combat the effects of tracheo-oesophageal fistula and/or to permit feeding. It remained to provide alimentary continuity and, having reached this step, to obtain survival. Ladd and Leven were to obtain survival, utilising the indirect and multi-stage approach. Many have referred to their epoch-making successes, none more concisely than Woolley in 1979 at the 5th Annual Lyman A. Brewer III Cardiothoracic Symposium in Los Angeles. In due course, Woolley [202] published his review under the heading "Esophageal Atresia and Tracheoesophageal Fistula: 1939–1979", and it is interesting to note that in review he refers to the fact that R. E. Gross "commonly expressed personal feelings and value judgments in his operative dictation. After one difficult anastomosis, he dictated: 'This is the worst esophageal anastomosis that I have ever done. As I proceeded through the chart review for that particular patient, I was surprised to find that the patient had no postoperative complications, the esophageal anastomosis healed without evidence of leak, and the patient was discharged from the hospital alive and swallowing well'". It is not without interest to note that in the same symposium, Belsey [12] gave a paper entitled "Gastro-Oesophageal Reflux", a condition which was to emerge as a very significant problem in the follow-up of patients with repaired oesophageal atresia.

Holder and Ashcraft, inter alios, referred to Ladd and Leven both in their erudite essay in 1969 and again in their collective review in 1970 [65]. But it is best to turn to the original description by Leven in 1941 and by Ladd in 1944. Firstly Leven: "That the surgical management of cases of congenital atresia of the oesophagus with tracheoesophageal fistula is a difficult problem is indicated by the many reports of various unsuccessful operative procedures". Leven goes on to give an excellent historical review, observing that "the following various methods have been attempted or suggested", and subsequently states: "I became convinced that the fistulous communication with the trachea must be attacked directly." Leven performed a preliminary gastrostomy, but pointed out that "it is important to pass the catheter through the pylorus into the duodenum or jejunum as suggested by Villemin [190]. ... By passing the catheter into the jejunum these patients have very little difficulty with regurgitation of gastric contents into the trachea if frequent small feedings are used". In his case report, gastrostomy was performed on the patient, a 2-day-old male infant admitted to University Hospital on November 28, 1939, on the following day. It was not until January 5, 1940 that extra-pleural ligation of the oesophagus at its fistulous communication with the trachea was carried out. At the time when he reported his experience, it was apparent he planned to perform "an ante-thoracic esophagoplasty". Apparently, Leven [96] ultimately interposed jejunum, completing the replacement in 1951.

Ladd's [88] article should be read in toto; in doing this, one appreciates the true historic significance of the pioneering efforts in surgery to find the "best" cure for oesophageal atresia. In addition, one notes the courtesy he accords Leven in writing:

> It is interesting to note that Leven, at almost the identical time, came to the same conclusion about methods of attacking this problem and adopted principles identical with ours with only minor variations of technic. So far as I know, he has the oldest living patient with esophageal atresia and a tracheo-esophageal fistula, his patient being twenty-four hours older than our oldest living one. In a recent personal communication, he states that he has 4 additional patients living who have been operated on according to principles similar to those about to be described.

It is clear from Ladd's article that he performed gastrostomy on his patient on the November 28, 1939, but did not attack the tracheo-oesophageal fistula until March 15, 1940; later he was to perform cervical oesophagostomy and antethoracic oesophagoplasty (Leven had actually performed cervical oesophagostomy on his patient on March 27, 1940). Ladd's summary in 1944 warrants repetition:

> From our experience and that of others, it seems fair to conclude that atresia of the esophagus with or without tracheoesophageal fistula should no longer be considered as a hopeless condition carrying with it a 100 per cent mortality. It also seems justifiable to predict that if obstetricians and pediatricians are on the alert from making an early diagnosis, the mortality will be further lowered.
>
> It should also be stated that the surgical methods for combating this condition are subject to change. At the present time, however, primary anastomosis

of the esophagus appears to be the operation of choice when the two ends of the esophagus can be approximated without too much tension. In other cases, where the ends of the esophagus are far apart, the three-stage operation with the ultimate construction of an anterior thoracic esophagus is a safer operation.

Ladd acknowledged the careful post-mortem operations of Sidney Farber and the help he received from Tague Chisholm in reviewing the literature and tabulating the statistics.

The difficulties in accurately recording the corrective operation for oesophageal atresia result from many factors, not the least of which has been confusion regarding the exact order of the steps as carried out by Ladd and by Leven. Their original articles provide the correct information, but basically this is unimportant; the important factor is that their patients were the first babies to be born with oesophageal atresia and a tracheo-oesophageal fistula and to survive.

Some years later, Robert Gross [51] was to summarize progress in the following manner:

In recent years there has been no more dramatic advance in surgery than that which has taken place in the treatment of congenital atresia of the esophagus. In spite of innumerable attempts by many surgeons to correct the malformation by operative means, the abnormality was uniformly fatal throughout the world prior to 1939. In the decade following this, improvements in the surgical handling of babies with this anomaly have been so remarkable that in many centres a high proportion of these children now can be saved and can be provided with a satisfactory pathway for the transport of food to the stomach.

Reference should also be made to Gross' comments on "multi-stage operations for building an antethoracic esophagus", which he commences as thus: "After stumbling through many dismal experiences and failures, a new ray of light dawned when in 1939 Ladd in Boston and simultaneously Leven in St. Paul, the activity of each being unknown to the other, developed a multi-stage attack for treatment of esophageal atresia."

Gross also stated:

While multiple-stage attacks on esophageal atresia and tracheo-esophageal fistula, with subsequent construction of an antethoracic esophagus, are no longer used by us, it might be well to summarize here some of the experiences gained from the 12 patients who have survived such procedures in this clinic. This brief resume in no way indicates the innumerable tribulations and infinite patience of Ladd in eventually getting these youngsters through the many complicated steps in the construction of antethoracic subcutaneous tubes.

Throughout the history of oesophageal atresia, particularly the history of surgical treatment, it is apparent that many of the advances were dependent upon skills developed in adult patients with oesophageal problems. In this context in 1948, Ivy, Hawthorne and Ritter [80] presented a paper to the Philadelphia Academy of Surgery entitled "Construction of Skin-Tube Esophagus, Following

Surgical Treatment of Tracheoesophageal Fistula". This paper contains an excellent review of the "various procedures ... proposed for reconstruction of the esophagus following resection for stricture due to caustic burns, malignant disease, or congenital anomalies", and should certainly be read in conjunction with Gross' comments.

Perhaps it is relevant at this stage to mention also Sweet [173, 174], whose interest in the surgical management of oesophageal carcinoma led him to the technique of "high intra-thoracic esophagogastric anastomosis", a technique which he was to use in oesophageal atresia when the gap precluded end-to-end oesophageal anastomosis.

Although others [92, 161] had effected satisfactory axial oesophageal anastomoses, with survival of up to 12 days, it was Cameron Haight who was to be the first surgeon to achieve long-term survival with preservation of the oesophagus. Before this, although attempts had been recorded by Shaw [161] and Lanman [92], most would agree that the latter's name stands supreme at this stage in the history of oesophageal atresia.

T. H. Lanman performed the first primary anastomosis of the oesophagus in 1936; the patient lived for only 3 h. He reported his experience in 1940 in a paper entitled "Congenital Atresia of the Esophagus. A Study of 32 Cases". Having had the opportunity to speak to present-day paediatric surgeons who knew Lanman, I feel sure that it is appropriate that extracts of his paper should be quoted. The following are some of his comments:

> In the past eleven years, 32 cases of congenital atresia of the esophagus have been observed. ... 30 patients were submitted to operation and complete autopsy was performed on the other 2 patients. In the 30 operative cases the surgical findings were supplemented by complete post-mortem examination in 22 instances. ... It is only since 1929 that a discussion of the forms of surgical treatment has been of value.

We come then to Lanman's description of case 16:

> M.C., a girl, entered the hospital Jan. 1, 1936, at the age of 2 days. There had been difficulty with breathing since birth and regurgitation of all fluid taken by mouth. On entrance there was some diminished resonance over the left side of the chest and many coarse rales were heard in both lungs. A catheter passed down into the esophagus met an obstruction at the level of the second dorsal vertebra. There was considerable gas in the stomach and the intestines.
>
> On January 2, the exploration of the mediastinum through the posterior extra-pleural approach was done (T.H.L.). About 1½ inches (3.7 cm) of the fourth rib was resected, and the third and fifth ribs were sectioned close to the transverse processes. In pushing the pleura laterally a small hole was made in it. Good exposure was obtained. The upper segment ended blindly, and the lower segment of the esophagus was found to communicate with the trachea just above the bifurcation. The anomaly was a type 3b. The fistulous tract was doubly tied and cut between the ties. The upper and lower segments were then freed; both ends were opened, and an end-to-end anastomosis was performed

with interrupted mattress sutures of fine silk. The wound was closed, a small rubber drain being left down to the mediastinum. The child's condition was good at the start but was rather poor at the end of the procedure, and she died three hours after the operation.

Post-mortem examination showed bilateral bronchitis and a moderate amount of pulmonary atelectasis. The anastomosis appeared to be tight and not under undue tension.

Lanman's paper provides a very clear description of the 32 patients he referred to and when, in 1972, I was able to hear something of Lanman, the man, from Lester Martin (currently Professor of Paediatric Surgery, University of Cincinnati), Lanman's approach to the problem was made even clearer. Lanman commented particularly on the merits of the extra-pleural approach, indicating that "the extra-pleural approach required a good deal of time so that in Case 25 a trans-pleural approach to the mediastinum was used as practised by Churchill". He also wrote: "The discouraging results in ... last 6 cases led in 1939 to the use ... of the procedure suggested by Gage and Oschner. Both patients died. It is felt that ligation of the cardiac end of the stomach will not accomplish its purpose, as secretions in the lower esophageal segment still can and do drain into the trachea."

Lanman also commented on the procedure advocated by Gamble, namely, division of the stomach, introduction of a gastrostomy tube into the distal segment for feeding, and exteriorization of the upper segment of the stomach to allow material in the esophagus to drain to the outside.

Lanman came to the following conclusion: "Anterior gastrostomy is futile ... unless the lower segment does not communicate with the trachea." He commented: "These types are rare; each occurred only once in this series."

Lanman further concluded:

> Regardless of what procedure is used for the lower segment (other than a direct anastomosis), the upper segment must be treated in such way to prevent aspiration of the overflow secretions from this blind pouch. ... Early exteriorization of this upper segment has been advocated and practised ... without success. ... Exteriorization of the upper segment commits the patient, if he survives, to some form of permanent exterior esophagus.
>
> Treatment of the lower segment ... must include measures to prevent contents from the lower segment from entering the trachea.
>
> ... If the infant is placed with the head up to allow dependent drainage of the lower segment, the upper segment fills, and the secretions will overflow into the trachea. If the patient is placed with the head lowered, drainage of the upper segment is facilitated, but secretions from the lower segment are allowed to gravitate through the fistula into the trachea.

At this point, Lanman was commenting on those methods aiming at exterior drainage of the lower segment, and he also stated:

> ... In the 2 cases in which these procedures were used it was noted that there was increased respiratory difficulty, which was thought to be due in part to

free escape of the inspired air through the tracheal fistula and out the exteriorized lower segment of the esophagus.

No method of attack that does not have as its first step direct closure of the fistula between the lower segment and the trachea has any reasonable chance of success, particularly as regards a primary anastomosis, which is the goal of surgical endeavour in this condition. Direct exposure of the site of the fistula by the extrapleural approach is by no means as formidable a procedure as has been thought. Indeed, with increasing experience and improvement in technique and anaesthesia, it seems to involve less shock – certainly no more – than the methods that include a gastrostomy with anterior drainage of the lower segment of the esophagus.

... If the gap is too wide to allow an anastomosis without tension, it is probably futile to attempt it. ... By using the extrapleural approach it is possible to drain the posterior mediastinum, and drainage is desirable. It is not feasible to drain the mediastinum when using the transpleural approach. With experience, it is possible to enter the mediastinum and to perform the anastomosis without opening the pleural cavity.

... If infection occurs when the extrapleural approach is used, it is likely that there is a far better chance for it to be taken care of by the extrapleural drainage of the mediastinum. If it occurs when the transpleural approach is used, both the mediastinum and the pleural cavities are likely to be involved, and there is no feasible method of drainage of either at the time of operation.

Finally, Lanman summarizes the situation thus:

In spite of the fatal outcome in all the 30 operative cases, it is felt that considerable progress along rational lines is being made. The successful operative treatment of a patient with this anomaly is only a question of time.

From the experience presented here, the extrapleural approach would seem to be safer than the transpleural.

If direct anastomosis is possible, it should be done. ... If direct anastomosis of the two segments is impossible or inadvisable, the tracheoesophageal fistula should be closed and nothing further done at that time. ... If the patient survives, construction of an exterior connection between the upper esophagostomy and the anterior gastrostomy can then be postponed until a suitable age. *One must remember that an exterior esophagus as a palliative procedure for an elderly patient with cancer is justifiable and endurable, but one dreads to commit an infant to the sort of existence it entails.* Every effort should be made to recognize these conditions in the first few hours of life as well as to improve surgical technic to such a degree that a direct anastomosis will be possible in an increasing number of cases.

Given a suitable case in which the patient is seen early, it is felt that, with greater experience, improved technic and good luck, the successful outcome to a direct anastomosis can and will be reported in the near future.

Lanman's prediction was to become a reality: Haight's success occurred in March 1941 and was subsequently reported by Haight and Towsley in 1943. The full report of the clinical findings, operative procedure and post-operative course appears in their article [53]. Fourteen years later in a subsequent contribution, Haight [56] was to comment thus:

> With knowledge of the 10 unsuccessful attempts to obtain a primary anastomosis ... we could not manifest undue encouragement when our next patient arrived on March 14th, 1941, twelve days after her birth. This infant was unusually robust, weight 8 pounds and 4 ounces upon admission. Roentgenograms obtained before admission had demonstrated a blind upper esophagus. The presence of air in the stomach indicated the existence of a communication between the trachea and the lower esophagus. On the day following the admission, the patient's tracheoesophageal fistula was ligated and divided through a left extrapleural approach; an end-to-end anastomosis was performed, employing a single layer of interrupted sutures of fine silk. Local anesthesia was administered until construction of the anastomosis was begun, when ether by drip method was required so that enough relaxation could be achieved to allow approximation of the esophageal segments. The wound was closed around a narrow rubber drain. Since penicillin was not then available, the only antimicrobial agent used post-operatively was sulfathiazole, administered rectally. Fortunately, the patient survived in spite of the fact that generalized edema had appeared on the third post-operative day as a result of excessive use of physiologic saline solution; and leakage of the anastomosis into the extrapleural wound had occurred on the seventh day after the operation. The parietal pleura had not been injured, however, at the time of operation, and the esophagocutaneous fistula remained localized and had healed by the twentieth post-operative day. In the interim, a gastrostomy to make feedings possible was performed on the tenth post-operative day. ... A stricture developed at the site of the anastomosis. As a result of this, accumulation of mucus in the pharynx and upper esophagus interfered greatly with the ability of the patient to swallow, and necessitated a prolonged period of convalescence in the hospital. Eventually, a single dilatation of the stricture was performed 17 months after the operation, and the patient was allowed to return home 20 months following the operation. She continued to improve and has developed normally.

It is appropriate to quote further from Cameron Haight; in 1943 he summarized the situation thus:

> In the surgical management of congenital atresia of the esophagus associated with tracheoesophageal fistula, two general plans of treatment have been used. One plan, the indirect attack, aims to circumvent the anomaly by the use of stage operations. In principle, the indirect plan consists of 1) a gastrostomy for permanent feedings, 2) ligation or exteriorization of the distal esophageal segment to prevent the regurgitation of gastric contents into the trachea and bronchi, and 3) exteriorization of the upper esophageal segment to allow for drainage of pharyngeal secretions onto the skin. ... The other plan of attack is the direct one whereby the continuity of the esophagus is restored. The operation consists of a one stage extrapleural exposure of the anomaly with ligation

of the tracheoesophageal fistula and simultaneous anastomosis of the two esophageal segments. The advantage of the direct plan is that, if successful, the patient is able to swallow normally.

In 1957, Haight wrote:

The development of a satisfactory approach to the correction of congenital atresia of the esophagus provides a stimulating example of the quest for a solution to a baffling problem. The pioneering efforts of many surgeons working in this field established the ground work for the satisfactory correction of this anomaly. Credit for their efforts should be generously paid to a list of names too long to be given in full; I should especially like to pay tribute, however, to H. M. Richter, N. Logan Leven, W. E. Ladd and to Thomas H. Lanman and Robert Shaw, the latter two being the first active proponents of the principle of esophageal anastomosis for the correction of atresia.

With Cameron Haight's success in 1941 a new era had commenced, and although alimentary continuity was being restored by other measures in a small percentage of patients, the technique of ablation of the tracheo-oesophageal fistula and primary end-to-end oesophageal anastomosis was to remain the cornerstone of treatment from that day on.

For a time, survivals following direct anastomosis of the oesophagus were sporadic, and then there were an increasing number of survivals from an increasing number of centres. Many of the early reports remain of historical significance; for example, in 1947 Longmire [103] reported "four consecutive cases of successful primary esophageal anastomosis" presenting these successes "to direct attention again to a congenital anomaly which if untreated is incompatible with life, but which can now frequently be satisfactorily corrected by surgical procedures". One of Longmire's babies weighed only 1.4 kg, and he commented: "It has previously been suggested that infants having this anomaly and weighing less than 4 pounds (1.8 kg) at birth probably should not be operated on. Operation should not be deferred solely because of the infant's weight."

History has recorded that the first survival in the United Kingdom occurred in 1947 at Hammersmith Hospital, and that the operating surgeon was Franklin [36]. Franklin's patient was born in Queen Charlotte's Hospital on January 10, 1947, and was seen in consultation by Professor Alan Moncrieff, who made a tentative diagnosis of oesophageal atresia and arranged for the baby to be transferred to Hammersmith Hospital "where the diagnosis was confirmed". It is interesting to note that at operation, performed on January 13, "the infant was secured in a prone position over a rubber water bottle, the head turned to the right and a folded towel placed over the right shoulder. The line of the skin incision was infiltrated with 1% Procaine. No other anaesthetic was used. On January 16th a salivary leak was noted and on January 19th a gastrostomy was performed".

Breast feeding was commenced on January 31 and it was observed on March 12 that "the child is taking food well by mouth". It is to be noted that Franklin's second case presented 3 months later and that in that baby "no leakage took place from the mediastinum wound at any time; consequently a gastrostomy was unnecessary".

The first survival in Australia (and I believe this is the first survival in the Southern hemisphere) was obtained in 1949 by Russell Howard [71] and reported in the *Medical Journal of Australia* in 1950. Russell Howard's interest in oesophageal atresia was to continue and as a result of his leadership, he and six surgeons at the Royal Children's Hospital, Melbourne, five of whom are still on the staff of this hospital and the sixth a consultant paediatric surgeon in England, accumulated experience with a total of 511 patients during the years 1948–1984. Russell Howard's first three survivals were in 1949; although the survival rate during the first 5 years of experience at the Royal Children's Hospital (1948–1952) was of the order of 30%, by 1972 it had risen to almost 100% in all but the "high-risk" babies, and it was this change in prognosis which led to oesophageal atresia being described by Myers [116] as "the epitome of modern surgery". Many large series have been reported which add emphasis to this description.

In the 1950s, series small and large were being reported, and reference has already been made to Humphreys' series from New York. In 1954, Oterdoom [128] of Groningen, reporting seven treated cases, drew attention to "the problem of oesophageal atresia", and with reference to diagnosis and assessment he recommended "both X-ray and fluoroscopy". He pointed out that "absence of air from the stomach is not absolutely incompatible with oesophagotracheal fistula", and that Haight had observed "a small fistular passage in 2 out of 5 patients without air in the stomach". Oterdoom asked the question "whether oesophagoscopy and bronchoscopy should be systematically carried out in these cases", a question which is still being asked and answered.

At about this time, from England, Roberts [148] presented "A Review of 36 Patients", and quoted Ladd: "Atresia of the oesophagus, with or without tracheo-oesophageal fistula, has been a baffling problem for the surgeon. If there is any surgeon who has attempted to save the lives of patients suffering from these malformations who has not had any disappointments and numerous trials and tribulations, I have not heard of him."

In 1947 Ladd and Swenson [89] reviewed the 82 cases of oesophageal atresia seen at the Children's Hospital, Boston, since 1939; 76 of these "have been operated on by Ladd". They concluded: "The time has obviously passed when obstetricians, or pediatricians should advise parents of infants with esophageal atresia that nothing can be done for them. The time has now come when alertness in making early diagnosis of this disease may lead to successful treatment. Obstetricians and pediatricians have the opportunity of seeing these patients first, and mortality in the future will depend to a large extent on their quick recognition of the condition and prompt transfer of the patient to a hospital equipped to care for the child properly." Their final sentence warrants repetition: "There undoubtedly will continue to be an appreciable mortality due to associated anomalies incompatible with life."

Classification

There are also many significant aspects in relation to the classification of oesophageal atresia; the incision, surgery of access, and technique of anastomosis also deserve historical review.

The history of the approach to classification showed that although there has been little or no argument regarding the types of anomalies encountered, there have been differences of opinion regarding the most appropriate terminology. Classifications have been numerical or alphabetical or both, and reference has already been made to Morell MacKenzie's contribution. In 1905, "A Case of Congenital Stenosis of the Lower End of the Oesophagus" was reported by Whipham and Fagge [199] from the Evelina Hospital for Sick Children in London, and the report includes remarks by the authors; they offered a classification which clearly included acquired lesions. In his *Manual of Antenatal Pathology and Hygiene,* Ballantyne [10] enumerated seven forms of malformation. The third in this classification was "termination of the oesophagus in a cul-de-sac, the lower rudiment of the canal communicating with the trachea or bronchi"; Ballantyne pointed out that "all these anomalies are rare with the exception of the third; I therefore choose this as the type of special description". His early references are of great interest.

Perhaps the classification most recently referred to in the literature is that of E. C. Vogt [194], a radiologist, who in 1929 recognised the following types:

Type 1: Absent oesophagus.
Type 2: Oesophageal atresia without accompanying tracheoesophageal fistula.
Type 3: Oesophageal atresia accompanied by tracheoesophageal fistula:
- 3a: Oesophageal atresia with proximal fistula; distal oesophagus ending blindly.
- 3b: Oesophageal atresia (blind proximal end) with distal tracheo-oesophageal fistula.
- 3c: Oesophageal atresia with fistulae between both oesophageal segments and the trachea.

Type 4: Isolated tracheoesophageal fistula with an intact oesophagus.

Although Vogt's classification is rarely used today, it was widely adopted in the years following its introduction, but there were many who suggested alternative forms of classification. At times, the classifications were not restricted to congenital anomalies; for example, Vincent [191] in 1923 and Abel [1] in 1929 suggested methods of classification. However, their inclusion of acquired lesions made Aberdeen [2] feel that he could not recommend the inclusion of Vincent's and Abel's classifications in a review of the classifications which had been offered.

In the decade 1930–1940 classifications included those of Fritz [38] in 1933. In 1944 Ladd introduced a numerical form of classification which was widely used, recognising five types and utilising Roman numerals. Some 10 years later, in altering the numerical system to an alphabetical one, Gross was to set the scene for that and subsequent decades. In 1952 Holinger [68] identified three major groups of oesophageal anomalies:

1. Those involving the oesophagus alone
2. Those in which the trachea is associated in the anomaly
3. Those in which anomalies of other structures influence the function of the oesophagus

In 1956 Stephens, Mustard and Simpson [168] brought considerable logic to their approach, giving pride of place to the most frequently encountered anomaly of proximal atresia and distal fistula, but in 1962 Swenson [176] returned to a numerical classification using Arabic numerals in preference to the Roman system. In recent years, there has been an increasing preference for descriptive terms and avoidance of the use of letters or numbers or both.

Many unusual types of oesophageal malformation were also described (and continued to be described) and reference can be made to O'Bannon [125], who in 1946 described partial duplication or diverticulum formation with stenosis but without atresia; to Overton [129] and Creech (1958), who described the common type but with an associated atretic membrane across the lower oesophagus; to Robb [147] (1952: tracheo-oesophageal fistula with oesophageal diverticulum); to Schwartz and Dale [154] (1955: tracheo-oesophageal fistula with an atretic membrane and some degree of mega-oesophagus); to Babbitt [9] (1957: double tracheo-oesophageal fistula without atresia); and to Devens [29] (1964: common anomaly with double fistulae of the lower oesophageal segment). There were many others, and reference should be made to the contributions of, inter alios, Petterson [130], Wiesema [200], Goldenberg [47], Minnis [113], Tugen [187], Humphreys [74], Sideway [162] and Yahr [203]. In a more recent communication (1973) Touloukian [183] reported "membranous oesophageal obstruction simulating atresia with a double tracheo-oesophageal fistula in a neonate", and he stressed that such cases are "reported to emphasise that completely or partially obstructed oesophageal webs accompanied by tracheo-oesophageal fistula are rare variants of the common form of oesophageal atresia which involves a distal tracheo-oesophageal fistula".

With reference to the uncommon types, many of which were reported as anecdotal experiences, the ultimate is to be found in the magnificent contribution of Kluth [84], which also highlights the various forms of classification. As one studies Kluth's contribution, one is impressed by the many gaps in any recorded history of oesophageal atresia.

Clearly, there are several important areas in the field of classification. First, with regard to classification of the most frequently encountered anomalies the classical contributions before and after Vogt are certainly of historical significance, but in the modern idiom one cannot but agree with the sentiments expressed by El Shafie, Klippel and Blakemore [34] in 1978: "We recommend avoiding the use of classification and ... using simple anatomic descriptions of the different congenital esophageal anomalies."

Remarks regarding classification would not be complete without reference to the classification of risk factors. From the Hospital for Sick Children, Great Ormond Street in London, Waterston, Bonham Carter and Aberdeen [195, 196] suggested that three groups of babies could be recognised – "good" risk, "moderate" risk and "high" risk – referring to these groups as A, B and C. Not only has their contribution been quoted and re-quoted, it has been a model which has enabled different large series from a variety of centres to be compared, and the introduction of the Waterston classification must be recognised as one of the major landmarks in the history of oesophageal atresia.

Incision, Approach and Technique of Anastomosis

In an excellent summary, Freeman [37] made "an attempt to trace the history of the thoracotomy incision currently used in the repair of esophageal atresia". He described the approach as performed by Richter in 1913, by Lanman, by Leven and by Haight. He also drew attention to the axillary approach as practised and taught by Denis Browne.

With regard to the technique of anastomosis, during the "early years" specific comments were made on the subject of anastomosis by Haight [54], Ladd [89], Lam [90], Humphreys [75], Daniel [28], Gross and Scott [50] and Swenson [175]. Haight was to popularise the telescopic type of anastomosis; Ladd described a single-layer anastomosis using interrupted mattress sutures with supporting tension sutures; and Lam also described a single-layer anastomosis using interrupted mattress sutures completing the anastomosis over an indwelling catheter. Humphreys' technique was essentially an ink-well inversion of the upper segment with a two-layer anastomosis, whereas Gross and Scott described an oblique oesophageal anastomosis with a single layer of interrupted sutures, but also with supporting tension sutures. In 1944 Daniel described a technique whereby an indwelling catheter was firmly tied to the lower segment and pulled upwards to reduce tension, and an end-to-side anastomosis of the upper to the lower segment was then effected. Many years later H. Noblett was to re-introduce this technique for use when a significant gap was present between the two oesophageal segments, her technique differing in that she used a Foley catheter. Swenson recommended a two-layer anastomosis using interrupted sutures, with the addition of tension sutures between the upper oesophageal segment and the paravertebral tissues, a technique also recommended by Denis Browne.

There were to be a whole host of variations, and two areas warrant mention. Firstly, several authors, including Gough [48] and Ten Kate [179], suggested alternative methods of anastomosis when difficulties were encountered, specifically the use of an anterior flap. Ten Kate's technique was somewhat different in that he used an anterior muscle flap to wrap around the mucosa.

However, of the variations, the one which has received the most attention is the end-to-side anastomosis, and the reader is referred to Sulamaa et al. [171] in 1951, to Berman and Berman [13] in 1953, to Sanderud [152] in 1960, and, at a later stage to Ty, Brunet and Beardmore [188]. The name Duhamel will also always be linked with this technique, credit being given to him by Ty and his co-authors.

The Less Frequently Encountered Anomalies

Many references have already been made to those anomalies which are of the most frequently encountered type, i.e. proximal atresia with distal fistula. Various authorities referred to oesophageal atresia without any accompanying fistula, and, as has already been mentioned, survival of such a case preceded survival of the more frequently encountered type. The first known survivor, a baby with oesophageal atresia without any accompanying fistula, was born on February 16, 1935 in New York State; a description of this patient appears in the article by Humphreys and Ferrer [76] in 1964, and is also referred to by Ashcraft and Holder [7]. The latter authors' excellent summary of the case of this patient reads thus:

> ... Contrast X-rays had demonstrated a blind proximal pouch. Gastrostomy was performed the next day by James Donovan of Newburgh. Ten days later, barium, placed through the gastrostomy tube, demonstrated a distal blind esophagus extending about 4 cm above the diaphragm. The tube gastrostomy was converted to a more permanent mucosal-tube gastrostomy when the child was 2 years of age.
>
> The child was presented to George H. Humphreys, II, at the Babies Hospital in New York City, at the age of 11 years. He was normally developed and well nourished. On August 14th, 1946, a long segment of jejunum was mobilized for interposition. The jejunogastrostomy was completed and the upper end closed and attached to the mediastinal pleura near the apex of the chest pending later esophagojejunostomy. The upper 3 to 4 inches appeared dusky but viable at the end of closure.
>
> Nearly 4 weeks later, the child underwent operation for completion of the upper anastomosis. Dr. Humphreys wrote, – 'To our great disappointment it was found that although there was no evidence of pleural infection, the upper 4 inches of jejunum was necrotic, and that viable jejunum could not be mobilized. The necrotic jejunum was excised and the chest closed with drainage. ... He went home to Marlboro and resumed his former way of life.'
>
> For 5 years more he took all food through the gastrostomy. He had noted an occasional cold sensation on putting cold liquids into his stomach. A barium study showed a coil of jejunum which filled readily from below. On August 14th, 1951, Humphreys freed this coil by dividing the dense pleural adhesions and anastomosed it easily to the cervical esophageal stump. Thus, the first patient to survive with esophageal atresia was able to take oral feedings at 16 years of age.

It is appropriate to proceed from this fascinating episode in the history of oesophageal atresia to certain aspects of history which have been specifically concerned with what has become to be known as the "problem of the long gap". In fact, no account of the history would be complete without reference to this aspect, and at two international meetings much time was spent in discussing "the problem of the long gap". The first of these meetings was held in Bremen, West Germany, in 1974, and the second in Perth, Australia, in 1984.

An early reference to the problem was discussed by Sweet in 1948 [174] advocating esophago-gastrostomy and describing "a new method of restoring continuity of the alimentary canal in cases of congenital atresia of the esophagus with tracheo-esophageal fistula not treated by immediate primary anastomosis". Despite many different approaches to the problem, it is still recognised that oesophageal atresia with a long gap has remained a surgical problem, but with the development of thoracic surgery and a wide variety of techniques of oesophageal reconstruction, many different operations have been successfully performed to combat this type of anomaly. Substitution by colon segments has been in greatest favour, and although many surgeons have worked in this field, credit should certainly be given to David Waterston [197] of the Hospital for Sick Children, Great Ormond Street, London, who with his technical skills standardised the operation utilising the transverse colon, based on the upper left colic artery, as a substitute for the oesophagus. As pointed out by Waterston in Pittsburgh in 1979, "Like most things in pediatric surgery, success depends upon perhaps minor methods, minor points in technique, minor points, perhaps in how to prepare the colon and so on and so forth. Postoperative care is important..." Others have preferred to use the right colon, e.g. Martin [108], and site the oesophageal substitute in the anterior mediastinum.

More recently, there has been renewed interest in the greater curvature tube described by Gavriliu [45], a method frequently referred to as the Hemlich tube. Considerable experience in this technique has been reported from Toronto by Stephens [21] and from Sydney by Cohen [25, 26].

The situation with reference to long-gap oesophageal atresia was summarized by Myers [117]:

> Although problems of the 'long gap' are of significance in the commonly encountered anomaly with proximal atresia and a distal tracheo-oesophageal fistula, they are of particular significance in the less frequently encountered anomalies...
>
> 1. Oesophageal Atresia Without Fistula.
> 2. Oesophageal Atresia With a Proximal Tracheo-Oesophageal Fistula and a Distal Blind Oesophageal Segment.

Myers went on to say: " Despite the presence of a very long gap between the two oesophageal segments in these types of anomaly, it is still possible to entertain the thought of achieving end-to-end oesophageal anastomosis and if this proves to be possible the patient is at an advantage if one believes that 'one's own oesophagus is the best oesophagus.'"

These statements were made in Bremen in 1974, and discussants at that time included many who were to make contributions on the problems of the long gap, including Woolley, Livaditis, Waterston, Soave and Shafer.

Recent history has highlighted the difference of opinion between those who have advocated oesophageal preservation (almost at all costs), and those who have opted for replacement. Although two of the papers presented at the Perth meeting described techniques of replacement rather than of oesophageal anastomosis, the consensus of opinion on that occasion was certainly in favour of oesophageal preservation. Among those who have described techniques to permit oesophageal preservation rather than replacement are Rehbein [139], Fuzeman [41], Hendren [58, 59], Shafer [157], Howard [72] and Livaditis [99–102]. Techniques described have included self-fistulisation, electromagnetic bougienage and circular myotomy. The impact of the Livaditis technique, "circular myotomy", has been profound, and recent literature contains many references, including those to Zigiotti [204], Ricketts [144], Vizas [193] and his co-authors, Takada [178] and Rosselo [151]. With regard to the suture fistula technique as described by Shafer and David, it is interesting to note that others have now contributed to the literature in the light of their experience, including Schullinger [153] and Brown and Nixon [20].

In the light of the many techniques which have been described, the differences of opinion, and the specific needs of case selection, there can be little doubt that much of the history of "long-gap oesophageal atresia" remains to be written.

Tracheo-Oesophageal Fistula Without Atresia

At different times, this has been referred to as an isolated tracheo-oesophageal fistula, as an H-fistula, or as an N-fistula. The initial description was by Lamb [91] in 1873, and the first operative success was reported by Imperatori [79] in 1939. Imperatori's patient was born in 1931 and had a long and complicated history of repeated episodes of respiratory infection; these are referred to in Imperatori's article, which should be read carefully.

Since then there have been many contributions to the literature on H-fistula, including an early reference from Cameron Haight [55], who commented: "The only recorded instance of an attempt to correct the anomaly is one described by Imperatori." In his excellent "Atlas of Esophageal Atresia" [84], Kluth also mentions Pinard [133] in 1873 and illustrated examples of double and triple fistulae as described by Hubner [73] in 1943, Leven [96] in 1952, and Eckstein and Somasundaram [32] in 1966. Many additional references in the literature are to be found in an article by Egami and Myers [33]. In 1969, Kappelman [81] reported that approximately 125 cases of H-fistula had been recorded in the "pediatric, surgical and otolaryngological literature". Most of the history of this anomaly relates to incidence, diagnosis and surgical approach. Those who have commented on incidence in large series include Haight, Holder, Waterston and Myers. Two schools of thought have developed in relation to diagnosis – those who have advocated radiological evaluation, and those who have a preference for endoscopy.

Operative correction of fistula has usually been via the neck, but again there has been difference of opinion regarding the merits of a left-sided or a right-sided approach.

Radiology

Diagnostic radiology was destined to play a vital role in the management of oesophageal atresia: a role which would include diagnosis, pre-operative evaluation and recognition of associated anomalies. In addition, radiology was to prove to be of great value in the early and late post-operative periods.

Despite this, in 1946 Holt, Haight and Hodges [70] were to comment:

> The relatively meagre roentgenological literature on the subject of congenital esophageal atresia has dealt almost exclusively with isolated case reports. The apparent reason why more comprehensive analyses of the subject have not appeared is that, until very recently, this interesting anomaly has been universally fatal and generally regarded as a distinct medical oddity. The condition is relatively uncommon, but through various improvements in surgical technic and post-operative care, it has been brought into the realm of surgically correctable anomalies, and greater interest is being taken in the establishment of its diagnosis. Many of the diagnostic and therapeutic problems which have arisen confront the roentgenologist directly because it is largely by his methods that the diagnosis of esophageal atresia, the recognition of its complications, and the results of surgical management are graphically recorded. It may be stated justifiably that roentgen examination is essential in the proper management of the condition, especially during the post-operative period.

Vogt, a radiologist from Boston, has already been mentioned; his classification and description of the X-ray findings in the various anatomical types of oesophageal atresia is often quoted, and no one would argue with his final two sentences: "If surgery is to be of any real value it is important to recognize the type of atresia. Roentgen-ray examination is most valuable in diagnosis and differentiation." Two early references in the radiological literature are those to Skinner [164] in 1921 and Brown [19] in 1926.

Others who have contributed to the literature include Sussman [172] in 1931 and Fuhrman, Dragutsky, Rook and Grossman [39, 40] in 1942. Their contribution was "Aero-esophography in Congenital Atresia of the Esophagus", and they had previously, and in the same year, suggested a "simple roentgenographic procedure to establish the diagnosis of congenital atresia of the esophagus without the use of a liquid contrast medium". Some years later, support for avoiding the use of a liquid contrast medium was emphasised by Koop from Philadelphia. Reitter's [140] contribution, previously referred to, concluded: "Upon submitting the patient to X-ray examination, the diagnosis is easily established."

Various articles appeared in the 1950s, including one from New York City entitled "Tracheoesophageal Fistula Unassociated With Atresia or Stenosis: Difficulties in Diagnosis and Suggestions for Greater Accuracy", and one from Atlanta, Georgia, entitled "Roentgenologic Considerations in Tracheo-Esophageal Fistula Without Esophageal Atresia", the authors being Leigh, Abbott and Hopkins [93].

Babbitt [9] from the department of radiology, Milwaukee Children's Hospital, described "Double Tracheoesophageal Fistula Without Atresia" in 1957, and in 1964 an article entitled "Congenital Esophageal Atresia with Tracheo-Esophageal Fistula: Associated Congenital Anomalies" was presented by Maddock [106], a resident in the department of radiology at the Children's Hospital of Michigan. Maddock's paper was largely concerned with the history, classification and results of treatment, indicating the "overlap" between the diagnostic and therapeutic services.

Finally, in this all too brief review of some of the radiological literature, reference can be made to the textbook by Swischuk [177] with an excellent list of references numbering 50 in all, of which 21 were from radiology journals or the like. A review article from Toronto by Cumming [27] was entitled "Esophageal Atresia and Tracheoesophageal Fistula", and commences with a strange quotation from Vogt: "If congenital esophageal atresia were as rare as it is fatal, we would as yet be unable to find the first recorded instance." Although we are not in any doubt as to Vogt's meaning, the phraseology is somewhat confusing. Cumming reviewed 10 years of experience at the Great Ormond Street Hospital for Sick Children; his comments on manometric oesophageal motility studies are to be noted, and his final statement emphasises:

> There is a typical esophageal motility pattern in patients with repaired atresia. Peristalsis starts normally in the proximal esophagus but stops a short distance above the site of the anastomosis. Contraction of the distal esophagus may be peristaltic or static and may or may not be accompanied by relaxation of the inferior esophageal sphincter. Intraluminal pressure studies may be helpful in clarifying distorted motility.

Where Next?

As previously quoted, Ashcraft and Holder suggested: "To those who are not satisfied with the present outlook there remains much of this story to be written."

For those who feel that this historical review is incomplete, it is suggested that there are many areas still to be explored, including the emergence of such problems as post-operative gastro-oesophageal reflux, tracheal instability and the surgical measures used to overcome it, the significance of the Vater association, and the various long-term follow-ups which have now been presented.

Advances in endoscopy have in themselves re-written many important areas and the excellent review by Gans and Berci [44] in 1971 expounds a philosophy which is particularly relevant to oesophageal atresia: "This paper represents what we hope is a new chapter in a work which will permit specialists to operate under superior conditions, contributing to improved patient care from increased diagnostic accuracy and more usefully applied therapy, with decreassed risk."

There have also been many other contributions relevant to anatomy and pathology, and more recently there has been an increasing interest in basic research. The history would certainly be incomplete if reference were not made to the impact of anaesthesia, intensive care and the role of intravenous nutrition.

In asking the question "What Next?" in 1979, Myers [119] referred to the description of oesophageal atresia as "the epitome of modern surgery", but also suggested that in many ways oesophageal atresia also epitomises modern paediatrics and modern investigative procedures. In attempting to answer the question "Where Next?", he suggested that consideration should be given to the following areas:

1. The timing of the operation
2. The pre-operative evaluation with particular reference to the presence of an associated cardiovascular abnormality
3. Case selection
4. The validity of the Waterston classification nearly 20 years after its introduction
5. Gastro-oesophageal reflux – its management and evaluation
6. Tracheal instability
7. The problems and management of the baby with the "long gap"
8. Diagnosis and management of the baby with an H-fistula

In referring [119] to the publication in that year (1979) of the third edition of the textbook *Pediatric Surgery* [3], he pointed out: "Among the problems requiring further investigation are:

i) The need to identify the cause of the faulty embryogenesis and the genetic implications for these families.
ii) Problems associated with the 'long gap' ...
iii) Life threatening respiratory tract obstruction from tracheal compression.
iv) Should all patients have a gastrostomy?
v) Are all the advantages claimed for gastrostomy combined with a transpyloric jejunostomy tube valid? ...
vi) What are the long-term results of end-to-side anastomosis, particularly in relation to oesophageal motility and the frequency of respiratory tract infection?"

These questions seemed particularly pertinent in 1979, which was "The International Year of the Child", and the next historian will find much to write about in relation to these questions.

History never ends but this story must, and in conclusion it would seem relevant to quote a few of the more meaningful statements made about oesophageal atresia or made in reference to related areas, and in this connection W. Thomson [181], discussing "gastrostomy" in 1878, concluded his comments thus:

> He who cannot take part in the friendly meal is half shut out from the society of man.

He had commenced his paper thus: "Our object in publishing cases should be to demonstrate something tending to the good of the human family; and although we may traverse the same ground which others have traversed, there is work still left, and our labours with this object in view will never be unrewarded."

Surely, Thomson and Koop would have had much to discuss when one recalls that 96 years later, in 1974, Koop [87] was to present the final paper at the symposium in Bremen, under the title "The Social, Physiological, and Economic Problems of the Patient's Family after Successful Repair of Esophageal Atresia."

That others also felt that oesophageal atresia epitomised modern surgery is indicated by reference to Pinus [134], who wrote in 1972: "Success in the surgical correction of oesophageal atresia was one of the most important steps in the acceptance of Pediatric Surgery as a speciality."

There seems no need for these quotations to be in chronological order, and therefore one passes next to Lam, who, in 1945, wrote: "The subject of the surgical repair of congenital atresia of the oesophagus is a pleasant one to discuss, because this operative procedure which has evolved after many trials and failures represents a bright milestone in the surgical progress of our day. ... If successful, the operation ... restores to an infant the probability of a lifetime of living when otherwise he faced certain death." This was a far cry from Brennemann's philosophy, previously quoted: "The physician who after making his diagnosis of congenital atresia of the oesophagus decides to let his little patient die unstirred ... can amply justify his course."

The accuracy of early descriptions is a highlight of the history, and O'Hare [127] in 1937 concisely stated: "It is interesting to note that Thomas Gibson described the first case in 1670 and left little to be said subsequently." Note that O'Hare was inaccurate in relation either to the name or the year.

During the discussion which followed O'Hare's paper, Ross of Erie commented: "The longest time any of may patients have lived with this condition was 12 days. They usually die of starvation or aspiration pneumonia or both. Theoretically, in the 10 per cent of cases in which there is no complicating fistula, life might be maintained by feeding through a gastrostomy opening. In February 1936, an article appeared in the press recording the first birthday of a baby so born and so fed. I wrote to the physician said to have had charge of the case asking for further particulars but received no reply." Surely this was the baby born in 1935 and subsequently reported by Humphreys.

In 1947 Ladd and Swenson wrote: "The time has obviously passed when obstetricians and paediatricians should advise parents of infants with oesophageal atresia that nothing can be done for them...", and: "[Mortality in the future will depend to a large extent on] ... prompt transfer of the patient to a hospital equipped to care for the child properly."

In 1963 Richardson [142] was to write: "Although the earliest survivors treated by Leven, Ladd and Haight are now of voting age, this congenital lesion, with or without tracheo-oesophageal fistula, continues to present a major challenge in surgical management."

Two years earlier, Koop [85] had stated: "... Management of atresia of the oesophagus has become a criterion of competence for both individual surgeon and institution in the field of pediatric surgery."

In 1972, Soave was to say: "Every experienced surgeon knows the difficulties encountered when one has to bridge the gap between the proximal and distal oesophageal segments in some cases of oesophageal atresia", and reference has already been made to the wide variety of techniques described and introduced to manage such problems.

One of the greatest paediatric surgeons of the twentieth century, Sulamaa of Finland, summarized the situation in 1951, when he stated: "The progress in treatment made in the 1940s has made this anomaly practically important." The contribution from the same centre made by Lindahl [97] over a quarter of a century later was in keeping with Sulamaa's prediction, because with Louhimo [105] he was able to present "Esophageal Atresia. Primary Results of 500 Consecutively Treated Patients".

The contributions of many have been recognised; the contributions of others have been indirectly recognised in relation to the hundreds of references available in the many writings. Although the major advances have come from paediatric, paediatric surgical, and para-paediatric areas, it is to be remembered that the forerunners of paediatric surgeons were general surgeons; the final comment comes from one of this group who achieved the first survival in the United Kingdom, namely R. H. Franklin, who, in 1947, provided a fitting epilogue: "The post-operative management is of the utmost importance, and without the co-operation of a skilled Paediatrician to take charge of the fluid requirements and the unstinted services of an intelligent and conscientious nurse, the most careful operation will be of no avail."

Summary

The history of oesophageal atresia commenced in the year 1670 with Durston's description of "A narrative of a monstrous birth at Plymouth". However, the most significant contribution in the 17th century was made by Gibson, who clearly described the clinical picture and necropsy findings in a baby with a proximal oesophageal atresia and a distal tracheo-oesophageal fistula. The 18th century was singularly lacking in contributions to the literature, but there were many important presentations during the 19th century. Early in that century Martin in France and Hill in United States of America contributed to the literature; subsequently, many anecdotal references can be found particularly in England, and ultimately a surgical attempt to correct the anomaly was made in 1888 by Steele in London. With this, the pre-surgical era gave way to the surgical era, and at a later stage pre-survival era was to give way to the survival phase. Reference will be made in the text to these various phases in the history and to the many pioneering surgical endeavours which took place in the earlier years of the 20th century. It will be seen that the surgical efforts employed palliative procedures, indirect attacks on the problem and finally direct attacks. The classic successes by indirect methods which were achieved by Ladd and Leven in babies born in 1939 were to be followed by the first successful end-to-end anastomosis which was achieved in Ann Arbor, Michigan, by Cameron Haight. Others had attempted primary anastomosis, and Lanman in particular deserves mention. However, it was Cameron

Haight who opened a new era in the history of the treatment of oesophageal atresia; the recent history is largely concerned with increasing experience and refinements in technique.

For the future historian many pathways can still be explored, including oesophageal replacement, the unstable trachea, follow-up studies and research projects.

This history also included comments on the history of the less frequently encountered anomalies and such aspects as classification and radiology.

The history of oesophageal atresia and tracheo-oesophageal fistula is a mini history of surgery – "oesophageal atresia is the epitome of modern surgery".

Résumé

L'histoire de l'atrésie de l'œsophage commence en 1670, date à laquelle Durston relate la "naissance d'un monstre à Plymouth". La contribution la plus importante au XVIIe siècle est due à Gibson. Il a décrit avec une remarquable clarté les constatations cliniques et les résultats de l'autopsie d'un nouveau-né présentant une atrésie de l'œsophage et une fistule œsophagotrachéale. Au XVIIIe siècle, très peu de cas sont décrits mais un grand nombre de descriptions datent du XIXe siècle. Au début du XIXe siècle, Martin en France et Hill aux Etats-Unis publient les premières observations suivies par un grand nombre de publications en Angleterre et en 1888, Steel à Londres, essaie pour la première fois une correction chirurgicale de cette malformation. C'est la fin de la phase pré-chirurgicale, à laquelle succède une phase chirurgicale sans survies, puis la phase avec survies. Ces phases sont décrites en détail dans ce chapitre et l'auteur insiste sur les travaux de pionniers au début du XXe siècle. Il montre que le traitement chirurgical se contenta d'abord de soulager puis chercha une solution indirecte au problème et finit par s'y attaquer directement. Les opérations des nouveaux-nés par Ladd et Leven en 1939 sont des exemples classiques de la méthode indirecte. Vint ensuite la première anastomose bout à bout réalisée par Cameron Haight à Ann Arbor, Michigan. D'autres avaient essayé de pratiquer des anastomoses primaires et dans ce contexte, il faut mentionner Lanman mais c'est Cameron Haight qui réussit à inaugurer une ère nouvelle en ce qui concerne le traitement de l'atrésie de l'œsophage. Ces derniers temps, cette technique n'a cessé d'être perfectionnée.

A l'avenir, un grand nombre de problèmes sont encore à résoudre: remplacement de l'œsophage, trachée instable, contrôles post-opératoires et recherche.

Ce chapitre traite aussi d'anomalies plus rares, propose une classification et n'oublie pas les aspects radiologiques.

L'histoire de l'atrésie de l'œsophage et de la fistule œsophagotrachéale est une micro-histoire de la chirurgie et l'atrésie de l'œsophage "un abrégé de la chirurgie d'aujourd'hui".

Zusammenfassung

Die Geschichte der Ösophagusastresie beginnt im Jahre 1670 mit Durstons *Bericht über die Geburt eines Monsters in Plymouth.* Der wichtigste Beitrag im 17. Jahrhundert jedoch wurde von Gibson geleistet. Er beschrieb mit großer Klarheit das klinische Bild und die Obduktionsergebnisse im Falle eines Säuglings mit proximaler Ösophagusatresie und distaler Ösophagotrachealfistel. Im 18. Jahrhundert wurden erstaunlich wenige Fälle beschrieben, aber aus dem 19. Jahrhundert stammen zahlreiche wichtige Beschreibungen. Am Anfang des 19. Jahrhunderts lieferten Martin in Frankreich und Hill in den USA die ersten Beiträge; später kamen zahlreiche Beschreibungen (besonders aus England), und 1888 versuchte Steele in London zum ersten Mal, diesen Fehler chirurgisch zu beheben. Damit war die vorchirurgische Phase beendet. Es folgte die chirurgische Phase, zunächst die Zeit ohne Überlebenserfolge, dann gab es zunehmend Überlebenserfolge. Diese Phasen werden beschrieben unter besonderer Berücksichtigung der Pionierarbeit am Anfang des 20. Jahrhunderts. Es wird gezeigt, daß sich die chirurgische Behandlung zuerst auf Linderung beschränkte, dann das Problem indirekt anging und später zu einem direkten Angriff überging. Klassische Beispiele von Erfolgen nach der indirekten Methode sind die Operationen von Säuglingen 1939 durch Ladd und Leven. Es folgte die erste erfolgreiche End-zu-End-Anastomose, die von Cameron Haight in Ann Arbor, Michigan, durchgeführt wurde. Andere hatten primäre Anastomosen versucht, wobei Lanman nicht unerwähnt bleiben darf. Es war jedoch Cameron Haight, dem es gelang, eine neue Ära der Behandlung der Ösophagusatresie einzuleiten. In jüngster Zeit wurde diese Technik fortwährend ausgefeilt.

Für die Zukunft stellen sich noch viele Aufgaben: Einsetzen einer neuen Speiseröhre, instabile Trachea, Nachsorgeuntersuchungen und Forschungsvorhaben.

Dieser Beitrag behandelt auch seltenere Anomalien sowie Klassifizierungs- und radiologische Probleme.

Die Geschichte der Ösophagusatresie und der Ösophagotrachealfistel ist eine Mikrogeschichte der Chirurgie, und die Ösophagusatresie ist „ein Abriß der Chirurgie von heute".

Acknowledgements. It is a pleasure to record my thanks to Peter Rickham, who waited patiently while I completed this review. As ever I am grateful to my mentor Russell Howard, who originally stimulated my interest in oesophageal atresia. Miss Ada Lewis typed the original text and Miss Janice Parfitt the final draft; I am grateful to both. Miss Marjorie Thomas accurately and painstakingly researched and checked the references.

References

1. Abel AL (1929) Oesophageal obstruction. London, pp 50–57
2. Aberdeen E (1968) Personal communication
3. Aberdeen E, Myers NA (1979) The esophagus. In: Ravitch MM, Welch KJ, Benson CD, Aberdeen E, Randolph JG (eds) Paediatric surgery, 3rd edn. Year Book Medical Publishers, Chicago, p 446

4. Alonso JM (1933) Les malformation congénitales de l'œsophage. Rev Laryngol Otol Rhinol 54:72
5. Anderson KD, Randolph JG (1973) The gastric tube for esophageal replacement in children. J Thorac Cardiovasc Surg 66:333
6. Annandale T (1868–69) Case of congenital malformation of the oesophagus. Edinburgh Med J 14:598
7. Ashcraft KW, Holder TM (1969) The story of oesophageal atresia and tracheo-esophageal fistula. Surgery 65:332
8. Atwell JD, Beard RC (1974) Congenital anomalies of the upper urinary tract associated with esophageal atresia and tracheo-esophageal fistula. J Pediatr Surg 9:825
9. Babbitt DP (1957) Double tracheo-esophageal fistula without atresia, report of a case. N Engl J Med 257:713
10. Ballantyne JW (1904) Manual of antenatal pathology and hygiene. Green, Edinburgh, p 462
11. Barry JE, Auldist AW (1974) The Vater Association: one end of a spectrum of anomalies. Am J Dis Child 128:769
12. Belsey RHR (1980) Gastroesophageal reflux. Am J Surg 139:775
13. Berman JK, Berman EJ (1953) Congenital atresia of the esophagus with tracheo-esophageal fistula. A simplified technique restoring continuity of the esophagus. Am J Surg 86:436
14. Blair VP (1938) Discussion of article by Gamble HA, "Tracheo-esophageal fistula. Description of a new operative procedure and case report". Ann Surg 107:701
15. Blasius (1674) Ger observata anatom pract in homine. Ludg Batav et amsterlod. Tab XV, Fig 6
16. Bowes GK (1897) Congenital obliteration of oesophagus with other malformations. Br Med J March:586
17. Brennemann J (1913) Congenital atresia of the oesophagus, with report of three cases. Am J Dis Child 5:143–150
18. Brennemann J (1918) Congenital atresia of the esophagus with report of four additional cases, with three necropsies. Am J Dis Child 16:143–153
19. Brown RM (1926) Congenital deformity of trachea and esophagus: report of a case. Radiology 6:166
20. Brown S, Nixon HH (1983) Spontaneous anastomosis of the esophagus in esophageal atresia. J Pediatr Surg 18:293
21. Burrington JD, Stephens CA (1969) Esophageal reconstruction with a gastric tube in infants and children. J Pediatr Surg 3:246
22. Cameron JA, Lightoller GS (1909) A case of congenital malformation of the oesophagus. Aust Med Gaz March:137–138
23. Cardullo HM, Berens DL (1950) Tracheo-esophageal fistula unassociated with atresia or stenosis. Difficulties in diagnosis and suggestions for greater accuracy. N Engl J Med 243: 853–856
24. Chang JHT (to be published) Esophageal atresia and tracheo-esophageal fistulas. In: History of pediatric surgery, chap 2
25. Cohen D (1970) Esophageal reconstruction using a gastric tube. A preliminary report. Aust Paediatr J 6:22–24
26. Cohen DH, Middleton AW, Fletcher J (1974) Gastric tube esophagoplasty. J Pediatr Surg 9:451
27. Cumming WA (1975) Esophageal atresia and tracheo-esophageal fistula. Radiol Clin North Am 13:277
28. Daniel RA Jr (1944) Congenital atresia of the esophagus: with tracheo-esophageal fistula. Ann Surg 120:764
29. Devens K, Ritz O (1965) Eine bisher unbekannte Form der Ösophagusatresie. Z Kinderchir 2:484
30. Duhamel B (1957) Technique chirurgicale infantile. Masson, Paris, pp 82–96
31. Durston W (1670) A narrative of a monstrous birth in Plymouth October 22, 1670; together with the anatomical observations taken thereupon by William Durston, Doctor of Physick, and communication to Dr Tim Clerk. Philosophical Transactions of the Royal Society V:2096

32. Eckstein HB, Somasundaram K (1966) Multiple tracheo-esophageal fistulas without atresia. Report of a case. J Pediatr Surg 1:381
33. Egami K (to be published) The "H" type tracheo-oesophageal fistula experience
34. El Shafie M, Klippel CH, Blakemore WS (1978) Congenital esophageal anomalies: a plea for using anatomic description rather than classifications. J Pediatr Surg 13:355
35. Flood HC (1926) Congenital obstruction of the oesophagus. Atlantic Med J 29:537–538
36. Franklin RH (1947) Congenital atresia of the oesophagus. Two cases successfully treated by anastomosis. Lancet 2:243
37. Freeman NV, Walkden J (1969) Previously unreported shoulder deformity following right lateral thoracotomy for esophageal atresia. J Pediatr Surg 4:627
38. Fritz E (1933) Eine seltene Mißbildung der oberen Luftwege (teilweiser Mangel der Luftröhre, Verschluß des Kehlkopfes und Ösophagotrachealfistel). Virchows Arch [A] 289:264
39. Fuhrman M, Dragutsky D, Rook G, Grossman L (1942) Congenital atresia of the esophagus. Radiology 38:326
40. Fuhrman M, Dragutsky D, Rook G, Grossman L (1942) Aero-esophography in congenital atresia of the esophagus. Radiology 39:100
41. Fuzeman V, Veleanu C, Duica C, Habenicht E, Socolius M (1975) The use of azygo-oesophagoplasty in the treatment of oesophageal atresia. Kind Chir [Suppl] 134
42. Gage M, Oschner A (1936) The surgical treatment of congenital tracheo-esophageal fistula in the newborn. Ann Surg May:725–737
43. Gamble HA (1938) Tracheo-esophageal fistula, description of a new operative procedure and case report. Ann Surg 107:701
44. Gans SL, Berci G (1971) Advances in endoscopy of infants and children. J Pediatr Surg 6(2):199–233
45. Gavriliu D (1975) Aspects of esophageal surgery, in current problems in surgery. Year Book Medical Publishers, Chicago
46. Gibson T (1697) The anatomy of humane bodies epitomized, 5th edn. Awnsham and Churchill, London
47. Goldenberg IS (1960) An unusual variation of congenital tracheo-esophageal fistula. J Thorac Cardiovasc Surg 40:114
48. Gough M (1980) Esophageal atresia: use of an anterior flap in the difficult anastomosis. J Pediatr Surg 15:310
49. Griffiths JPC, Lavenson RS (1909) Congenital malformation of the esophagus with the report of a case. Pediatr March:161–169
50. Gross RE, Scott HW Jr (1946) Correction of esophageal atresia and tracheo-esophageal fistula by closure of the fistula and oblique anastomosis of the esophageal segments. Surg Gynecol Obstet 82:518
51. Gross RE (1953) Surgery of infancy and childhood. Saunders, Philadelphia, chap 6, p 75
52. Guy's Hospital Reports (1858) London
53. Haight C, Towsley HA (1943) Congenital atresia of the esophagus with tracheo-esophageal fistula. Extrapleural ligation of fistula and end-to-end anastomosis of esophageal segments. Surg Gynecol Obstet 76:672–688
54. Haight C (1944) Congenital atresia of the esophagus with tracheo-esophageal fistula. Ann Surg 120:623
55. Haight C (1948) Congenital tracheo-esophageal fistula without esophageal atresia. J Thorac Surg 17:600
56. Haight C (1957) Some observations on esophageal atresia and tracheo-esophageal fistulas of congenital origin. J Thorac Surg 34(2):141–172
57. Heimlich HJ (1959) Esophageal replacement with a revised gastric tube. Dis Chest 36:478
58. Hendren WH, Hale JR (1975) Electromagnetic bougienage to lengthen esophageal segments in congenital esophageal atresia. N Engl J Med 293:428–432
59. Hendren WH, Hale JR (1976) Esophageal atresia treated by electromagnetic bougienage and subsequent repair. J Pediatr Surg 11(5):713
60. Hill TP (1840) Congenital malformation. Boston Med Surg J 21:320
61. Hirsch IS (1921) Congenital atresia of the esophagus. Report of two cases. JAMA 76(22):1491–1493

62. Hirschsprung H (1861) Den medfodte tillerkning of spiseroret (4 cases) (Congenital destruction of the oesophagus). Medico-Chirurg Rev 30:437
63. Hoffman S (1976) Emergency repair of esophageal atresia with lower fistula and segment elongation in cases with large gap between segments. J Pediatr Surg 11(2):257
64. Hoffman W (1899) Atresia oesophagi congenita et communicatio inter oesopagiu et tracheon. PhD dissertation, Greifswald
65. Holder TM, Ashcraft KW (1970) Esophageal atresia and tracheo-esophageal fistula. Ann Thorac Surg 9:445
66. Holder TM, Cloud DT, Lewis JE, Pilling GP (1964) Esophageal atresia and tracheo-esophageal fistula. A survey of its members by the surgical section of the American Academy of Pediatrics. Pediatrics 34:542
67. Holderman HH (1927) Congenital atresia of the esophagus with esophageal diverticulum and tracheo-esophageal fistula. Arch Surg 14:917–920
68. Holinger PH, Johnson KC, Potts WJ (1952) Congenital anomalies of the esophagus. Acta Otolaryngol (Stockh) 10:100
69. Holmes T (1869) The surgical treatment of diseases of infancy and childhood, 2nd edn. Lindsay and Blakiston, Philadelphia
70. Holt JF, Haight C, Hodges FJ (1946) Congenital atresia of the esophagus and tracheo-esophageal fistula. Radiology 47:457
71. Howard R (1950) Oesophageal atresia with tracheo-oesophageal fistula: report of six cases with two successful oesophageal anastomoses. Med J Aust 1:401–404
72. Howard R, Myers NA (1965) Esophageal atresia: a technique for elongating this upper pouch. Surgery 58(4):725–727
73. Hubner O (1943) Doppelte angeborene Ösophagotrachealfistel ohne Ösophagusatresie. Zentralbl Allg Pathol 80:358–362
74. Humphreys GH (1944) The surgical treatment of congenital atresia of the esophagus. Surgery 15:801–823
75. Humphreys GH, Hogg BM, Ferer J (1956) Congenital atresia of esophagus. J Thorac Surg 32:332
76. Humphreys GH, Ferrer JM Jr (1964) Management of esophageal atresia. Am J Surg 107: 406
77. Hunter J (1793) A case of paralysis of the muscles of deglutition, cured by an artificial mode of conveying food and medicines into the stomach. Transactions of a Society for the Improvement of Medical and Chirurgical Knowledge 1:182
78. Huntington JL, Young JH, Foote NC (1919) Report of a case of congenital atresia of the esophagus. Boston Med Surg J March:354–358
79. Imperatori CJ (1939) Congenital tracheo-esophageal fistula without atresia of the esophagus. Report of a case with plastic closure and cure. Arch Otolaryngol 30:352–359
80. Ivy RH, Hawthorne HR, Ritter JA (1948) Construction of skin tube esophagus following surgical treatment of tracheo-esophageal fistula. Plast Reconstr Surg 3:173
81. Kappelman MM, Dorst J, Haller A, Stambler A (1969) H-Type tracheo-esophageal fistula. Am J Dis Child 118:568
82. Kastner AL (1920) Congenital atresia of the esophagus. Arch Pediatr 37:670
83. Kelly A (1931) Congenital abnormalities at or near the upper end of the oesophagus. J Laryngol Otol 46(8):521–531
84. Kluth D (1976) Atlas of esophageal atresia. J Pediatr Surg 11:901
85. Koop CE, Verhagen AD (1961) Early management of atresia of the esophagus. Surg Gynec Obstet 113:103
86. Koop CE, Hamilton JP (1965) Atresia of the esophagus. Increased survival with staged procedure in the poor risk infant. Ann Surg 162:389
87. Koop CE, Schnaufer L, Thompson G, Haecker T, Dalrymply D (1975) The social, psychological and economic problems of the patient's family after successful repair of oesophageal atresia. Z Kinderchir 17:125
87a. Kreuter E (1905) Die angeborenen Verschließungen und Verengungen des Darmkanals im Lichte der Entwicklungsgeschichte. Dtsch Z Chir 79:1–89

88. Ladd WE (1944) The surgical treatment of esophageal atresia and tracheo-esophageal fistulas. N Engl J Med 230: 625–637
89. Ladd WE, Swenson O (1947) Esophageal atresia and tracheo-esophageal fistula. Ann Surg 125: 23–40
90. Lam CR (1945) The surgical treatment of congenital atresia of the esophagus with tracheo-esophageal fistula. Q Bull Indiana Univ Med Center 32
91. Lamb DS (1873) A fatal case of congenital tracheo-esophageal fistula. Philadelphia Med Times 3: 705
92. Lanman TH (1940) Congenital atresia of the esophagus. A study of thirty-two cases. Arch Surg 41: 1060–1983
93. Leigh TF, Abbott OA, Hopkins WH (1951) Roentgenologic consideration in tracheo-esophageal fistula without esophageal atresia. With report of two cases. Radiology 57: 871
94. Leven NL (1936) Surgical management of congenital atresia of the esophagus with tracheo-esophageal fistula. Report of two cases. J Thorac Surg 6: 30
95. Leven NL (1941) Congenital atresia of the esophagus with tracheo-esophageal fistula. Report of successful extrapleural ligation of fistulous communication and cervical esophagostomy. J Thorac Surg 10: 648–657
96. Leven NL, Varco RL, Lannin BG, Tongen LA (1952) Congenital atresia of esophagus and tracheo-esophageal fistula. J Thorac Surg 136: 701
97. Lindahl H (1984) Esofagusatresia ja trakeosofageaalinen fisteli (Oesophageal atresia and tracheo-oesophageal fistula). Helsinki
98. Lilienthal (1926) Imperforate esophagus. Saunders, Philadelphia (Thoracic surgery, vol 1, p 317)
99. Livaditis A (1973) Esophageal atresia; a method of overbridging large segmental gaps. Z Kinderchir 13: 298
100. Livaditis A et al (1972) Esophageal end-to-end anastomosis. Scand J Thorac Cardiovasc Surg 6: 206
101. Livaditis A (1969) End-to-end anastomosis in esophageal atresia. A clinical and experimental study. Scand J Thorac Cardiovasc Surg [Suppl] 2
102. Livaditis A, Bjorck G, Kangstrom LE (1969) Esophageal myectomy. An experimental study in piglets. Scand J Thorac Cardiovasc Surg 3: 181
103. Longmire WP (1947) Congenital atresia and tracheo-esophageal fistula. Arch Surg 55: 330
104. Losee JR (1914) A report of two cases of oesophago-tracheal fistula. Bull Lying In Hosp NY 9: 209
105. Louhimo I, Lindahl H (1983) Esophageal atresia. Primary results of 500 consecutively treated patients. J Pediatr Surg 18(3): 217
106. Maddock GE (1964) Congenital esophageal atresia with tracheo-esophageal fistula. Associated congenital anomalies. Harfer Hosp Bull: 246
107. Martin M (1821) Observateur des sciences médicales Marseille. Exposé des Traveaux de la Soc Roy de Med de Marseille: 44
108. Martin LW (1972) The use of colon for oesophageal replacement in children. Aust NZ J Surg 42: 160
109. Mathieu A, Goldsmith HE (1933) Congenital atresia of the esophagus with tracheo-esophageal fistula. Am J Surg 22: 233–238
110. Meeker IA, Weitzman JJ, Brennan LP (1967) Double gastrostomy for poor risk newborns with esophageal atresia and distal tracheo-esophageal fistula (type C). Meeting of British Association of Paediatric Surgeons, Bremen
111. Mellor T (1846) Malformation of the oesophagus. Lond Med Gaz 2: 542
112. Mercer RD (1945) Laryngeal stridor with temporary cardiac and respiratory arrest. Am J Dis Child 70: 336
113. Minnis JF, Burko H, Brevetti G (1962) Segmental duplication of the esophagus associated with esophageal atresia and tracheo-esophageal fistula. Ann Surg 156: 271–275
114. Mixter CE (1936) Discussion of article by Gage and Oschner. Ann Surg 103: 736
115. Mondière JT (1833) Notes sur quelques maladies de l'œsophage. Arch Gerer Med II(2): 504
116. Myers NA (1974) Oesophageal atresia: the epitome of modern surgery. Ann R Coll Surg Engl 54: 277–287

117. Myers NA (1975) Large gap between the segments. Kind Chir [Suppl] 65
118. Myers NA (1977) Oesophageal atresia with distal tracheo-oesophageal fistula – a long term follow-up. Progr Pediatr Surg 10:5–17
119. Myers NA (1979) Oesophageal atresia. Where next? Presented at the Annual Meeting of the Greek Association of Paediatric Surgeons
120. Myers NA (1979) Oesophageal atresia and/or tracheo-oesophageal fistula… A study of mortality. Progr Pediatr Surg 13:141–165
121. Myers NA (to be published) Oesophageal atresia and tracheo-oesophageal fistula, experience with 514 patients
122. McClellan RH, Elterich TF (1921) Atresia of the esophagus with tracheo-esophageal fistula. Am J Dis Child 21:339
123. Mackenzie M (1880) Malformations of the esophagus. Arch Laryngol 1(4):301–315
124. Mackenzie M (1884) Manual of diseases of the nose and throat, vol 2. William Wood, New York, p 156
125. O'Bannon RP (1946) Congenital partial atresia of the esophagus. Report of a case. Radiology 47:471
126. Ogle JW (1955–56) Malformed trachea and oesophagus: congenital communication between them. Trans Pathol Soc Lond 7:52
127. O'Hare HA (1937) Esophageal atresia. Penn Med J 40(11):914–917
128. Oterdoom HJ (1954) The problem of oesophageal atresia. Arch Chir Neerl 6:229
129. Overton RC, Creech O (1958) Unusual esophageal atresia with distant membranous obstruction of the esophagus. J Thorac Surg 35:674–677
130. Petterson G (1955) Inhibited separation of largynx and upper part of trachea from oesophagus in newborn. Report of case successfully operated upon. Acta Chir Scand 110:250
131. Piekarski DH, Stephens FD (1974) The association and embryogenesis of tracheo-oesophageal and anorectal anomalies. Progr Pediatr Surg 9:63–76
132. Pietsch JB, Stokes KB, Beardmore HE (1978) Esophageal atresia with tracheo-esophageal fistula. End-to-end versus end-to-side repair. J Pediatr Surg 13:677–681
133. Pinard (1873) Vices de conformation. Absence d'anus, communication de l'intestin et de l'uréthre; fistule trachéo-oesophagienne. Bull Soc Anat (Paris) VIII:682
134. Pinus J (1972) Contribution to the study of extra-parietal arterial blood supply of the thoracic portion of the normal and the atresic esophagus in the newborn. PhD dissertation, Escola Paulista de Medicina Department of Surgery, Sao Paulo
135. Plass ED (1919) Congenital atresia of the esophagus with tracheo-esophageal fistula; associated with a fused kidney case report and a survey of the literature on congenital anomalies of the esophagus. Johns Hopkins Hosp Rep 18:259
136. Putnam D (1909) Discussion of paper by Griffiths JPC and Lavenson RS. Congenital malformation of the esophagus with the report of a case. Arch Pediatr March:161–169
137. Randolph JC, Tunnell WP, Lilly JR, Altman RP (1971) Gastric division: a surgical adjunct in selected problems with esophageal anomalies. J Pediatr Surg 6:657–663
138. Ravdin I (1933) Cited in Tucker G, Pendergrass ED. Congenital atresia of the esophagus: a new diagnostic technique. JAMA 101:1726
139. Rehbein F, Schweder N (1972) Neue Wege in der Rekonstruktion der kindlichen Speiseröhre. Dtsch Med Wochenschr 19:757
140. Reitter GS (1933) A case of congenital atresia of the upper end of the esophagus with tracheo-esophageal fistula. Radiology 587–589
141. Reynolds RP, Morrison WW (1921) Congenital malformation of the esophagus. Am J Dis Child 21:339–346
142. Richardson WR, Brown IH, Williams GR (1963) Congenital atresia of the esophagus. Am Surg 29:166–178
143. Richter HM (1913) Congenital atresia of the esophagus, an operation designed for its cure. Surg Gynecol Obstet 17:397
144. Ricketts RR, Luck SR, Raffensperger JG (1981) Circular esophagomyotomy… for primary repair of long gap esophageal atresia. J Pediatr Surg 16:365
145. Rickham PP (1969) In: Johnston JH (ed) Neonatal surgery, 1st edn. Butterworth, London, p 133

146. Rickham PP, Stauffer UG, Cheng SK (1977) Oesophageal atresia: triumph and tragedy. Aust NZ J Surg 47:138–143
147. Robb D (1952) Congenital tracheo-oesophageal fistula without atresia but with large oesophageal diverticulum. Aust NZ J Surg 22:120–122
148. Roberts KD (1958) Congenital oesophageal atresia and tracheo-esophageal fistula: a review of 36 patients. Thorax 13:116
149. Rosenthal AH (1931) Congenital atresia of the esophagus with tracheo-esophageal fistula. Report of 8 cases. Pathol 12:756
150. Rosenthal AH, Himmelstein U (1932) Congenital atresia of the esophagus with tracheo-esophageal fistula. Arch Pediatr 49:444
151. Rossello PJ, Lebron H, Franco AAR (1980) The technique of myotomy in esophageal reconstruction. An experimental study. J Pediatr Surg 15:430
152. Sanderud A (1960) Treatment of oesophageal atresia: a modification in technique. Acta Chir Scand 119:339
153. Schullinger JN, Vinocur CD, Santulli TV (1982) The suture fistula technique in the repair of selected cases of esophageal atresia. J Pediatr Surg 17:234–236
154. Schwartz SE, Dale WA (1955) Unusual tracheo-esophageal fistulae with membranous obstruction of the esophagus and post-operative pyloric stenosis. Ann Surg 142:1002
155. Scott WJM (1936) Some problems in esophageal atresia. Ann Otol Rhinol Laryngol 45:1122
156. Sédillot M (1868–69) Quoted by Annandale T. Case of congenital malformation of the oesophagus. Edinburgh Med J 14:598
157. Shafer AD, David TE (1974) Suture fistula as a means of connecting upper and lower segments in esophageal atresia. J Pediatr Surg 9:669
158. Shattock CE (1922) Specimen of congenital malformation of the esophagus. Proc R Soc Med Sect Dis Child 15:2
159. Shattock SG (1890) Congenital atresia of the esophagus. Trans Pathol Soc Lond XL1:87
160. Shaw HLK (1920) Congenital atresia of the esophagus with report of a case. Am J Dis Child 20:507–515
161. Shaw RC (1939) Surgical correction of congenital atresia of the esophagus with tracheo-esophageal fistula. J Thorac Surg 9:213
162. Sideway ME (1964) Duplication of the oesophagus. Ann Radiol 7:400
163. Singleton AO, Knight MD (1944) Congenital atresia of the esophagus with tracheo-esophageal fistulae. Transpleural operative approach. Ann Surg 119:556
164. Skinner EH (1921) Congenital atresia of the esophagus. Am J Roentgenol 8:319
165. Smith ED (1923) The treatment of congenital atresia of the esophagus. Am J Surg 37:157–158
166. Soave F (1972) Intra-thoracic transposition of the transverse colon in complicated oesophageal atresia. Progr Pediatr Surg 4:91
167. Steele C (1888) Case of deficient oesophagus. Lancet 2:764
168. Stephens CA, Mustard WT, Simpson JS (1956) Congenital atresia of the esophagus with tracheo-esohageal fistula. Surg Clin North Am 36:1465
169. Stewart W, Thomson J (1899) Congenital malformation of the esophagus. Lancet 1:378
170. Strong RA, Cummins H (1943) Congenital atresia of the esophagus with tracheo-esophageal fistula. Am J Dis Child 47:1299
171. Sulamaa M, Gripenberg L, Ahvenlainen EK (1951) Progress and treatment of congenital atresia of the oesophagus. Acta Chir Scand 102:141
172. Sussman ML (1931) Congenital atresia of the esophagus: case report. Am J Roentgenol 26:894
173. Sweet RH (1946) Carcinoma of the midthoracic esophagus; its treatment by radical resection and high intra-thoracic esophago-gastric anastomosis. Ann Surg 124:653
174. Sweet RH (1948) A new method of restoring continuity of the alimentary canal in case of congenital atresia of the esophagus with tracheo-esophageal fistula not treated by immediate primary anastomosis. Ann Surg 127:757
175. Swenson O (1947) End-to-end anastomosis of the esophagus for esophageal atresia. Surgery 22:324

176. Swenson O, Lipman R, Fisher JH, De Luca FG (1962) Repair and complications of oesophageal atresia and tracheo-oesophageal fistula. N Engl J Med 267:96
177. Swischuk LE (1980) Radiology of the newborn and young infants, 2nd edn. Williams and Wilkins, Baltimore
178. Takada Y, Kent G, Filler RM (1981) Circular myotomy and esophageal length and safe oesophageal anastomosis. An experimental study. J Pediatr Surg 16(3):343
179. Ten Kate J (1952) Method of suturing in operations for congenital oesophageal atresia. Arch Chir Neerl 4:43
180. Thomas W (1904) On congenital occlusion of the oesophagus. Lancet 1:361
181. Thompson W (1878) Notes on gastrostomy in stricture of the esophagus. Lancet 2:284
182. Time Magazine (1974) The hardest choice
183. Touloukian RJ (1973) Membranous esophageal obstruction simulating atresia with a double tracheo-esophageal fistula in a neonate. J Thorac Cardiovasc Surg 65:191
184. Touloukian RJ, Pickett LK, Spackman T, Biancani P (1974) Repair of esophageal atresia by end-to-side anastomosis and ligation of the tracheo-esophageal fistula: a critical review of eighteen cases. J Pediatr Surg 9:305–310
185. Trump FA (1933) Congenital esophagotracheal fistula. Report of a case living 37 days on glucose intraperitoneally. J Pediatr 2:212
186. Tucker G, Pendergrass EP (1933) Congenital atresia of the esophagus: a new diagnostic technic. JAMA 101:1726
187. Tugan NA (1962) Annular stricture of the esophagus distal to congenital tracheo-esophageal fistula. Surgery 52:394–395
188. Ty TC, Brunet C, Beardmore NE (1967) A variation in the operative technic for the treatment of esophageal atresia with tracheo-esophageal fistula. J Pediatr Surg 2:118–126
189. Verneul (1876) Observation de gastrotomie paraique avec succés pour un rétrécissement cicatriciel infranchissable de l'œsophage. Bull Acad Med 44
190. Villemin (1904) Imperforation de l'œsophage. Arch Med Enfants VII:511
191. Vincent (1905) Cited in Kreuter E, ref 87a
192. Vinson PP (1923) Congenital strictures of the esophagus. JAMA 80:1754–1755
193. Vizas D, Ein SH, Simpson JS (1978) The value of circular myotomy for esophageal atresia. J Pediatr Surg 13:357
194. Vogt EC (1929) Congenital esophageal atresia. Am J Roentgenol 22:463
195. Waterston DJ, Bonham Carter RE, Aberdeen E (1962) Oesophageal atresia: tracheo-esophageal fistula. A study of survival in 218 infants. Lancet 1:819–822
196. Waterston DJ, Bonham Carter RE, Aberdeen E (1963) Congenital tracheo-oesophageal fistula in association with oesophageal atresia. Lancet 2:55–57
197. Waterston DJ (1979) Colon transplant in long term follow-up in congenital anomalies. Paediatric Surgical Symposium. The Children's Hospital of Pittsburgh, p 7
198. Weiss E (1923) Congenital atresia of esophagus with esophago-tracheal fistula. JAMA 80: 16–18
199. Whipham TRC, Fagge CH (1905) A case of congenital stenosis of the lower end of the oesophagus; with remarks. Lancet 1:22
200. Wiersema JA (1956) Partial reduplication of the oesophagus with oesophageal atresia and oesophago-tracheal fistula. Arch Chir Neerl 8:97–101
201. Willard HB (1922) Congenital atresia of the esophagus. JAMA 78:649
202. Woolley MM (1980) Esophageal atresia and tracheo-oesophageal fistula. Am J Surg 139:771
203. Yahr WZ, Azzoni AA, Santulli TV (1962) Congenital atresia of the esophagus with tracheo-esophageal fistula. An unusual variant. Surgery 52:937
204. Zigiotti GL, Domini R (1974) La miotomia cincolare del moncone superiore secondo livaditis nell'anastomosi primari per atresia esofagea. Riv Chir Pediatr 16:49

Historical Aspects of Hydrocephalus

E. Ring-Mrozik[1] and T. A. Angerpointner[1]

Anatomy and Physiology

Hydrocephalus was described by even the earliest medical authors because of its grotesque appearance. Hippocrates (460–377 B.C.) recognized that fluid was responsible for the enlargement of the head [95, 231]. One can conclude from his texts, which are difficult to interpret, that he imagined the fluid to be extracerebral, and he thus recommended treating the condition by means of frontal decompression trephination. Although Herophilus [93] and Erasistratus [51, 231] found enlarged cavities in the brains of hydrocephalics, they were unable to clarify the anatomy of the ventricular system. Galen (131–201 A.D.) was the first to determine that the brain ventricles communicate with each other, but he had no insights into their function [63, 231]. According to his doctrine, the ventricles were inhabited by the soul, the *"spiritus animalis,"* which underwent a process of purification therein. The purified products would then pass to the brain pores and would be excreted as "pituita" by the pituitary body (hypophysis) into the nasal cavity. Galen fitted the fluid-filled cavities into his doctrine of body juices and deduced that hydrocephalus could be affected by diet [26, 198, 230, 231]. Galen's doctrines were held to be valid until the late Middle Ages.

Oribasius classified three types of hydrocephalus [162, 231]. In the first type, the fluid was located between the skin and pericranium, between pericranium and skull in the second, and between the skull and the dura mater in the third. He advised incision in the first two types, but advised against treatment in the third. Paul of Aegina (seventh century) also disapproved of surgical intervention and allowed only the resection of a small piece of bone for trepanation [166, 231]. In accordance with Rhazes, the Arabs used a sort of cautery for trepanation at the suture lines and the temporal veins [192, 231].

During the next 500 years, knowledge about hydrocephalus increased only slightly, until Vesalius (1514–1564 A.D.) denied the existence of the *spiritus animalis* in 1543 and described internal hydrocephalus in detail: "The water had not collected between the skull and its outer surrounding, or the skin (where the doctors' books teach that water is depositioned in other cases), but in the cavity of the brain itself, and actually in the right and left ventricles of the brain. The cavity and breadth of these had so increased – and the brain itself was so dis-

[1] Pediatric Surgical Clinic, Dr. von Haunerschen Kinderspital of the University of Munich, Lindwurmstr. 4, D-8000 München 2, FRG

Progress in Pediatric Surgery, Vol. 20
Ed. by P. P. Rickham

tended – that they contained about 9 pounds of water or three Augsburg wine measures (so help me God)" [25, 187, 229, 231].

The true shape of the cerebral ventricles was determined by Leonardo da Vinci in 1505 by means of a wax mold: "Make two air holes in the horns of the large ventricles, inject the molten wax by boring a hole into the ventricle of Memoria, and, through this hole, fill the three cerebral ventricles. As soon as the wax has hardened, take the brain out, and you will be able to recognize exactly the form of the three ventricles. Before this, though, insert thin tubes into the airholes, that the air in these ventricles may escape and make room for the wax to flow into the ventricles" (*Quaderni* V, 7r). The object of investigation was obviously an ox brain (Fig. 1).

Two centuries later, Morgagni (1682–1771) confirmed that the massive dropsy in hydrocephalus originates from the ventricular system, and he pointed out that infantile hydrocephalus is always associated by distention of the head, whereas this is possibly absent in adults [148]. Drawing on the findings of 20 autopsies (probably for tuberculous meningitis), Robert Whytt gave a clear definition in 1768 of internal and external hydrocephalus in his "Observations of dropsy of the brain" [240].

He believed a fluid imbalance between a "sweating" artery and an absorbing vein to be the cause of hydrocephalus. At the same time, however, he denied that a patient could be ever cured by removal of the fluid.

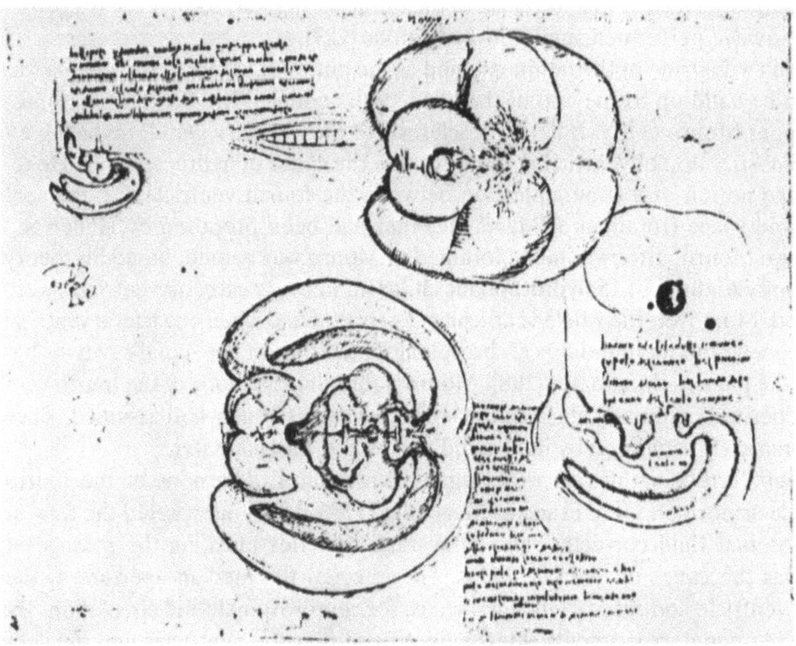

Fig. 1. Sketch by Leonardo da Vinci of cerebral ventricles detected by means of a wax mould (*Quaderni* V, 7r, about 1500 A.D.)

By end of the eighteenth century, physicians started to doubt idiopathic dropsy as it had been proposed by the ancients. Quin assumed in 1790 that hydrocephalus was analogous to dropsy of the body and that rickets or other debilitating conditions were responsible for it [182]. Rush (1809) of Philadelphia agreed with Quin's assumptions, blaming hydrocephalus on intermittent, remittent, and continuous fever, rheumatism, pulmonary consumption, eruptive fevers, and worms [200]. He suggested always keeping the head in a higher position than the rest of the body.

Many theories concerning the contents of the ventricles have been put forward since the rejection of Galen's idea of the *spiritus animalis.* At different times, water, air, vacuum, or vapour were successively considered, until fluid was generally accepted as the substance contained in the ventricles.

Although Haller (1762) was aware that cerebrospinal fluid was contained in the ventricles and subarachnoid space, he was not able to analyse its nature and consistency. He therefore developed his vapour theory [73], according to which the vapour was sweated out by arteries and reinhaled by veins. The impetus for his theory was a controversy with Verduc, who had stated in 1700 that normal ventricles could never contain fluid (cited by [28]). At that time, every fluid was regarded as a result of pathological processes or postmortem vapor condensation. For this reason, the theories of Cotugno, who in 1770 first proved the existence of the subarachnoid space, were not accepted either. He found that structure to contain cerebrospinal fluid in living fish and turtles, but not in dogs, since in that species the spinal cord was too close to the dural sac [22, 26, 231]. Valsalva (1741) is said to have performed similar investigations [227].

Galen's doctrine of the pituitary gland as the outlet of ventricular contents was held to be valid up to the end of the eighteenth century. The Scottish anatomist Alexander Monro (1733–1807) took sclerosis of the pituitary gland, involving effective obstruction of ventricular outlets, to be the cause of hydrocephalus. He refuted the notion of a communication between the fourth ventricle and the subarachnoid space (foramen of Magendie) that had been proposed by Haller and Cotugno. Monro, after whom the foramen of Monro was named, based his theory on autopsy findings of 15 hydrocephalic children; in every case, all ventricles were enlarged. Moreover, the whole ventricular system emptied when one lateral ventricle was opened, and he found no cerebrospinal fluid either in the spinal cavity or between the pia and dura mater [198]. Monro noted that the floor of the fourth ventricle does not communicate with the spinal cavity, as Haller had assumed, since it is completely separated by its choroid plexus and the pia mater.

Monro erred in this, since he regarded arachnoid adhesions of the fourth ventricle as normal. Only François Magendie (1783–1855) interpreted the flow of cerebrospinal fluid correctly, suggesting that a barrier blocking the passage of fluid was the cause of hydrocephalus. He detected the median aperture of the fourth ventricle and realized its significance for cerebrospinal fluid circulation. By means of animal experiments, Magendie proved that the ventricles and the subarachnoid space are filled with fluid, that these structures communicate freely with each other, that the subarachnoid spaces of the brain and the spinal cord are uniform, and that aqueduct of Sylvius and foramen of Magendie were obstructed in several cases of hydrocephalus [138, 139]. He did not recognize, however, why an obstruction of these pathways should cause hydrocephalus, since in his opinion the cerebrospinal fluid was excreted by the pia mater and then passed in some way into the ventricles. For some unknown reason, he believed the passage back was obstructed, leading to an accumulation of cerebrospinal fluid in the ventricles and, subsequently, to hydrocephalus [26].

Circulation of Cerebrospinal Fluid

The German anatomist Hubert von Luschka (1820–1875) confirmed Magendie's findings and went on to describe a lateral aperture [133, 134]. Its existence, however, was doubted by many anatomists, even after the publications of the Swedish scientists Ernst Axel Key (1832–1901) and Gustav Magnus Retzius (1842–1919) in 1875, whose observations on the circulation of cerebrospinal fluid are essentially still valid today [118].

Vincent Bochdalek of Prague (1801–1883) also discovered the lateral aperture of the fourth ventricle [134] which was recognized by von Luschka as the pathway from the fourth ventricle to the cisterna magna (apertura lateralis rhombencephali; foramen of Luschka). All subsequent research, particularly experimental investigations, are based on these findings.

Production of Cerebrospinal Fluid

Faivre suggested in 1854 that the cerebrospinal fluid is produced in the choroid plexus [53]. The embryological studies of Weed in 1920–23 [233, 234] and the observations of Cushing on the "sweating" of the choroid plexus in 1905, 1914 and 1926 [23–25] confirmed his suggestions.

In 1913, Dandy and Blackfan showed that the lateral ventricles do not become enlarged in the case of an obstruction of the foramen of Monro, if the plexus has already been removed, but that it does become enlarged, if the plexus is intact [31]. By means of intravenous fluorescence studies performed in 1927, Schaltenbrand and Putnam directly observed the production of cerebrospinal fluid by the choroid plexus of the lateral ventricles in the cat [206]. Nevertheless, in 1930, Hassin questioned the finding that the cerebrospinal fluid is produced by the choroid plexus [79]. There are many reviews on the physiology of the choroid plexus in the literature [111]. Particularly during inflammatory episodes, both the meninges and the ependyma are able to excrete cerebrospinal fluid [65, 195, 119].

Absorption of Cerebrospinal Fluid

Only if absorption mechanisms of the cerebrospinal fluid are elucidated can the pathogenesis of hydrocephalus be entirely understood. Key and Retzius concluded in 1872 from their dye injection studies that pacchionian bodies would absorb cerebrospinal fluid [118]. However, they also showed that pacchionian bodies are not present in children and higher primates. Demme pointed out (1956) that pacchionian bodies appear only with increasing age [41].

It was therefore evident that different structures must be able to absorb the cerebrospinal fluid. Weed supposed that the cerebrospinal fluid passes through the arachnoid villi, which, through the microscope, look very much like pacchionian bodies [233]. Moreover, he regarded the latter as pathological enlargements of microscopic arachnoid villi [235].

According to Gerlach et al. (1967), the whole arachnoides is capable of absorbing the cerebrospinal fluid in newborns and infants [65]. Weed proved in 1922 that the cerebrospinal fluid passes through the arachnoid villi into the veins [234]. Based on their experiments with phenolsulphonphthalein Dandy et al. also concluded that the cerebrospinal fluid is absorbed by the arachnoid villi [27].

Pathogenesis of Hydrocephalus

Current knowledge of the pathogenesis of hydrocephalic ventricular enlargement is founded on Dandy's experimental work from 1913–1922 [31, 32]. Accordingly, there is no doubt that an obstruction of the passage of cerebrospinal fluid may effect a hydrocephalic enlargement of the region lying above that obstruction. Thus, hydrocephalus might be due to a blockage of the foramina of Monro, Magendie and Luschka as well as of the aqueduct of Sylvius. Inflammatory adhesions of the basal cisternae and impaired absorption of cerebrospinal fluid may also cause hydrocephalus. In 1914, Dandy et al. subdivided hydrocephalus into an obstructive type, which usually results from a closure of the aqueduct of Sylvius or the foramina Magendie and Luschka, and a communicating type, resulting from impaired absorption of the cerebrospinal fluid at the brain surface. This subdivision was necessary after studies with intravenous injection of phenolsulphonphthalein, yielded results that could be obtained by lumbar punction in communicating hydrocephalus but not in obstructive hydrocephalus [27]. A table of possible pathological conditions resulting in hydrocephalus was published by Russell in 1949 [201]. Experiments on the pathogenesis of this conditioned were performed by many other investigators [71].

Conservative Treatment

The possibility of spontaneous cure must be kept in mind in the treatment of hydrocephalus. This occurs in 10% of all cases, according to Bucy (1950) [17], whereas Laurence reported 46% spontaneous cures [126–128] in 1958 and 1962 and Riley 45% [187] spontaneous cures in children with communicating hydrocephalus [112, 184].

The helplessness as far as hydrocephalus is concerned became particularly evident in methods of treatment. Madame de Fouquet, for instance, wrote in her *Hauß-Artzneyen* (presumably dating from the first half of the eighteenth century):

"Now and then, headaches stem from a water-filled sac containing a thick fluid that forms in the cavity of the brain or above it, and no remedy for it is known except fasting, and these things are very dangerous" [230].

In 1790, Quin recommended bleeding, purging, diuretics, the local application of cold, blisters and cupping [182]. Kausch (1908) was of the opinion that conservative treatment would fail unless the hydrocephalus were of luetic origin [112]. In such cases, complete cure of even severe cases by iodine or mercuric therapy was reported by Haller in 1892 and 1898 [88, 89], Neumann in 1901 [153], Immerwol in 1901 [102] and others. Soma reported cure in four of five cases by systematic solar radiation [190]. His results, however, were unreproducible.

By the beginning of the nineteenth century, the idea that external pressure would be of benefit in the treatment of hydrocephaly, came into fashion, as described by Blane in 1821 [14]. Girdlestone and Costerton (1822) also used compression therapy in several cases of hydrocephalus [66], as did Barnard 3 years later [6]. Several sporadic reports on compression treatment were published over the next 50 years. Muslin bandages were readjusted daily and kept wet for proper compression. Adhesive plasters were also in use; rubber bandages were preferred, however, for they provided stronger tension and constant pressure. This concept has recently been reintroduced because of the idea that the higher intracranial pressure created by head bandages would open the absorption pathways, thus reducing dependence on shunts [50].

By increasing intracranial pressure, however, this compression only served to hamper cerebrospinal fluid circulation, leading to convulsions and even fracture of the skull, according to Von Bruns [112].

In 1916, Frazier suggested treating the condition with thyroidal extracts [61], and Mariott (1924) proposed theobromine sodium salicylate [140]. Both methods turned out to be a failure. Furthermore, an attempt was made to inhibit the production of cerebrospinal fluid by isosorbide and acetazolamide (Diamox) [3, 13, 132, 242]. If Diamox is administered intravenously, intracranial pressure rises significantly [5]; if it is given orally, intracranial pressure is reported to drop in some cases. Whereas Epstein was able to reduce cerebrospinal fluid production by 40% [50], Ransohoff (1960) found that the clinical course in hydrocephalics was not influenced by Diamox [187]. The effects of isosorbide and Diamox are also subject to considerable individual variation as to duration and side effects [144, 199]. These drugs are only useful as a temporary or adjuvant measure in relative shunt insufficiency, for instance, and are dangerous if applied as an alternative to shunt treatment [11]. Osmotic therapy by administration of 40% sorbitol solution combined with diuretics such as frusemide or ethacrynic acid is effective for only a short time, if at all. In 1952, Hemmer described intravenous administration of highly concentrated glucose and saline infusions, combined with oral or rectal saline purgatives (magnesium sulfate, Carlsbad salts, etc.) and a saline- and water-reduced diet as a short-term stosstherapy [90]. Umbach (1959) regarded these methods only as emergency measures [226].

X-ray irradiation did not inhibit plexus activity, as Sgalitzer had assumed [90, 110]. To achieve a selective irradiation effect on the plexus and ventricular ependyma, Riechert (1963) used trace doses of radioactive phosphorus (^{32}P) injected intraventricularly, which brought about a short-term inhibition of excretion, but no lasting success [196]. Mundinger obtained growth inhibition of cells producing cerebrospinal fluid by dye injection in individual cases in 1960 [149].

Surgical Treatment

Because of the hopelessness of conservative treatment, a large variety of operative techniques for the treatment of hydrocephalus were developed [37] (Fig. 2).

Puncture of Cerebrospinal Fluid

The first operative intervention consisted of repeated lumbar and ventricular punctures [8]. Puncture of the lateral ventricles represents the oldest method of

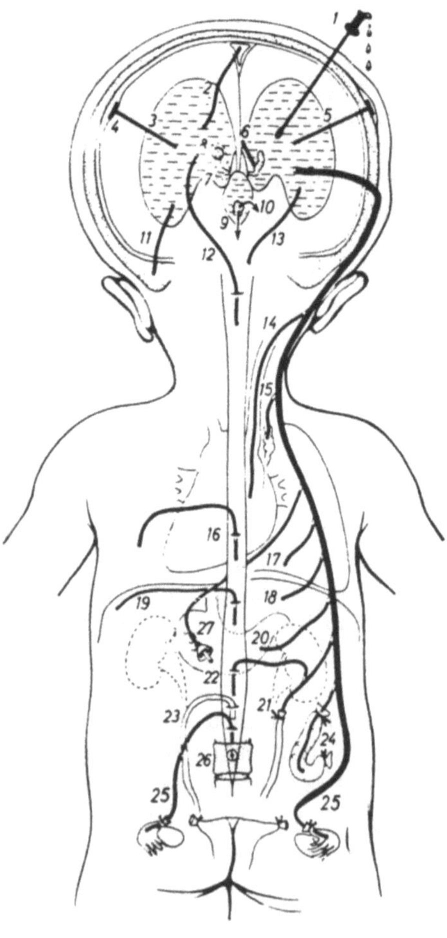

Fig. 2. Various surgical techniques for correcting hydrocephalus [65]. *(1)* Ventricular puncture [164]; *(2)* ventriculosinostomy with transplanted blood vessels [167]; *(3)* ventriculoarachnoidostomy [167]; *(4)* ventriculosubdurostomy [58]; *(5)* ventriculosubgaleostomy [167]; *(6)* callosal puncture [4]; and permanent drainage [129]; *(7)* extirpation of the choroid plexus or coagulation [32]; *(8)* lateral ventriculostomy [99]; *(9)* posterior ventriculostomy (third ventricle) [30]; *(10)* anterior ventriculostomy (third ventricle) [218]; *(11)* ventriculomastoidostomy [157]; *(12)* ventriculocisternostomy [225]; *(13)* transtentorial ventriculocisternostomy [195]; *(14)* ventriculoauriculostomy with Holter and Pudenz valves [178]; *(15)* ventriculolymphangiostomy [247]; *(16)* spinopleurostomy; *(17)* ventriculopleurostomy [85]; *(18)* ventriculosubdiaphragmatostomy [106]; *(19)* lumboperitonostomy [54]; *(20)* ventriculoperitonostomy [112]; *(21)* ventriculoureterostomy [142]; *(22)* lumboureterostomy [142]; *(23)* duroureterostomy [86]; *(24)* ventriculoileostomy [152]; *(25)* lumbo-(ventriculo)-salpingostomy [78]; *(26)* transdural shunt to vertebral bone marrow [249]; *(27)* ventriculogastrostomy [2]

surgical treatment hydrocephalus in infants with open fontanelles, one used already in ancient times. The Greeks attempted to treat hydrocephalus by incision and drainage. Fabricius Hildanus reported puncture by means of a trocar in 1646 [52]. In 1745, Stevens advised trephining the head of Dean Swift [193]. By the middle of the eighteenth century, the Monros were of the opinion that incisions should be made with a lancet, which made it possible to avoid injuring cranial arteries or veins [146, 147].

In 1888, Keen considered the posterior temporal region as ideal for puncture [113], as did Broca, who is said to have performed ventricular drainage for the first time in France in 1891 [16].

Chipault (1894), on the contrary, differentiated between subarachnoid and ventricular hydrocephalus and performed punctures on all regions of the head, even through the nose [20].

For a while, tappings were combined with compression bandages and intraventricular injection treatment in the middle of the nineteenth century. Compression bandages often caused a decubitus and were useful only if the fontanelle was still open. In 1894, Bilhaut recommended combining trepanopuncture with circular craniectomy and compression [12].

An intraventricular injection of iodine tincture was tried by both Boinet and Hayden in 1856 [15], as well as by others. The results were to no avail [80, 186]. In 1829, Greatwood claimed to have achieved a cure by intraventricular injection of potassium hydroiodate [69].

Quinke's lumbar puncture represents the simplest operative method (1891) but can be performed only if the ventricles and subarachnoid communicate [18]. However, this method also yielded unsatisfactory results [154, 173]. A logical step was to combine ventricular and lumbar puncture or to alternate the procedures. This procedure, recommended among others by Nölke (1897) [156] and Cassel (1897) [18], was unsuccessful. Chater advised drainage by means of a seton in 1845 [19]. Ricketts (1904) [193] and Grantham (1854) [68] applied this method of drainage as well, after repeated ventricular punctures had failed. The seton method was rejected in 1882 despite several successes.

According to Pampus (1953), temporary ventricular drainage using a closed system might be of benefit by allowing simultaneous intraventricular application of antibiotics [164].

If repeated punctures are necessary over a longer time, the subcutaneous ventriculostomy cerebrospinal fluid reservoir described by Rickham (1965) may be efficacious [194].

Open Ventricular Drainage

A consequence of repeated ventricular punctures was that sometimes the penetration points did not close immediately and cerebrospinal fluid leaked for several days. This "natural" drainage was to some degree effective. Therefore, in 1881, Wernicke advised a permanent open drain [239]. Initially, a large tube was used for drainage [9] permitting such a rapid outflow of cerebrospinal fluid that the patient quickly died. Keen (1891) thus began using a thin cord of horse hairs, which he successively replaced with thicker bundles and finally, with a rubber drain [114, 115]. Illingworth reported in 1891 successful trephination and drainage by means of a Southey trocar and cannula, which was removed 8 days later [101]. This was the precursor of the Frazier needle and the technique of ventricular drainage by catheter recommended by Ingraham and Campbell in 1941 [103].

Closed Ventricular Drainage

Shunt to Subcutis. Since external, open drainage was often associated with infections, several methods of internal drainage were developed to avoid infection. Von Miculicz (1896) was the first to try internal drainage of the lateral ventricles [143]. He inserted a nail-shaped mass of glass wool into the lateral ventricle and put the end of the drain below the positioned periostal flap. Later, he used gold and glass tubes, but achieved poor results.

Shunt to Subdural Space. Von Miculicz also attempted intracranial drainage from the ventricles to the subarachnoidal and the subdural spaces in 1896 [153]. However, the experiments were a failure. Sutherland and Cheyne made similar efforts in 1898 [219, 220].

In 1903, Senn described ventriculosubdural drainage by means of a perforated rubber tube [210, 211], and Krause and Heymann drained the ventricles in 1917 by means of a flanged silver tube extending to the pericranium [121]. Shortly thereafter, Taylor reported ventriculosubdural drainage with a catgut suture covered by a Cargile membrane [223, 224]. In 1957, Forrest et al. used a shunt which diverted the cerebrospinal fluid from the ventricles to the subdural space above, thus achieving an arrest of hydrocephalus in 50% of cases. The remaining patients died of progressive hydrocephalus intracranial infections or other complications [58, 59].

Diversion of cerebrospinal fluid from the lateral ventricles to the subgaleal space had been attempted by many surgeons by the turn of century [112] (Fig. 3). This procedure did not yield satisfactory results, and yet, as recently as 1977, it was recommended by Perret and Graf, who employed subgaleal shunts in 173 patients for transitory treatment of hydrocephalus or drainage of subdural hematoma [171].

Vascular Shunts. The idea of diverting the cerebrospinal fluid into the venous blood stream or lymphatic channels is an old one. Gärtner suggested at the *Lübeck Naturforscherversammlung* in 1895 using an artificial connection between the ventricles and the lymphatic or venous systems for intracranial drainage [62].

Drawing on animal experiments, Payr, a surgeon from Leipzig, succeeded in the clinical application of this idea, and he reported his revolutionary technique for drainage of the ventricles by means of transplanted blood vessels at the 1908 Surgeons' Congress. He linked the lateral ventricle and the longitudinal sinus by

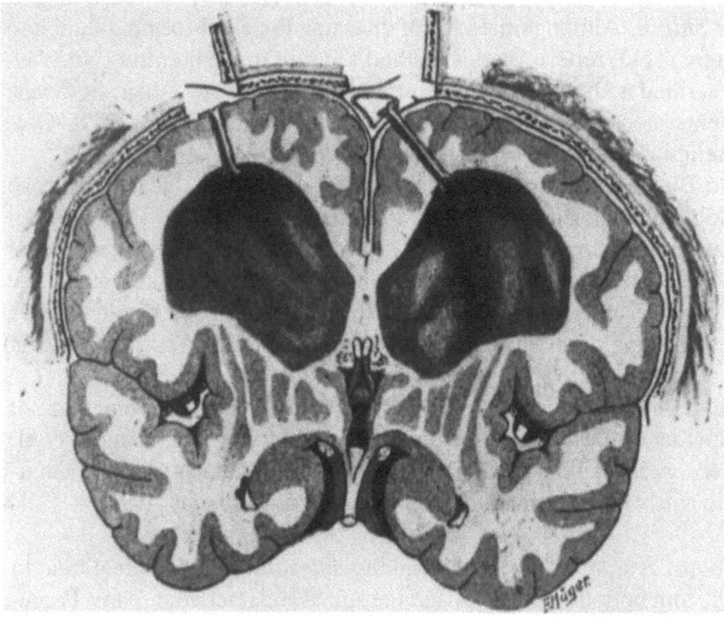

Fig. 3. *(Right)* Ventriculosinostomy (sinus sagittalis sup.); *(left)* ventriculosubarachnoidostomy [167]

a saphenous vein graft [167, 170] (Fig. 2). However, the patients treated with this method died within 4 months. Payr (1911) also used heterologous, denatured arteries of dogs and calves (anterior and posterior tibial arteries) for drainage of cerebrospinal fluid. The calf arteries were formaline fixed, paraffin impregnated and covered by autogenous saphenous vein. In addition, Payr described drainage via the internal jugular vein [168]. Eight of 15 patients survived, and four improved.

Imitators of Payr established connections between the lateral ventricles or the cisterna magna and the intracranial venous sinuses or the cervical veins, though without success [49, 81, 82, 136]. Four decades passed before the work of Payr was expanded on.

Nulsen and Spitz initiated the first shunting system with a working ball valve [160]. In 1949, they implanted a ball valve in a 14-month-old child with hydrocephalus and were thereby able to arrest the condition.

Sikkens also reported satisfactory results in 1957 following implantation of shunting systems between the lateral ventricles and the caval vein with an integrated ball valve imbedded in methyl methacrylate [213].

In 1950 Gupta described his technique of diversion from the lateral ventricle into the proximal segment of an obstructed facial vein or the external jugular vein [47, 72].

Thoracic Duct Shunts. Although the idea of diverting the cerebrospinal fluid into the lymph system is old, reports on this method are rare in the literature. In 1959, Yokoyama described a shunt from the ventricles to the thoracic duct; however, the three patients died within 2 weeks of an obstruction in the duct [247]. Olds published a preliminary case report in 1962 [161].

Kempe and Blaylock published a report in 1977 on their 12-year experience with ventriculolymphangiostomy performed on 16 patients [116]. They also described the anatomical circumstances in 51 adults who had undergone cervical sympathectomy. Thanks to the competence of the valves of the thoracic duct, they simply used a silicone tube without a valve. After achieving good results in 62% of the patients, Kempe and Blaylock recommended employing this method in infants and children also [116].

In animal experiments, Ingraham et al. (1949) observed valve incompetence of the thoracic duct as well as a tendency for the lymph to clot [105]. Jaques et al. (1978) however, were unable to confirm the clotting tendency in ventricular-ductal shunts in cats with experimentally produced hydrocephalus [109].

Abdominal Shunts. Attempts have been made to divert the cerebrospinal fluid to the *peritoneum* from both the ventricles and the spinal subarachnoid space. Ferguson (1898) did a laminectomy of the fifth lumbar vertebra and, after moving the spinal cord to one slide, drilled through the vertebral body into the peritoneal cavity. He then moved a sling of silver wire through the hole and directed the end down to the cauda equina [54, 106]. The three patients treated in this fashion survived only a few months. Nicoll (1905) drew a tip of the omentum through a paravertebral incision and fixed it below the spinal dura mater [155].

Cushing (1905) anastomosed the spinal subarachnoid space with the peritoneal cavity or the retroperitoneal space [24]. By means of combined laparotomy and laminectomy, he drilled a hole through the fourth lumbar vertebra and inserted a silver cannula. Heile (1908) passed two silk threads from the dura mater to the peritoneal cavity of a child who did well for 2 years after surgery, but then died of an infection [84]. In addition, in 1914, he described a connection between the spinal subarachnoid space and the abdominal cavity by means of a transplanted saphenous vein, which had to be replaced with a rubber tube due to a malfunction [85]. This shunt continued to work 12 years later [86]. In 1919, Payr reported on a lumbar peritoneal shunt [169].

Kausch is said to have performed the first ventriculoperitoneal shunt in 1908 using a rubber tube [112]. The patient died 20 h after the operation of overdrainage. Other surgeons also had unsatisfactory experiences with ventriculoperitoneal shunting, and this method thus fell into disuse until it was revived by Cone et al. in 1949 [21, 106–108, 144]. Scarff published the results of ventriculoperitoneal shunting in 230 patients in 1963, reporting a hydrocephalic arrest rate of 55% and a mortality rate of 13% (Fig. 4) [203].

Since that time, many improvements in both shunt systems and surgical techniques have been introduced. Ventricular catheters that are less prone to obstruction by the choroid plexus, brain tissue or ventricular walls and valves with vary-

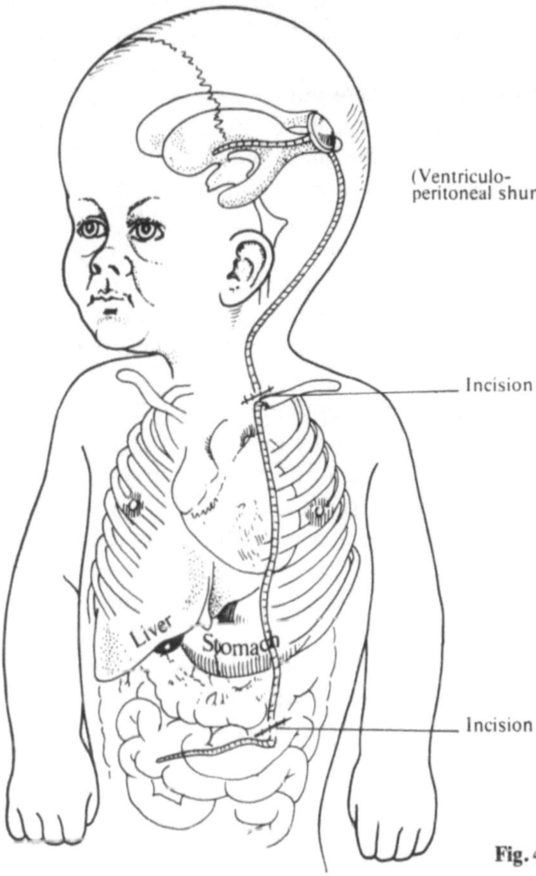

Fig. 4. Ventriculoperitoneal shunt [216a]

ing pressure ranges have been developed. Antisiphon devices were constructed to prevent overdrainage, the first one being devised by Portnoy and Schulte in 1971 [137, 175, 244]. Furthermore, distal catheters that do not bend and that are constructed with or without terminal slit valves are available today [185]. To prevent the spreading of metastases via a shunt systems in brain tumors, millipore filters were constructed [96].

The lumbar subarachnoid-peritoneal shunt was simplified by the introduction of percutaneous techniques [45, 123, 209, 216]. These methods are particularly useful for evaluating shunt efficiency in cases of so-called "normal-pressure" hydrocephalus, cerebrospinal fluid rhinorrhea and transitory secondary hydrocephalus following subarachnoid bleeding.

Despite all these improvements, however, there is a large variety of minor and major complications, as Davidson pointed out in 1976 [38]. Obviously, peritoneal shunting has only limited long-term efficiency in spite of the simple operative technique [38, 100, 107, 117, 131, 144, 150, 208].

Picaza described his technique of diverting the cerebrospinal fluid to the *omental bursa* from the lumbar subarachnoid space into the retro-omental region in 1956 [172], a method he developed to prevent obstruction of the shunt by the major omentum. Comparing his results with those of anterior peritoneal shunts, he found a significantly higher rate of hydrocephalic arrest. Dodge et al. (1957) diverted the cerebrospinal fluid directly into the omental bursa with good results [42]. Pudenz (1981) also employed the omental bursa shunt successfully with five children. Using a right-sided subcostal approach, a slit-valve catheter is inserted through Winslow's foramen into the omental bursa and is attached to the posterior peritoneum [176]. Since clinical experience with this method is still limited, it remains to be seen whether this method is to be preferred over peritoneal shunts. A simplification of this technique by means of a peritoneoscope for insertion of the catheter has been discussed.

Alther (1965) used a shunt from the ventricles to the *stomach* [2], and other reports on the same method have been published by Lamesch in 1972 [125] and Weiss et al. in 1975 [238]. Alther constructed his own gastric valve system, while Weiss et al. employed commercially available shunt devices, whereby the distal catheter tip is fixed in the gastric cavity. The authors report an acceptable complications rate. Duff (1977), however, pointed out that neither function tests nor repair of obstructions at the distal catheter tip could be carried out without gastroscopy [43].

Smith et al. described *ventriculocholecystostomy* in 1959 [214]. Following previous experiments in dogs, they implanted a specially designed valve system in ten patients. Whereas six patients survived for at least 2 years, in the four deceased patients the shunts worked only up to 8 months.

A further method is shunting from the lumbar subarachnoid space to the *ileum* via a diverted and sterilized ileal loop and a synthetic tube, as described by Neumann et al. (1959) in an 8-month-old infant with rapidly progressing hydrocephalus [151, 152].

Heile's anastomosis of the subarachnoid space with the renal pelvis following nephrectomy became well known in 1925 [86, 87]. He reported success in 75% of the patients treated with this method. In Europe, the technique was employed frequently, whereas it was not used often in North America until Matson described a modification in 1949 [141] (Fig. 5).

While Heile linked the renal pelvis to the dura mater, Matson connected the lumbar subarachnoid space and the ureter by means of a molded polyethylene drain. Matson (1956) considered the *ureteral shunt* as the most satisfying method he had ever used [142], since there was no surgical mortality in 108 patients. The complications reported involved meningitis, mechanical obstruction and, in particular, dehydration because of electrolyte and fluid losses associated in intercurrent infections. Matson first used ventrico-uretral shunting (Fig. 6) and later abandoned ventriculoperitoneal shunting. He declared that he would only use lumbar subarachnoid ureteral shunting, but only if the patient had two good kidneys, parents with a sense of responsibility, a well-trained physician and an excellent hospital nearby [177].

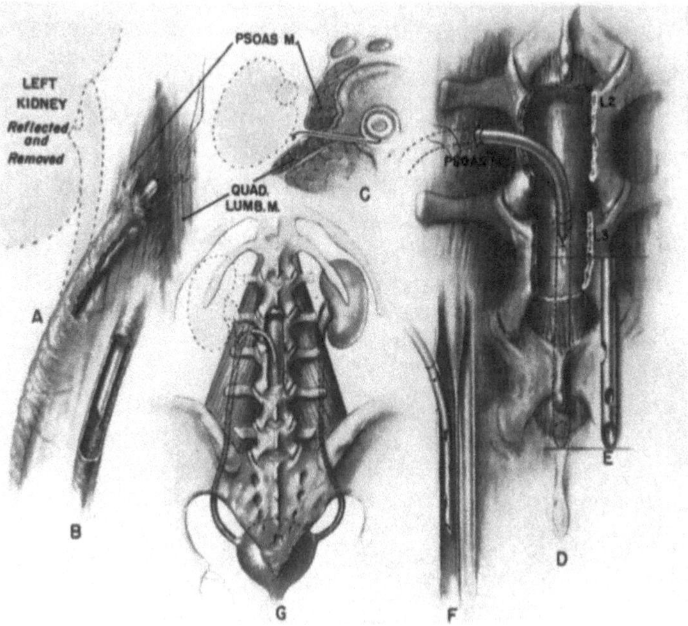

Fig. 5. Arachnoidureterostomy [142a]

Smith et al. (1980) developed an improved technique of ventriculoureteral shunting in which nephrectomy was unnecessary [215]. They transsected the ureter near the bladder, reimplanted the proximal part into the bladder wall and connected the distal segment to the shunt catheter. The results so far have been good, if vesicoureteral reflux, which can lead to ascending infection, is avoided prior to surgery.

Harsh described a shunt from both ventricles and the lumbar subarachnoid space to the *fallopian tubes* in 1954 [78]. All eight salpingothecal anastomoses and three of four ventriculosalpingostomies worked satisfactorily. However, this technique has been employed by only a few operators such as Resnikoff [191] and McCarthy et al. [135] with good results.

Shunt to Epidural Space. Hakim et al. reported on a method of shunting to the epidural space in 1955 [74]. During a cervical laminectomy, they had observed that 300 ml saline injected into the epidural space seeped rapidly away. Subsequently, they diverted the cerebrospinal fluid from the spinal subarachnoid space into the epidural space in four children with communicating hydrocephalus. The results during a follow-up period of 11–27 months were satisfactory. Furthermore, Hakim et al. modified Torkildsen's ventriculocisternostomy by placing the distal catheter tip into the epidural space.

Successful epiduroarachnoidostomy was also reported by Wallman and Donaghy (1958) in two cases [232]. Hakim, however, who was the first to note the syn-

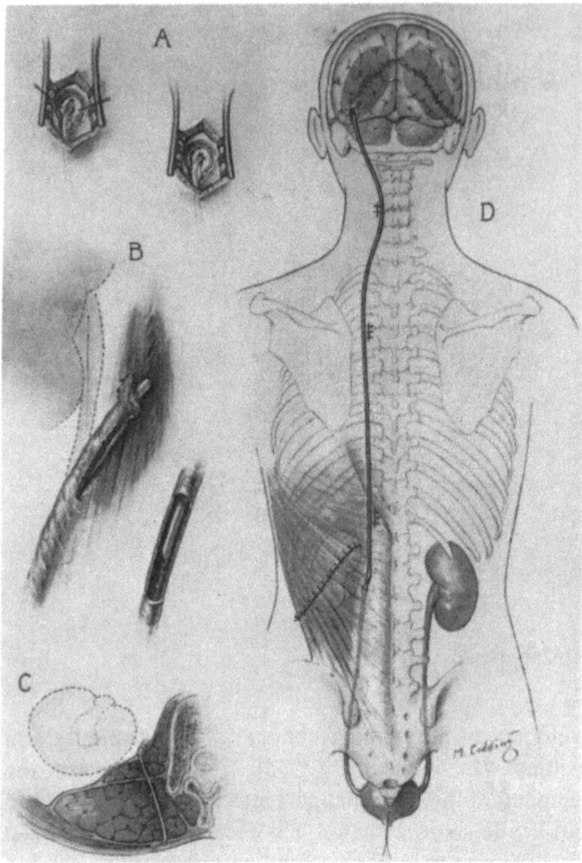

Fig. 6. Ventriculoureterostomy [142a]

drome of normal-pressure hydrocephalus found long-term results with spinal epidural shunting to be poor [1, 75–77]. He thus began to devise his valve system, which is widely used today.

Shunt to Bone Marrow. Subarachnoidintravertebral anastomosis was reported by Ziemnowicz in 1950 for treatment of communicating hydrocephalus [249]. He connected the lumbar subarachnoid space with the vertebral bone marrow by means of a hollow metal screw in a 14-year-old girl with metainfective hydrocephalus. He had observed that 500 ml normal saline were absorbed within 1 h when a pressure of 60 cm H_2O was applied. He achieved good results, whereas Schulze (1956) reported unsatisfactory results after applying this method on five patients [207].

Thoracic Shunts. The method of shunting to the *pleural cavity* was first described by Heile in 1914 [37, 85, 188] and later by Ransohoff in 1954 [187]. Recent publications by Ransohoff et al. (1960) and Milhorat (1976) have shown an initial success-rate of 65% [144, 188]. This method is occasionally used today, even though numerous shunt revisions are required.

Pudenz performed animal experiments in 1955 to investigate the feasibility of shunting to the systemic circulatory system [177, 178]. These experiments resulted in the use of silicone as a tubing material. Pudenz was able to demonstrate that good shunt function was provided only if the cerebrospinal fluid was diverted into a large venous pool, such as the *right atrium*.

Ventriculoatrial shunting was first employed in 1955 in a child with stenosis of the aqueduct of Sylvius. Initially, the child did well (Fig. 7), but died 2 years after surgery of acute shunt dysfunction [178].

At the same time, Holter, a precision tool maker whose daughter had been born with myelomeningocele, worked indefatigably on the construction of a valve system for shunting into the jugular vein or the right atrium. Today, his valve is in worldwide use for ventriculoatrial and ventriculoperitoneal shunting [176] (Fig. 8).

During the 1960s, ventriculoatrial shunting became the preferred method for the treatment of both obstructive and communicating hydrocephalus. A variety of shunt devices and surgical techniques have been developed since then [7, 46, 91, 98, 159]. Implantation of the distal catheter was also carried out via the direct approach to the heart [144, 163, 237].

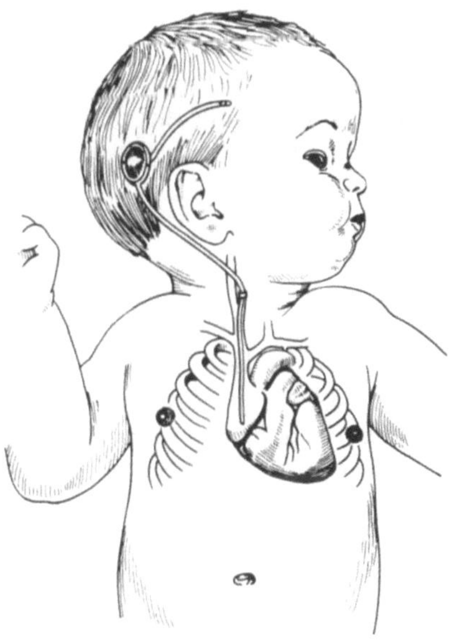

Fig. 7. Ventriculoatrial shunt [216a]

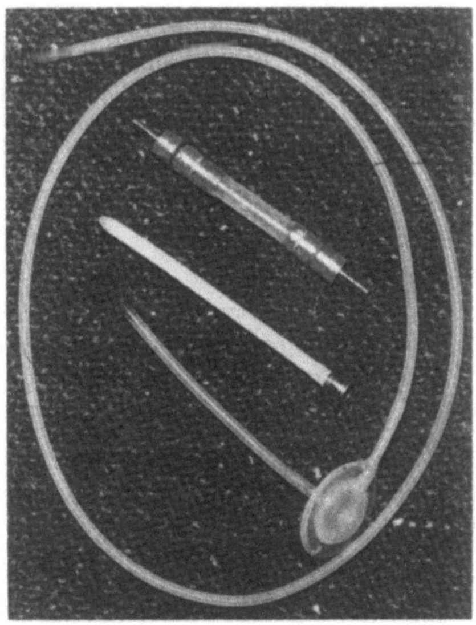

Fig. 8. Pudenz-Heyer ventriculoperitoneal shunting device with Holter valve and Rickham reservoir [216a]

Initial enthusiasm for this method was restrained by the occurrence of severe complications, such as thrombosis of the distal catheter, pulmonary embolism with subsequent cor pulmonale and a multitude of mechanical problems [56, 67, 91, 100, 117, 131, 144, 158, 159].

In 1979, George et al. reported infection rates in 840 patients with ventriculoatrial and 410 patients with ventriculoperitoneal shunts over 25 years; the infection rates were 11.4% and 12.0% respectively and thus roughly equal, being higher in very old and very young patients. Furthermore, the authors investigated the value of antibiotic prophylaxis, finding it questionable owing to bacterial resistance. Two-thirds of infections occurred within the 1st postoperative month. Infections occurred more frequently after revisions than after initial implantations and were furthermore related to the surgeon's technique and degree of experience [64].

Callosal and Cisternal Puncture. Once the pathogenesis of obstructive hydrocephalus had been elucidated, the development of surgical techniques for the recanalization of the cerebrospinal fluid circulation was attempted. In 1908, Anton and Von Bramann attempted the puncture of the corpus callosum by establishing a broad link between the third ventricle and the subarachnoid space. For that purpose, they trephined the skull in the median line and made a hole through the corpus callosum into the third ventricle [4]. This method soon was abandoned, since the pathways did not remain open.

The technique of suboccipital or cisternal puncture recommended by Anton and Schmieden should also be mentioned, whereby the membrane between the cisterna magna and the fourth ventricle was perforated in order to restore or enlarge the foramen of Magendie [122].

In 1921 and 1922, ventriculostomy of the third ventricle was described by Dandy [29, 30], who employed it in isolated stenosis of the aqueduct of Sylvius. Via a lateral, subfrontal approach, the floor of the third ventricle was opened and the optic nerve transsected [35].

By means of a surgical cystoscope, Mixter punctured the floor of the third ventricle in 1923 [145]. Stookey and Scarff (1936) recommended an approach through the lamina terminalis to the floor of the third ventricle for shunting [218]. All these methods were unsuccessful, since the drainage pathways closed. The procedure of interventriculostomy was reattempted by Leksell in 1949 [130].

Other techniques for shunting cerebrospinal fluid from the third ventricle to the regional subarachnoid cisternae have been described, among them transcallosal ventriculostomy by Lazorthes in 1953 [129], transcallosal shunting by Kluzer and Geuna in 1955 [120] and pericallosal ventriculostomy by Yelin and Ehni in 1969 [246].

Ventriculostomy of the third ventricle seems to be particularly well suited to the treatment of obstructive hydrocephalus, as shown by Guiot et al. in 1968 [70], Forjaz et al. in 1968 [57] and Sayers and Kosnik in 1976 [202]. That procedure was simplified by the introduction of a percutaneous technique with radiographic control, stereotaxis and specially designed instruments, such as the leukotoma.

Sayers and Kosnik achieved a remission rate of 90%–100% in 46 shunt-dependent children [202]. Hoffmann et al employed a stereotactical approach in 22 patients with good results [96, 97].

Ventriculocisternostomy. Ventriculocisternostomy was suggested by Torkildsen in 1939 for the treatment of obstructive hydrocephalus [92, 225]. He inserted a rubber tube with a freely floating end into the posterior horn of the lateral ventricle. The opposite end was attached to the posterior cisternal wall, taking care to connect the subarachnoid space and not the subdural space with the lateral ventricle. When both foramina of Monro are obstructed, Torkildsen recommended bilateral ventriculocisternostomy [225] (Fig. 9).

Hyndman suggested another technique of ventriculocisternostomy in 1946, recommending it for the treatment of both congenital and acquired hydrocephalus [99]. He established a shunt from the ventricles to the cisternal vv. parvae. This technique was modified by Strewler in 1948 [55], Graf and Hamby in 1957 [67], Matson in 1949 [141] and Ehni in 1976 [44].

Nosik described a simple variant of ventriculomastoidostomy in 1950, advancing a small catheter from the ventricles to the tympanum, which resulted in a flow of cerebrospinal fluid to the pharynx via the auditory tube [157].

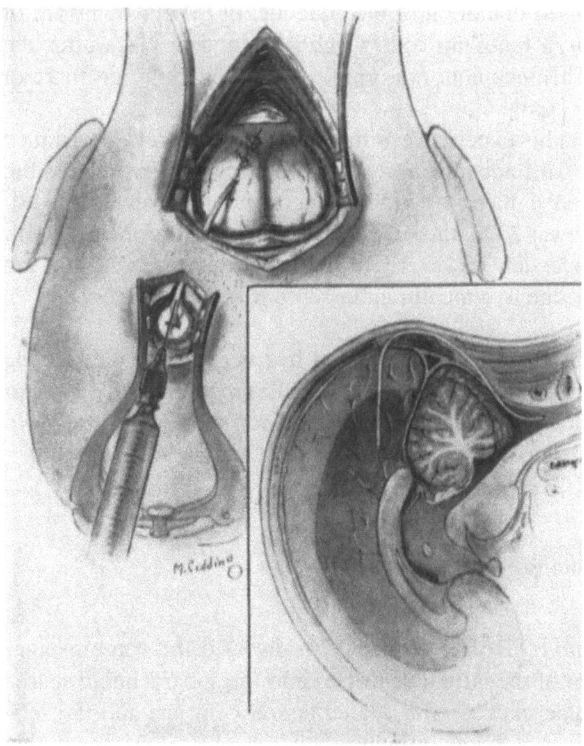

Fig. 9. Ventriculocisternostomy according to Torkildsen [142a]

Choroid Plexus Operations. Techniques implementing the choroid plexis are grounded in the belief that this structure is mainly responsible for the production of the cerebrospinal fluid. Lespinasse, a urologist, coagulated the choroid plexus for the first time by means of a surgical cystoscope in 1910 [39]. Dandy advised this technique as well in 1922; however, his clinical trial was a failure [30].

In the years to follow, Putnam (1934, 1943), Stookey and Scarff (1936) and Scarff (1963, 1970) reported coagulation of the choroid plexus by means of a ventriculoscope [179, 181, 218, 203, 204]. This technique was frequently employed by neurosurgeons up to the 1950s.

Operative removal of the choroid plexus was attempted by Dandy in 1918 and 1945 [32, 36]. Further reports were given by Hildebrand in 1923 [94], Laewan in 1922 [124], Putnam in 1935 [180], Dandy in 1938 [33] and Klein in 1957 [119]. Success was only sporadic with this method, and the mortality rate was high. The failure of these methods is explained by the fact that the cerebrospinal fluid is not produced mainly by the choroid plexus [10, 221, 222].

Canalization of the Aqueduct of Sylvius. Dandy reported dilating the aqueduct of Sylvius in 1920 by means of a metal probe and thereafter inserted a rubber catheter which permitted flow of the cerebrospinal fluid for 2–3 weeks [34, 48]. Two patients were treated in this manner, one of whom did well for a year, while the other child died of pneumonia 7 weeks after surgery.

Leksell (1949) also advised dilatation of the aqueduct of Sylvius by means of a rubber catheter wired by a tantalum coil, which remained in place after the catheter was withdrawn. This technique was employed on ten children, three of whom died postoperatively [130].

Elvidge reported in 1966 his experience with interventriculostomy performed on ten adults and children with aqueductal stenosis, in which he first dilated the aqueduct and then inserted a piece of rubber, tygon or a portex tube [48]. Whereas surgical mortality was 20%, the survivors had no shunt problems at all. This technique was controversial, however, since it was later revealed that the aqueductal obstruction was due to a membranous septum and not stenosis.

Other Operative Techniques. Parkin (1893) treated hydrocephalus by dissecting adhesions in the region of the posterior fossa [165]. Stiles recommended ligation of both carotid arteries in 1896 in order to reduce the blood supply to the choroid plexus [217]. This procedure was also used by Fraser and Dott in 1922–1923 [60].

Modern Experimental Methods

Ventriculosubarachnoid Shunts. DeFoe et al. (1976) diverted the cerebrospinal fluid from the anterior horn of the lateral ventricles into the subarachnoid space. They thus established fistulae between the dilated lateral ventricle and the subarachnoid space above in dogs with kaolin-induced hydrocephalus. Although this method seems to be promising, clinical application has not yet been attempted [40].

A similar technique was employed by Wong et al. in 1979 on monkeys [241]. Specially designed catheters connect the ventricles and the subarachnoid space. Radioisotope examinations confirmed the absorption of cerebrospinal fluid.

Omental Transplantation. By means of microsurgical techniques, Yasargil and Yonekawa et al. (1974, 1977) transplanted the major omentum in dogs to achieve revascularisation of the brain and absorption of cerebrospinal fluid [245, 248]. They tested the absorption capacity of the omentum and the possibility of using it to treat cerebral ischemia.

Significant advances have been made in our knowledge of physiology and the hydrodynamics of cerebrospinal fluid circulation, in the introduction of new materials, valve systems, and improved diagnostic techniques such as radioisotope cisternography or computerized axial tomography, as well as in the improvement of pre- and postoperative care. Yet, at the end of the twentieth century we are still far from a definite solution of many problems affecting hydrocephalic patients. As long as therapy is merely symptomatic, without taking into account the causes of the disorder and depends on foreign materials and mechanical devices, therapy of hydrocephalus will remain problematic, as shown by the high complication rate.

Summary

From early days on physicians took interest in hydrocephaly because of its grotesque appearance. Already Hippocrates recommended decompression-trepanation for the treatment of hydrocephalus. Only since anatomy and pathophysiology of hydrocephalus as well as production and absorption of the cerebrospinal fluid was clarified, more effetive operative techniques could be developed. Conservative treatment was unsuccessful or was useful only as temporary or adjuvant therapy supporting surgical procedures. A great variety of operative methods was described since the middle of 19th century which yielded, however, unsatisfactory results in most instances. Results improved since the introduction of effective valve systems in combination with ventriculoatrial and ventriculoperitoneal shunts. Despite of improved results, the treatment of hydrocephalus remains problematic as is shown by the still high complication rate and the restless search for more effective ways of treatment.

Résumé

L'hydrocéphalie a depuis toujours attiré l'attention des médecins, et Hippocrate recommandait déjà de procédér à une trépanation pour apporter un certain soulagement. Il a toutefois fallu d'abord avoir des connaissances plus approfondies en anatomie et physiopathologie et avoir éclairci le mécanisme de l'accumulation du liquide céphalorachidien et de sa résorption pour mettre au point une technique d'opération. Un traitement non-chirurgical, seul, n'a jamais donné satisfaction et doit toujours être accompagné d'un traitement chirurgical. Il existe un grand nombre de techniques opératives depuis la seconde moitié du XIXe siècle mais la plupart n'ont pas été couronnées de succès. Les résultats s'améliorèrent quand on parvint à mettre en place un système de dérivation par valve associé à une ventriculo-atriostomie et une ventriculo-opéritonéostomie. Les résultats sont meilleurs mais le traitement des hydrocéphalies ne donne toujours pas entière satisfaction. Les complications post-opératoires sont encore trop nombreuses et un traitement plus efficace reste à trouver.

Zusammenfassung

Der Hydrozephalus fand wegen seines grotesken Aussehens von alters her das Interesse der Mediziner. Schon Hippokrates empfahl die Entlastungstrepanation als Therapie. Erst durch Klärung der Anatomie und Pathophysiologie des Hydrozephalus sowie der Liquorproduktion und -absorption konnten wirksamere Operationsmethoden entwickelt werden. Die konservativen Therapieversuche waren erfolglos oder konnten nur temporär und adjuvant zu operativen Verfahren eingesetzt werden. Eine Vielfalt von Operationstechniken wurde seit der Mitte des 19. Jahrhunderts beschrieben, die jedoch meist keine guten Erfolge brachten. Erst mit Einführung wirksamer Ventilsysteme Ende der 50er Jahre in Kombination mit ventrikuloatrialen und ventrikuloperitonealen Ableitungen wurden die Ergebnisse besser. Die Behandlung des Hydrozephalus bleibt trotz dieser Verbesserungen problematisch, wie die noch hohe Komplikationsrate und die fortdauernde Suche nach wirksameren Verfahren zeigen.

References

1. Adams RD, Fisher CM, Hakim S, Ojemann RG, Sweet WH (1965) Symptomatic occult hydrocephalus with "normal" cerebrospinal fluid pressure: a treatable syndrome. N Engl J Med 273:117
2. Alther E (1965) Das Magenventil: eine neue Operationsmethode zur Behandlung des kindlichen Hydrocephalus. Schweiz Med Wochenschr 95:234
3. Ames A, Higashi K, Nesbett FB (1965) Effects of pCO_2 acetazolamide and onabain on volume and composition of choroid plexus fluid. J Physiol (Lond) 181:516
4. Anton, Von Bramann (1908) Balkenstich bei Hydrocephalien, Tumoren und Epilepsie. Münch Med Wochenschr 55:1673
5. Atkinson JR, Ward AA Jr (1958) The effect of diamox on intracranial pressure and blood volume. Neurology 8:45
6. Barnard JF (1838) Compression in chronic hydrocephalus. Lancet I:376
7. Becker DP, Nulsen FE (1968) Control of hydrocephalus by valve-regulated venous shunt: avoidance of complications in prolonged shunt maintenance. J Neurosurg 28:215
8. Bergmann E von (1907) Verletzungen und Krankheiten des Gehirns etc. Angeborene chirurgische Krankheiten. Handbuch der Chirurgie, 3rd edn. Enke, Stuttgart, vol 1, p 154
9. Bergmann E von (1899) Die chirurgische Behandlung von Hirnkrankheiten, 2nd edn. Hirschwald, Berlin

10. Bering EA Jr, Sato O (1965) Hydrocephalus: changes in formation and absorption of cerebrospinal fluid within the cerebral ventricles. J Neurosurg 20:1050
11. Bettex M, Genton N, Stockmann M (1982) Kinderchirurgie. In: Kaiser G (ed) Hydrocephalus. Thieme, Stuttgart, pp 2.52–2.71
12. Bilhaut (1894) Traitement chirurgical de l'hydrocéphalie. Rev Chir (Paris) 14:920
13. Birzis L, Carter CH, Maren TH (1958) The effect of acetazolamide on CSF pressure and electrolytes in hydrocephalus. Neurology 8:522
14. Blane G (1821) On the effect of mechanical compression of the head, as a preventive and cure in certain cases of hydrocephalus. Med Physiol (Lond) 46:353
15. Boinet AA (1856) De l'alimentation iodée comme moyen préventif et curatif dans toutes les maladies où l'iode est employé à l'interview comme médicament. Masson, Paris, p 24
16. Broca A (1891) Drainage des ventricules cérébraux pour hydrocéphalie. Rev Chir (Paris) 11:37
17. Bucy PC (1950) In: MacQuarrie J (ed) Brennemann's practice of pediatrics. Prior, Hagerstown, vol 4, chap 3
18. Cassel (1897) Discussion remark. Dtsch Med Wochenschr 23:231
19. Chater G (1845) Case of hydrocephalus; treatment by puncture and seton; autopsy. Prov Med Surg J 599–602
20. Chipault A (1894–95) Chirurgie opérative du système nerveux. Rueff, Paris, vol 1, p 734, vol 2, pp 1–799
21. Cone WF, Lewis RD, Jackson IJ (1949) Shunting of cerebrospinal fluid into the peritoneal cavity. Presented at the meeting of the American College of Physicians, Montreal, Canada
22. Cotugno D (1762) De ischiade nervosa commentarius. Simoniana, Naples
23. Cushing H, Weed LH, Wegefath (1914) Studies on the cerebrospinal fluid and its pathology. J Med Res 31:1
24. Cushing H (1905) The special field of neurological surgery. Cleve Med J 4:1
25. Cushing H (1926) Studies in intracranial physiology and surgery. Oxford University Press, London
26. Dandy WE, Blackfan I, Kenneth D (1914) Hydrocephalus internus. Eine experimentelle klinische und pathologische Untersuchung. Bruns Beitr Klin Chir 93:392
27. Dandy WE, Blackfan I, Kenneth D (1914) Internal hydrocephalus. An experimental, clinical and pathological study. Am J Dis Child 8:406
28. Dandy WE (1919) Experimental hydrocephalus. Ann Surg 70:129
29. Dandy WE (1921) The diagnosis and treatment of hydrocephalus due to occlusions of the foramina of Magendie and Luschka. Surg Gynecol Obstet 32:112
30. Dandy WE (1922) An operative procedure for hydrocephalus. Bull John Hopkins Hosp 33:189
31. Dandy WE, Blackfan I, Kenneth D (1913) An experimental and clinical study of internal hydrocephalus. JAMA 61:2216
32. Dandy WE (1918) Exstirpation of the choroid plexus of the lateral ventricles in communicating hydrocephalus. Ann Surg 37:569
33. Dandy WE (1938) The operative treatment of communicating hydrocephalus. Ann Surg 108:194
34. Dandy WE (1920) The diagnosis and treatment of hydrocephalus resulting from strictures of the aqueduct of Sylvius. Surg Gynecol Obstet 31:340
35. Dandy WE (1932) Surgery of the brain. In: Lewis D (ed) Lewis' practice of surgery. Prior, Hagerstown, pp 1–682
36. Dandy WE (1945) Diagnosis and treatment of strictures of the aqueduct of Sylvius (causing hydrocephalus). Arch Surg 51:1
37. Davidoff LM (1929) Treatment of hydrocephalus: historical review and description of a new method. Arch Surg 18:1737
38. Davidson RJ (1976) Peritoneal bypass in the treatment of hydrocephalus: historical review and abdominal complications. J Neurol Neurosurg Psychiatry 39:640
39. Davis I (1939) Neurological surgery. Lea and Febiger, Philadelphia, p 429
40. DeFoe D, Foltz E, Lederhaus S (1976) Hydrocephalus: possible role of an internal cerebrospinal fluid fistula in therapy. Surg Neurol 6:271

41. Demme H (1956) Der Liquor. Fortschr Neurol 24:113
42. Dodge HW, Remine WH, Leavens MD (1957) The treatment of hydrocephalus by spinal subarachnoid-omental bursa shunt. Minn Med 40:227
43. Duff TA, Rosenthal J, Jane JA (1977) Evaluation and revision of ventriculo-gastric shunts by gastrostomy. Neurochirurgia (Stuttg) 20:28
44. Ehni G (1976) Torkildsen's ventriculocisternostomy: some complications and their prevention. Clin Neurol Neurosurg 79:119
45. Ehni G (1953) Lumbar subarachnoid-peritoneal and -ureteral shunts. A simple method of implantation of the spinal end of the catheter. Meeting of the neurosurgical society of America, London
46. Eisenbrey AB (1975) The zig-zag tube in the treatment of hydrocephalus. Surg Neurol 3:21
47. El Shafei IL (1975) Ventriculo-venous shunt to the proximal segment of an occluded neck vein: a new method for the shunting of cerebrospinal fluid to the venous circulation. Surg Neurol 3:237
48. Elvidge AR (1966) Treatment of obstructive lesions of the aqueduct of Sylvius and the fourth ventricle by interventriculostomy. J Neurosurg 24:11
49. Enderlen E (1911) Zur Behandlung des Hydrocephalus. Beitr Klin Chir 76:889
50. Epstein M, Hydrocephalus. Progr Pediatr Surg
51. Erasistratus (1823) In medicorum graecorum opera quae extant. In: Kühn DCG (ed). Cnoblochius, Leipzig, vol 5, p 914. Cited in Walker AE (1967)
52. Fabricius Hildanus G (1646) Observationum et curationum medico-chirurgicarum. Opera quae extant omnia. Beueri, Frankfurt, pp 112, 1044, 104
53. Faivre (1854) Recherches sur la structure du conarium et des plexus chorioides chez l'homme et les animaux. Compt Rend Acad Sci 39:424
54. Ferguson AH (1898) Intraperitoneal diversion of the cerebrospinal fluid in cases of hydrocephalus. NY Med J I 67:902
55. Fincher EF, Strewler GJ, Swanson HS (1948) The Torkildsen procedure: a report of 19 cases. J Neurosurg 5:213
56. Foltz EL, Shurtleff DB (1966) Conversion of communicating hydrocephalus to stenosis or occlusion of the aqueduct during ventricular shunt. J Neurosurg 24:520
57. Forjatz S, Martinelli N, Latuf N (1968) Hypothalamic ventriculostomy with catheter. J Neurosurg 29:655
58. Forrest DM, Laurence KM, Macnab GH (1957) Ventriculosubdural drainage in infantile hydrocephalus. Selection of patients by subdural dye excretion test. Lancet II:827
59. Forrest DM, Laurence KM, Macnab GH (1957) Ventriculosubdural drainage in infantile hydrocephalus: analysis of early results. Lancet II:1274
60. Fraser J, Dott NM (1922–23) Hydrocephalus. Trans Med Chir Soc Edinburgh 102:1
61. Frazier CH (1916) Types of hydrocephalus, their differentiation and treatment. Am J Dis Child 11:95
62. Gärtner (1895) Discussionsbemerkung. 67. Naturforscherversammlung, Lübeck, part 2, sect 2, p 146
63. Galen. In: Baillière JB (ed) Oeuvres anatomiques, physiologiques et médicales de Galien. Daremberg, Paris, cited in Walker AE (1967) [Ref 231]
64. George R, Leibrock L, Epstein M (1979) Long-term analysis of cerebro-spinal fluid shunt infections. J Neurosurg 51:804
65. Gerlach J, Jensen H-P, Koos W, Kraus H (1967) Frühkindlicher Hydrocephalus. In: Pädiatrische Neurochirurgie. Thieme, Stuttgart, pp 296–339
66. Girdlestone T, Costerton C (1822) On the benefit arising from pressure applied to the head in certain cases of hydrocephalus. Med Physiol J 47:183
67. Graf CJ, Hamby WB (1957) A modification of Torkildsen's ventriculostomy. J Neurosurg 14:470
68. Grantham J (1854) A case of hydrocephalus externus treated with repeated puncturing and the seton. Med Times Gaz 9:110
69. Greatwood H (1829) Hydrocephalus cured by puncture. Lancet II:238
70. Guiot G, Derome P, Hertzog E, Bomberger C, Akerman M (1968) Ventriculocisternostomie sous contrôle radioscopique pour hydrocephalie obstructive. Presse Med 76(40):1823

71. Guleke N (1930) Über die Entstehung des Hydrocephalus internus. Arch Klin Chir 162:533
72. Gupta SM (1950) New surgical treatment for idiopathic hydrocephalus. Indian J Med Sci 4:85
73. Haller A (1762) Elementa physiologiae corporis humani. Grasset, Lausanne, vol 4, p 596. Cited in Dandy WE [Ref 28]
74. Hakim S, Jimenez A, Rosas F (1955) Drainage of cerebrospinal fluid into the spinal epidural space. Acta Neurochir (Wien) 4:224
75. Hakim S (1953) Hidrocefalia en el adulto conpresión "normal" del L.C.R. Hospital Militar, Bogotà
76. Hakim S (1964) Some observations on CSF-pressure. Hydrocephalic syndrome in adults with "normal" CSF-pressure (recognition of a new syndrome). Thesis No 957, Javeriana University, School of Medicine, Bogotà, Colombia
77. Hakim S, Adams RD (1965) The special clinical problem of symptomatic hydrocephalus. J Neurol Sci 2:307
78. Harsh GR (1954) Peritoneal shunt for hydrocephalus utilizing the fimbria of the Fallopian tube for entrance to the peritoneal cavity. J Neurosurg 11:284
79. Hassin GB (1930) Hydrocephalus. Studies on the pathology and pathogenesis, with remarks on the cerebrospinal fluid. Arch Neurol Psychiatr 24:1164
80. Hayden T (1856) Hydrocephalus in which paracentesis was repeatedly performed and a solution of iodine injected. Dublin Hosp Gaz 3:168
81. Haynes JS (1913) Congenital internal hydrocephalus: its treatment by drainage of the cisterna magna into the cranial sinuses. Ann Surg 57:449
82. Haynes JS (1916) Further experiences in the treatment of hydrocephalus by cisterna-sinus drainage (author's operation). NY State J Med 16:174
83. Heile B (1910) Zur chirurgischen Behandlung der Spina bifida mit Hydrocephalus. Berl Klin Wochenschr 47:2298
84. Heile B (1908) Zur Behandlung des Hydrocephalus. Dtsch Med Wochenschr 34:1468
85. Heile B (1914) Zur chirurgischen Behandlung des Hydrocephalus internus durch Ableitung der Cerebrospinalflüssigkeit nach der Bauchhöhle und nach der Pleurakuppe. Arch Klin Chir 105:501
86. Heile B (1925) Über neue operative Wege zur Druckentlastung bei angeborenem Hydrocephalus (Ureter-Duraanastomose). Zentralbl Chir 52:2229
87. Heile B (1927) Zur Behandlung des Hydrocephalus mit Ureter-Duraanastomose. Zentralbl Chir 54:1859
88. Heller J (1892) Ein Fall von chronischem Hydrocephalus bei hereditärer Syphilis. Dtsch Med Wochenschr 18:608
89. Heller J (1898) Weitere Mitteilungen über einen Fall von chronischem Hydrocephalus bei hereditärer Syphilis. Dtsch Med Wochenschr 24:74
90. Hemmer R (1952) Der Hydrocephalus: III. Therapie des Hydrocephalus. Zentralbl Neurochir 12:108
91. Hemmer R (1964) Erfahrungen mit der modernen operativen Hydrocephalusbehandlung. Enke, Stuttgart, p 64
92. Herlin L (1950) Ventriculosternostomy according to Torkildsen. A report of 22 cases. J Neurosurg 7:403
93. Herophile (1822) In medicorum graecorum opera quae extant. In: Kühn DCG (ed). Cnoblochius, Leipzig, vol 3, p 939. Cited in Walker AE (1967)
94. Hildebrand O (1923) Eine neue Operationsmethode zur Behandlung der durch Tumorschädel bedingten Sehnervenatrophie. Arch Klin Chir 124:199
95. Hippocrate (1953) Oeuvres complètes d'Hippocrate. Baillière, Paris, vol 8:40, p 676. Cited in Walker AE (1967)
96. Hoffman HJ, Hendrick EB, Humphreys RP (1976) Metastasis via ventriculoperitoneal shunt in patients with hydrocephalus. J Neurosurg 44:562
97. Hoffman HJ, Harwood-Nash D, Gilday DL (to be published) Percutaneous third ventriculostomy in the management of noncommunicating hydrocephalus. Neurosurgery
98. Hooper R (1969) A lengthening procedure for ventriculoatrial shunts. J Neurosurg 30:93
99. Hyndman OR (1946) Hydrocephalus: a contribution related to treatment. J Neurosurg 3:426

100. Ignelzi RJ, Kirsch WM (1975) Follow-up analysis of ventriculoperitoneal and ventriculoatrial shunts for hydrocephalus. J Neurosurg 42:679
101. Illingworth CR (1891) Tapping the ventricles. Br Med J 1:755
102. Immerwol (1901) Beitrag zur Heilung des Hydrocephalus. Arch Kinderheilkd 32:329
103. Ingraham FD, Campbell JB (1941) An apparatus for closed drainage of the ventricular system. Ann Surg 114:1096
104. Ingraham FD, Matson DD, Alexander E Jr, Woods RP (1948) Studies in the treatment of experimental hydrocephalus. J Neuropathol Exp Neurol 7:123
105. Ingraham FD, Sears RA, Woods RP, Bailey OT (1949) Further studies on the treatment of experimental hydrocephalus: attempts to drain the cerebrospinal fluid into the pleural cavity and the thoracic duct. J Neurosurg 6:207
106. Jackson JJ (1951) A review of the surgical treatment of internal hydrocephalus. J Pediatr 38:1
107. Jackson JJ, Snodgrass SR (1955) Peritoneal shunts in the treatment of hydrocephalus and increased intracranial pressure: a 4-year-survey of 62 patients. J Neurosurg 12:216
108. Jackson JJ, Thompson RK (1959) Pediatric neurosurgery. Thomas, Springfield, Ill, pp 143–165
109. Jaques S, Shelden Ch, Pudenz RH, Fort J (1978) Microsurgical cannulation of the thoracic duct in cats. J Immunol Methods 21:383
110. Kahn EA, Luros JT (1952) Hydrocephalus from overproduction of cerebrospinal fluid (and experiences with other papillomas of the choroid plexus). J Neurosurg 9:59
111. Katzman R, Pappius HM (1973) Brain electrolytes and fluid metabolism. Williams and Wilkins, Baltimore, pp 14–32
112. Kausch W (1908) Die Behandlung des Hydrocephalus der kleinen Kinder. Arch Klin Chir 87:709
113. Keen WW (1888) Exploratory trephining and puncture of the brain almost to the lateral ventricle, for intracranial pressure supposed to be due to an abscess in the temporosphenoidal lobe: temporary improvement; death on the fifth day; autopsy; meningitis with effusion into the ventricles, with a description of a proposed operation to tap and drain the ventricles as a definite surgical procedure. Med News 53:603
114. Keen WW (1891) Tapping the ventricles. Br Med J 1:486
115. Keen WW (1891) Surgery of the lateral ventricles of the brain. Verhandlungen, 10th Int med Congr III Chirurg, Berlin
116. Kempe LG, Blaylock R (1977) Ventriculolymphatic shunt. J Neurosurg 47:86
117. Keucher TR, Mealey J Jr (1979) Long-term results after ventriculoatrial and ventriculoperitoneal shunting for infantile hydrocephalus. J Neurosurg 50:179
118. Key EAH, Retzius MG (1872) Studier i nervsystemets anatomi. Norstedt and Soneo, Stockholm, p 68
119. Klein MR (1957) L'hydrocéphalie du nourisson. Etude clinique et traitement. Marson, Paris
120. Kluzer G, Geuna E (1959) Considerazoni sul trattamento palliativo dell' idrocefalo da occlusione tumorale del terzo ventricolo: indicazioni della ventriculocisternostomia diretta transcallosa posteriore. Minerva Chir 10:681
121. Krause F, Heymann E (1917) Textbook of surgical operations, illustrated by clinical observations for physicians and students. Rebmann, New York, vol 2, p 715
122. Kuettner H (1921) Hydrocephalus congenitus. II. Chirurgie des Gehirns. In: Handbuch der praktischen Chirurgie, 5th edn. Enke, Stuttgart
123. Kuwana N, Kuwabara T, Hosoda H (1977) A new technique for lumbar subarachnoid peritoneal shunting for communicating hydrocephalus. Yokohama Med Bull 28:3
124. Laewen A (1922) Über Operationen an den Plexus chorioidie der Seitenventrikel und über offene Fensterung des Balkens bei Hydrocephalus internus. Beitr Klin Chir 125:1
125. Lamesch AJ (1972) Ventriculogastrostomy by means of a gastric tube for the treatment of hydrocephalus: a preliminary report. J Pediatr Surg 7:55
126. Laurence KM (1958) The natural history of hydrocephalus. Lancet II:1152
127. Laurence KM, Coates S (1962) The natural history of hydrocephalus: detailed analysis of 182 unoperated cases. Arch Dis Child 37:345

128. Laurence KM, Coates S (1962) Further thoughts on the natural history of hydrocephalus. Dev Med Child Neurol 4:263
129. Lazorthes G (1953) La ventriculocisternotomie transcalleuse (technique nouvelle pour hydrocéphalie obstructive). Presse Med 61:1210
130. Leksell L (1949) A surgical procedure for atresia of the aqueduct of Sylvius. Acta Psychiatr Neurol Scand 24:559
131. Little JR, Rhoton AL Jr, Mellinger JF (1972) Comparison of ventriculoperitoneal and ventriculoatrial shunts for hydrocephalus in children. Mayo Clin Proc 47:396
132. Lorber J (1971) Medical and surgical aspects in the treatment of congenital hydrocephalus. Neuropediatrics 2:239
133. Luschka H von (1851) Die Struktur der serösen Häute des Menschen. Laupp and Siebeck, Tübingen, p 98
134. Luschka H von (1855) Die Adergeflechte des menschlichen Gehirns. Reimer, Berlin
135. McCarty CS, Pratt JH, Ewert JC (1957) Congenital communicating hydrocephalus: treatment by subarachnoid-fallopian tube peritoneal shunt for a patient with unusually high intelligence. Proc Staff Meet Mayo Clin 32:23
136. McClure RD (1909) Hydrocephalus treated by drainage into a vein of the neck. Johns Hopkins Hosp Bull 20:110
137. McCullogh DC, Fox JL (1974) Negative intracranial pressure hydrocephalus in adults with shunts and its relationship to the production of subdural hematoma. J Neurosurg 40:372
138. Magendie F (1842) Recherches philosophiques et cliniques sur le liquide céphalorachidien ou cérébro-spinal. Méquinon, Paris, p 40
139. Magendie F (1825) Mémoire sur le liquide qui se trouve dans le crâne et l'épine de l'homme et des animaux vertébraux. J Physiol Exp 5:27
140. Mariott WM (1924) The use of theobromin-sodio-salicylate (Diuretin) in the treatment of hydrocephalus. Am J Dis Child 28:479
141. Matson DD (1949) New operation for the treatment of communicating hydrocephalus: report of a case secondary to generalized meningitis. J Neurosurg 6:238
142. Matson DD (1956) Current treatment of infantile hydrocephalus. N Engl J Med 255:933
142a. Matson DD (1969) Neurosurgery in infancy and childhood. Thomas, Springfield
143. Miculicz J (1896) Beitrag zur Pathologie und Therapie des Hydrocephalus. Mitt Grenzgeb Med Chir 1:264
144. Milhorat TH (1976) Structures and function of the choroid plexus and other sites of cerebrospinal fluid formation. In: Bourne GH, Danielli JF (eds) International review of cytology. Academic, New York, vol 47, pp 225–288
145. Mixter WJ (1923) Ventriculoscopy and puncture of the floor of the third ventricle: preliminary report of a case. Boston Med Surg J 188:277
146. Monro A (1783) Observations of the structure and functions of the nervous system. Creech-Johnson, Edinburgh, p 176
147. Monro D (1755) An essay of the dropsy and its different species. Wilson and Durham, London, p 170
148. Morgagni GB (1769) The seats and causes of diseases investigated by anatomy: in five books, containing a great variety of dissections, with remarks. Miller, Cadell, Johnson and Payne, London, vol 1, p 868
149. Mundinger F (1960) Die intraventrikuläre Injektion basischer Vitalfarbstoffe als neue Methode zur Behandlung des frühkindlichen Hydrocephalus hypersecretorius communicans. Arch Psychiatr Nervenkr 200:462
150. Murtagh F, Lehman R (1967) Peritoneal shunts in the management of hydrocephalus. JAMA 202:1010
151. Neumann CG, Hoen TL, Davis DA (1959) The adaptation of ileo-eutectrophy to the control of congenital communicating hydrocephalus. Plast Reconstr Surg 23:159
152. Neumann CG, Richman H, Aridizone R (1959) Reconstructive surgery for hydrocephalus: anastomosis of an isolated ileal segment to the lumbar subarachnoid space (modified ileo-eutectropy). Surg Clin North Am 39:491
153. Neumann H (1901) Ein Fall von geheiltem Wasserkopf. Dtsch Med Wochenschr 27:39
154. Neurath (1898) Die Lumbalpunktion. Zentralbl Grenzgeb Med Chir 1:457

155. Nicoll JH (1905) Case of hydrocephalus in which peritoneo-meningeal drainage has been carried out. Glasgow Med J 63:187
156. Nölke (1897) Beobachtungen zur Pathologie des Hirndruckes. Dtsch Med Wochenschr 23:618
157. Nosik WA (1950) Ventriculomastoidostomy: technique and observations. J Neurosurg 7:236
158. Nugent GR, Lucas R, Judy M, Bloor BM, Warden H (1966) Thromboembolic complications of ventriculo-atrial shunts. Angiocardiographic and pathologic correlations. J Neurosurg 24:34
159. Nulsen FE, Becker DP (1967) Control of hydrocephalus by valve-regulated shunt: infections and their prevention. Clin Neurosurg 14:256
160. Nulsen FE, Spitz EB (1952) Treatment of hydrocephalus by direct shunt from ventricle to jugular vein. Surg Forum 2:399
161. Olds JM (1962) Surgical drainage of hydrocephalus via the thoracic duct and subclavian vein. Can Med Assoc J 86:696
162. Oribasius (1851–76) Oeuvres d'Oribase. Baillière, Paris. Cited in Walker AE (1967) [Ref 231]
163. Overton MC, Snodgrass SR, Derrick JR (1965) Direct atrial and vena caval shunting procedures for hydrocephalus. Surg Gynecol Obstet 124:819
164. Pampus F (1953) Zur Technik der Ventrikeldrainage. Zentralbl Neurochir 13:219
165. Parkin A (1893) The relief of intracranial pressure by the withdrawal of cerebrospinal fluid from the basal subarachnoid cavity. Lancet II:21
166. Paul of Aegina: The seven books of Paulus Aegineta. Cited in Walker AE (1967)
167. Payr E (1908) Drainage der Hirnventrikel mittels frei transplantierter Blutgefäße: Bemerkungen über Hydrocephalus. Arch Klin Chir 87:801
168. Payr E (1911) Über Ventrikeldrainage bei Hydrocephalus. Verh Dtsch Ges Chir 40:515
169. Payr E (1919) Elfjähriger Dauererfolg einer Ventrikeldrainage bei Hydrocephalus. Med Klin 49:1247
170. Payr E (1908) Drainage der Hirnventrikel mittels frei transplantierter Blutgefäße. Ref Zentralbl Chir 35
171. Perret GE, Graf CJ (1977) Subgaleal shunt for temporary ventricle decompression and subdural drainage. J Neurosurg 47:590
172. Picaza JA (1956) The posterior-peritoneal shunt technique for the treatment of internal hydrocephalus in infants. J Neurosurg 13:289
173. Pilcz A (1899) Die Behandlung des Hydrocephalus. Zentralbl Grenzgeb Med Chir 2:681
174. Pollay M (1977) Review of spinal fluid physiology: production and absorption in relation to pressure. Clin Neurosurg 24:254
175. Portnoy HD, Schulte RR, Fox JL, Croisaant P, Tripp L (1973) Antisiphon and reversible occlusion valves for shunting in hydrocephalus and preventing post-shunt subdural hematomas. J Neurosurg 38:729
176. Pudenz RH (1981) The surgical treatment of hydrocephalus – an historical review. Surg Neurol 15:15
177. Pudenz RH (1961) The surgical treatment of infantile hydrocephalus. In: Disorders of the developing nervous system. Proceedings of the Houston Neurological Society. Thomas, Springfield, pp 486–489
178. Pudenz RH (1958) Experimental and clinical observations on the shunting of cerebrospinal fluid into the circulatory system. In: Clinical neurosurgery. Congress of neurological surgeons. Williams and Wilkins, Baltimore, pp 98–115
179. Putnam TJ (1943) The surgical treatment of infantile hydrocephalus. Surg Gynecol Obstet 76:171
180. Putnam TJ (1935) Results of the treatment of hydrocephalus by endoscopic coagulation of the choroid plexus. Arch Pediatr 52:676
181. Putnam TJ (1934) Treatment of hydrocephalus by endoscopic coagulation of the choroid plexus: description of a new instrument and preliminary report of results. N Engl J Med 210:1373

182. Quin CW (1790) A treatise on the dropsy of the brain, illustrated by a variety of cases to which are added observations of the use and effects of the digitalis purpurea in dropsies. Murray, London, p 227
183. Quincke H (1891) Die Lumbalpunktion des Hydrocephalus. Berl Klin Wochenschr 28: 929–933, 965–968
184. Radionowa (1891) Ein Fall von spontaner Heilung eines Hydrocephalus chronicus congenitus. Jahrb Kinderheilkd 32:177
185. Raimondi AJ, Matsumoto S (1967) A simplified technique for performing the ventriculoperitoneal shunt: technical note. J Neurosurg 26:357
186. Von Ranke (1895) Jodinjection in den Gehirnventrikel bei einem 10 Monate alten, an fortgeschrittenem Hydrocephalus chron. int. leidendem Kinde. Jahrb Kinderheilkd 39:359
187. Ransohoff J, Shulman K, Fishman RA (1960) Hydrocephalus. A review of etiology and treatment. J Pediatr 56:399
188. Ransohoff J (1954) Ventriculo-pleural anastomosis in treatment of midline obstructional neoplasms. J Neurosurg 11:295
189. Rapoport SJ (1975) The blood-brain barrier in physiology and medicine. Raven, New York, pp 43–86
190. Rehn (1886) Über einfache chronische Hydrocephalie im ersten Kindesalter. Verh Congr Inn Med 5:489
191. Resnikoff SS (1975) External hydrocephalus caused by cysticercosis treated by subarachnoid-peritoneal anastomosis utilizing the fallopian tube. J Neurosurg 12:520
192. Rhazes (1511) Continens. Ferrari, Lugduni, p 284. Cited in Walker AE (1967)
193. Ricketts BM (1904) Surgery of hydrocephalus: a historic review. Am Med 7:983
194. Rickham PP, Penn JA (1965) The place of the ventriculostomy reservoir in the treatment of myelomeningoceles and hydrocephalus. Dev Med Child Neurol 7:296
195. Riechert T, Umbach W (1960) Die operative Behandlung des Hydrocephalus. In: Krenkel W, Olivecrona H, Tönnis W (eds) Klinik und Behandlung der raumbeengenden intrakraniellen Prozesse. Springer, Berlin Göttingen Heidelberg (Handbuch der Neurochirurgie, vol IV/1)
196. Riechert T (1963) Die Behandlung des Hydrocephalus. Med Welt, pp 771–776
197. Deleted in production
198. Rubenbauer H (1969) Zur atrio-ventrikulären Drainage des kindlichen Hydrocephalus mit dem Spitz-Holter-Ventil. Dissertation, Munich
199. Rubin RC, Henderson ES, Ohmaya AK, Walker MD, Rall DP (1966) The production of cerebro-spinal fluid in man and its modification by acetazolamide. J Neurosurg 25:430
200. Rush B (1809) Medical inquiries and observations: an inquiry into the causes and cure of the internal dropsy of the brain, 3rd edn. Kite and Hopkins, Philadelphia, vol 2, pp 453
201. Russell DS (1949) Observations on the pathology of hydrocephalus. Medical Research Council Special Report Series No 265. His Majesty's Stationery Office, London, p 138
202. Sayers MP, Kosnik EJ (1976) Percutaneous third ventriculostomy: experience and technique. Childs Brain 2:24
203. Scarff JE (1963) Treatment of hydrocephalus: an historical and critical review of methods and results. J Neurol Neurosurg Psychiatr 26:1
204. Scarff JE (1970) The treatment of nonobstructive (communicating) hydrocephalus by endoscopic cauterization of the choroid plexus. J Neurosurg 33:1
205. Scarff JE (1936) Endoscopic treatment of hydrocephalus: description of ventriculoscope and preliminary report of cases. Arch Neurol Psychiatr 35:853
206. Schaltenbrand G, Putnam T (1927) Untersuchungen zum Kreislauf des Liquor cerebrospinalis mit Hilfe intravenöser Fluorescineinspritzungen. Dtsch Z Nervenheilkd 96:123
207. Schulze HE (1956) Die Behandlungsmöglichkeit des Hydrocephalus communis durch intervertebrale Schraubendrainage im Lumbarbereich. Chirurg 27:420
208. Scott M, Wycis HT, Murtagh F, Reyes V (1955) Observations on ventricular and lumbar-subarachnoid peritoneal shunts in hydrocephalus in infants. J Neurosurg 12:165
209. Selman WR, Spetzler RF, Wilson CB, Grollmus JW (1980) Percutaneous lumboperitoneal shunt: review of 130 cases. Neurosurgery 6:255

210. Senn N (1903) Subcutaneous drainage in the surgical treatment of hydrocephalus internus. Alienist Neurol 24:317
211. Senn N (1903) Internal hydrocephalus. Int Clinics 13(1):131
212. Sgalitzer M (1926) Neue Erkenntnisse auf dem Gebiete der Röntgenstrahlenwirkung bei Hirntumoren. Strahlentherapie 22:701
213. Sikkens TB (1957) Traitment de l'hydrocéphalie du nourrison par ventriculo-jugulo-stomie. Neurochirurgie 3:65
214. Smith GW, Moretz WH, Pritchard WL (1959) Ventriculobilliary shunt. A new treatment for hydrocephalus. Surg Forum 9:701
215. Smith JA, Lee RE, Middleton RG (1980) Ventriculoureteral shunt for hydrocephalus without nephrectomy. J Urol 123:224
216. Spetzler R, Wilson CB, Schulte R (1977) Simplified percutaneous lumbo-peritoneal shunting. Surg Neurol 7:25
216a. Stark GD (1977) Spina bifida: problems and management. Blackwell, Oxford
217. Stilles HJ (1896) Contribution to the morbid anatomy and pathogenesis of chronic internal hydrocephalus. Trans Edinburgh Hosp Rep 4:517
218. Stookey B, Scarff JE (1936) Occlusion of the aqueduct of Sylvius by neoplastic and non-neoplastic processes with a rational surgical treatment for relief of the resultant obstructive hydrocephalus. Bull Neurol Inst NY 5:348
219. Sutherland GA, Cheyne WW (1898) The treatment of hydrocephalus by intracranial drainage. Br Med J 2:1155
220. Sutherland GA (1898) Case of chronic hydrocephalus treated by intracranial drainage. Lancet I:791
221. Sweet WH, Locksley HB (1953) Formation, flow and resorption of cerebrospinal fluid in man. Proc Soc Exp Biol Med 84:397
222. Sweet WH, Locksley HB, Brownell GL, Scholl JA, Bowsher DR, Benda P, Stickley EE (1956) The formations, flow and absorptions of cerebrospinal fluid: newer concepts based on studies with isotopes. Res Publ Assoc Nerv Met Dis 34:101
223. Taylor AS (1909) Subdural autodrainage in internal hydrocephalus. J Nerv Ment Dis 36:422
224. Taylor AS (1904) The treatment of chronic internal hydrocephalus by autodrainage. Am J Med Sci 2:255
225. Torkildsen A (1939) A new palliative operation in cases of inoperable occlusion on the Sylvian aqueduct. Acta Chir Scand 82:117
226. Umbach W (1959) Zweckmäßige Verfahren für die Diagnose und Therapie des Hydrocephalus im Kindesalter. Neurochirurgia 2:1
227. Valsalva AM (1741) Joannis Baptistae Morgagni epistolarum anatomicarum duodeviginti ad scripta pertinentium celeberrimi viri Antonii Marie Valsalvae pars altera. Pitterns, Venice, p 319. Cited in Walker AE (1967)
228. Deleted in production
229. Vesalius A (1725) Opera omnia anatomiba et chirurgica. Vivie and Verbeck, Batavorum, vol 1, pp 1611, 572; vol 2, pp 311, 577–1156
230. Voth D, Henn M (1983) Hydrocephalus im frühen Kindesalter. Enke, Stuttgart, chap III/1 (Historischer Überblick über die Behandlungsverfahren des Hydrocephalus internus im Kindesalter)
231. Walker AE (1967) A history of neurological surgery. Facsimile edn (Williams and Wilkins, Baltimore, 1951). Hafner, New York, pp 334–347
232. Wallman LJ, Donaghy P (1958) Experience with epiduroarachnoidostomy. J Maine Med Assoc 49:177
233. Weed LH (1920) The experimental production of internal hydrocephalus. Carnagie Inst Contr Embryol 9:425
234. Weed LH (1922–23) The absorption of cerebrospinal fluid into the venous system. Am J Anat 31:191
235. Weed LH (1914) Studies on cerebrospinal fluid: III. The pathways of escape from the subarachnoid spaces with particular reference to the arachnoid villi. J Med Res 31:51

236. Weed LH (1935) Certain anatomic and physiologic aspects of the cerebrospinal fluid and meninges. Brain 58:383
237. Weinman D, Paul ATS (1967) Ventriculoauriculostomy for infantile hydrocephalus using a direct cardiac approach. J Neurosurg 27:279
238. Weiss MH, Jane JA, Apuzzo MLJ, Heiden JS, Kurze T (1975) Ventriculogastrostomy, an alternate means for CSF diversion: a preliminary study. Bull Los Angeles Neurol Soc 40:140
239. Wernicke C (1881) Lehrbuch der Gehirnkrankheiten für Ärzte und Studierende. Fischer, Berlin, vol 3, pp 253–572
240. Whytt R (1768) Observations on the most frequent species of the hydrocephalus internus: the dropsy of the ventricles of the brain. The Works of Robert Whytt, MD. Balfour, Edinburgh, p 762
241. Wong T, Lee LS, Shen ALY, Huang CJ (1979) A research on ventriculo-subarachnoid shunt. 5th Asian Australien Congress of neurological surgery, Manila, Philippines, Nov 1979
242. Wood JH. Physiology, pharmacology and dynamics of cerebrospinal fluid
243. Wright EM (1978) Transport processes in the formation of cerebrospinal fluid. Rev Physiol Biochem Pharmacol 83:1
244. Yamada H, Funakoshi T, Ando T, Sakai N, Sakata K (1979) Clinical studies on prevention of overdrainage syndrome after ventriculo-peritoneal shunt by use of an antisiphon ball valve. 7th Scientific meeting of the International Society for Paediatric Neurosurgery, Chicago
245. Yasargil MG, Yonekawa Y, Denton J, Piroth D, Benes J (1974) Experimental intracranial transplantation of autogenic omentum majus. J Neurosurg 39:213
246. Yelin FS, Ehni G (1969) Percallosal sump ventriculostomy for shunt-dependent hydrocephalic patient with small ventricles. Case report. J Neurosurg 31:570
247. Yokoyama J, Aoki H, Takebayashi K, Hirai T, Matsumoto T, Fukushima T (1959) Ventriculo-lymphangiostomy: a shunting operation for hydrocephalus to drain cerebrospinal fluid into the thoracic duct. Folia Psychiatr Neurol Jpn 13:305
248. Yonekawa Y, Yasargil MG (1977) Brain vascularization by transplanted omentum: a possible treatment of cerebral ischemia. Neurosurgery 1:256
249. Ziemnowicz S (1950) A new trail of operative treatment of hydrocephalus communicans progressivus. Zentralbl Neurochir 10:11

The History of Colostomy in Childhood*

W. F. Schärli[1]

Until the midnineteenth century, the only forms of anal atresia accessible by perineal operation were those situated low down. Successes with blind puncture by trochar remained a matter of chance, and often peritonitis or perforation of the peritoneal cavity led to fatalities after apparent initial success. Patients with rectal cancer or colonic obstructions inevitably died of ileus. Injuries of the colon were left to follow a natural course and almost invariably resulted in death.

Intestinal Injuries

Nevertheless, a few descriptions of bowel injuries exist in ancient literature. One of the earliest references is found in Judges 3: 19–22, describing an incident in which Ehud stabbed Eglon, king of the Moabites, "and the dirt ran out and he died" [6]. Hippocrates regarded all bowel injuries as fatal, and Celsus left their cure to nature [15]. According to Coelius Aurelianus, in the 4th century B.C., Praxagoras opened the belly of a patient with intestinal obstruction, removed the contents of the bowel, and closed the incision [15]. In 1602, Fabricius Hildanus (1560–1634) described an adolescent whose intestines protruded from the inguina and whose stools were discharged through an intestinal opening (Fig. 1) [24].

Years before, this boy had fallen onto a pile of wood, cutting open his belly and intestines. Laurentius Heister [23] advocated that patients with intestinal wounds not be left untreated, recommending that the perforated bowel instead be stitched and closed or fixed to the abdominal wall (Fig. 2).

Inguinal Colostomy

The earliest proposal for a deliberate colostomy was made in 1710 by Alexis Littré (1658–1726) [27], a renowned anatomist in Paris during the reign of Louis XIV. While present at the autopsy of a child with anal atresia, he explained to the bystanders, who consisted of physicians and medical students: "It would be necessary to make an incision in the abdomen and place the two parts of bowel together after reopening them, or at least to bring the superior part of the bowel to the ab-

* This chapter is based on a lecture given to the Greek Paediatric Association, Chios, 1983

[1] Department of Pediatric Surgery, Children's Hospital, Lucerne, Switzerland

Progress in Pediatric Surgery, Vol. 20
Ed. by P. P. Rickham

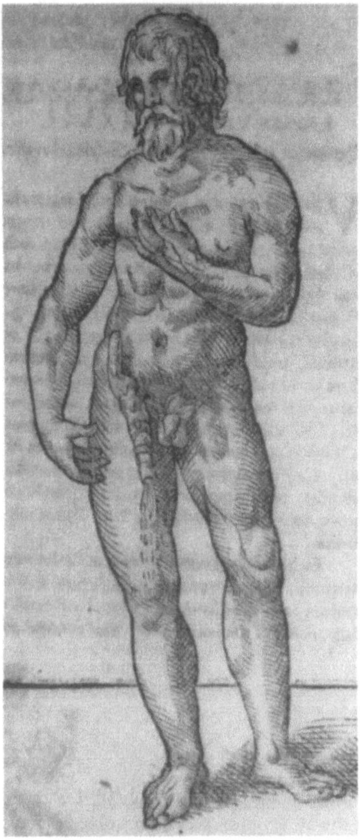

Fig. 1. Fabricius Hildanus described an adolescent who had fallen onto a pile of wood in 1602. The intestines protruded, and the stools were discharged through an intestinal opening [24]

dominal wound, which should never be closed and which would perform the function of the anus."

This excellent idea awaited realization until Pillore [31], a surgeon in Rouen, performed a colostomy 66 years later. In the year 1776, a certain Mr Morel, wine merchant from Vert-Gallant, turned to Pillore because of difficulty in moving bowels due to advanced rectal carcinoma. Purgatives and 2 pounds of mercury had not succeeded in improving Morel's condition. Pillore at last performed a colostomy which was functioning well until the patient died 28 days later of severe gangrene of the ileum, caused by the enormous weight of the mercury that lay in this loop.

The first surgeon who decided to perform a colostomy on a child with anal atresia was Antoine Dubois in the year 1783 [16]. Following Littré's idea, he constructed an inguinal colostomy in the child, who was 3 days old. Unfortunately, the child died on the 10th day. The colostomy was described as functioning and the edges of the wound as healed. A similar, unsuccessful attempt was made by Desault 1 year later on a 2-day-old child with imperforate anus [14]. The child

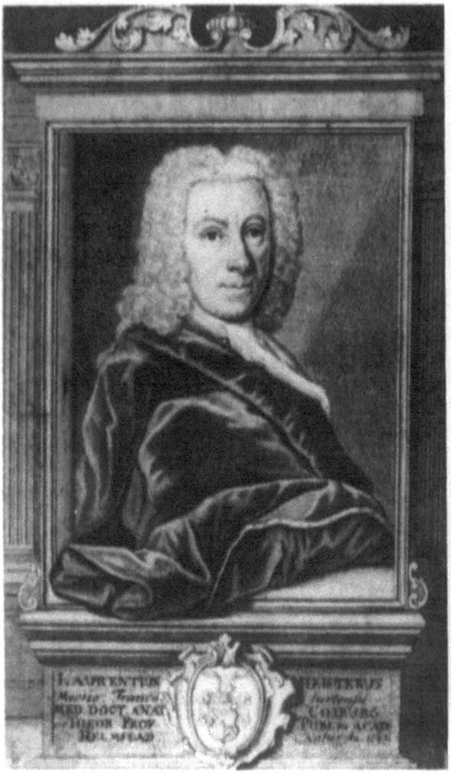

Fig. 2. In 1719, Laurentius Heister recommended that intestinal wounds always be stitched and closed. If this were to prove impossible, he felt they ought to be fixed to the abdominal wall [23]

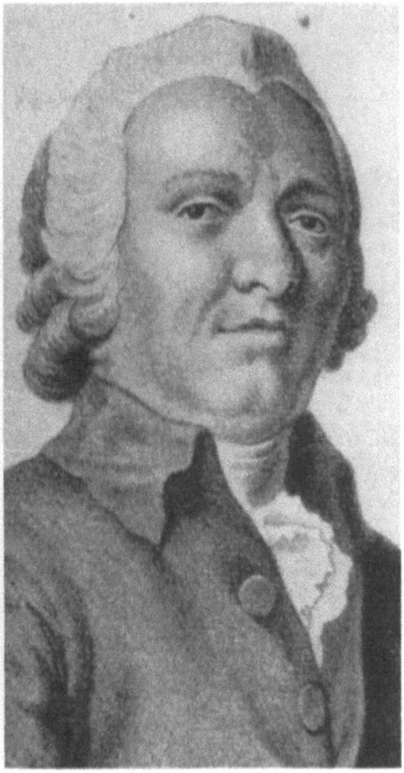

Fig. 3. Pierre Joseph Desault (1744–1795), one of the most famous surgeons of his time, was unsuccessful with Littré's procedure, but modified the operation later [14]

died 4 days later, and the specimen was modelled in wax (Fig. 3). In the hands of Duret [18], however, this procedure was successfully used for the time on a newborn child 10 years later: On October 18, 1793, the wife of Michel Sedrèves in Brales bore a son with imperforate anus. Duret, a ship's surgeon in Brest, decided on a perineal operation, at which the rectum could not be found. Duret then attempted to establish a lumbar colostomy of a cadaver from the poorhouse of Brest. The attempt failed. The next day Duret called all available physicians in Brest together in consultation and ventured an inguinal sigmoidostomy which was declared a complete success. Amussat [2] was able to report that this patient was still living 45 years later.

Up to 1825, this operation was employed in another 11 newborns, seven of these in Brittany. The only successes were noted among the patients of ship's surgeons [3, 28, 30].

Outside of Brittany, however, Littré's operation remained essentially fruitless. The case of Schlagintweit (1826) in Munich was the only one before 1850 in which

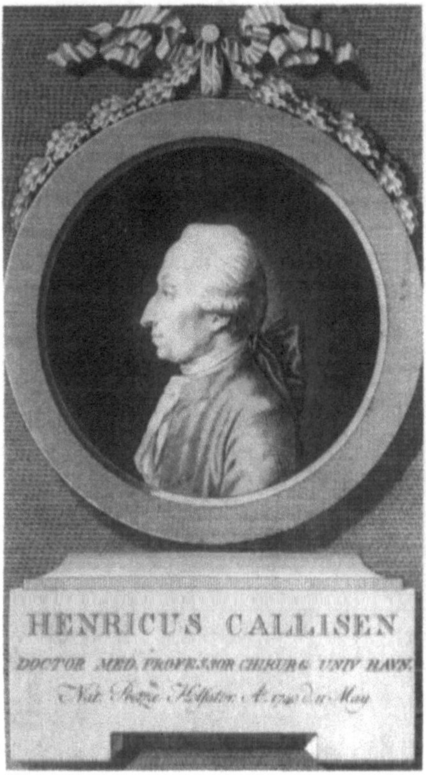

Fig. 4. Henry Callisen (1800) suggested using a retroperitoneal approach to the cecum or descending colon [9]

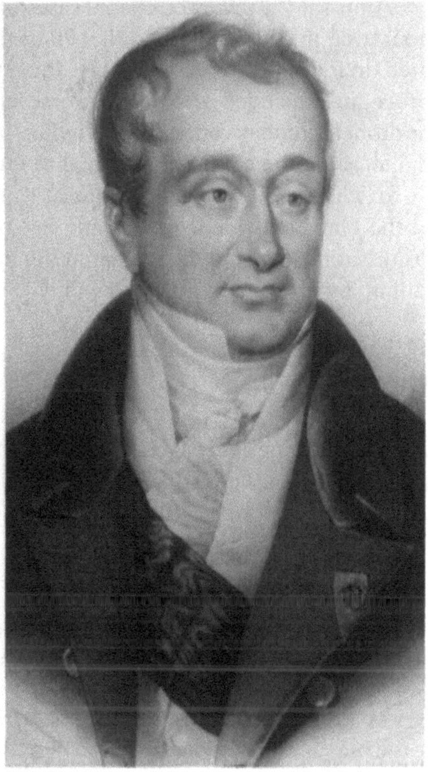

Fig. 5. G. Dupuytren (1778–1835) was one of the eminent proponents of lumbar colostomy [17]

a patient with imperforate anus survived a Littré colostomy. The chief risk of abdominal colostomy was seen to be in the opening of the peritoneum and the subsequent infection [33].

Lumbar Colostomy

In the year 1800, Callisen [9], who was professor of surgery in Copenhagen, suggested approaching the cecum or descending colon from the lumbar area, whenever the rectum could not be reached with either the knife or a trocar (Fig. 4). It is not known whether Callisen ever actually carried out a lumbar colostomy on a living child, but he attempted the operation on the corpse of a child with imperforate anus. However, his idea was decisive for Dupuytren [17] in 1818 (Fig. 5) and for Bougon [7] in 1828. Both cases ended lethally, and the lumbar approach came to be viewed in an unfavorable light.

Amussat [2] reviewed the 29 cases of colostomy in the 63 years after Pillore's operation in 1776 and found that 20 of the patients died. Of the 21 patients operated on for imperforate anus only, four survived, all in Brest (Table 1). Amussat's procedure included a long transverse incision to expose the colon by the retroperitoneal lumbar route, thus avoiding injury to the peritoneum. After longitudinal incision, the colon was stitched to the skin (Fig. 6).

Erichsen [19] witnessed Amussat's first operation and introduced this method at the University College Hospital in London. Friedberg [21] from Berlin visited Amussat in 1856 and disseminated the method in Germany. In 1876, Curling was still in favor of the lumbar colostomy [11].

Laparocolostomy

As surgical experience increased toward the end of the nineteenth century, the inguinal colostomy again gained importance, particularly through the advocacy of Allingham [1], Cripps [10], and Reeves [32].

Table 1. Review of colostomies between 1776 and 1839

29 cases	21 imperforate anus	17 dead
		4 survivors (in Brest)
	8 adults	3 dead
		5 survivors

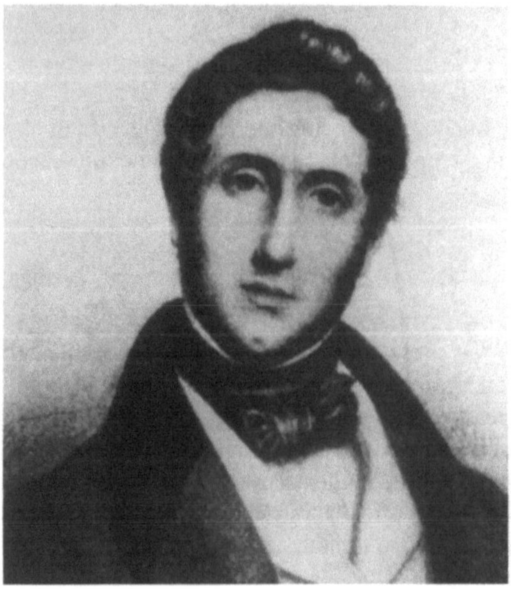

Fig. 6. Jean Zuléma Amussat (1796–1852) modified lumbar colostomy and was successful in treating several patients. After witnessing his operation, surgeons from England and Germany propagated his method in countries other than France [2]

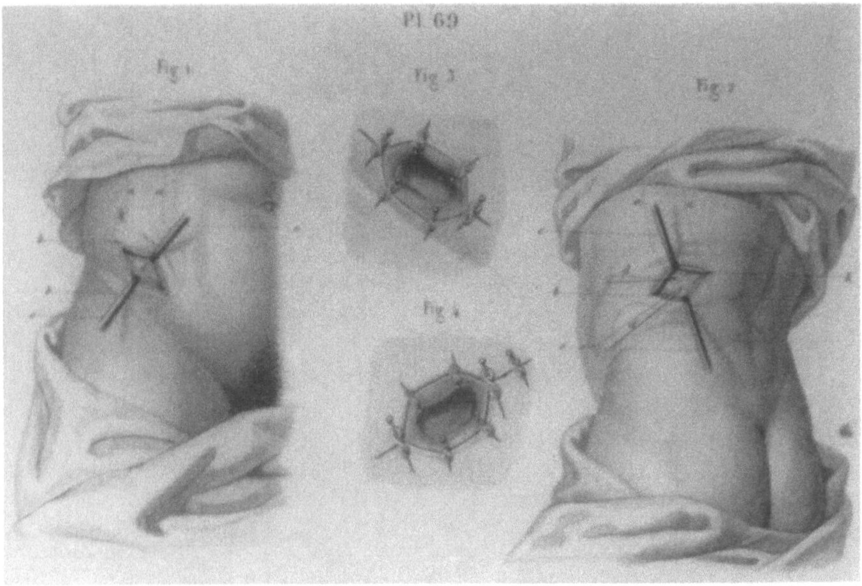

Fig. 7. Illustration of Littré's and Callisen's operation according to Hoffmann [9a]

Ball [4] advised against pulling down any part of the colon blindly and suggested the laparocolostomy. In his experience, the abdomen should be inspected, and the optimal site for the colostomy selected. The colostomy has been preserved in this form up to the present.

Modifications of Technique

Reviewing the literature, we can see that two distinct methods of performing a colostomy have evolved. The first involves the division of the bowel, with or without closure of the distal end. The other method is to construct a spur which prevents the overflow of feces into the distal colon [1, 18, 25, 29] (Fig. 7).

Ball [4] and Allingham [1] stitched the mesocolon to the skin in order to obtain complete separation of the two colonic parts. Maydl [29] used a rod to ensure that the colon would not fall back into the abdominal cavity (Fig. 8).

Davies-Colley [12], surgeon at Guy's Hospital made an important and original suggestion, consisting of utilizing a delayed opening of the bowel after the colon is sealed to the skin. This operation *"à deux temps"* prevents bacterial contamination and peritonitis.

Colostomy as an Aid for Pull-Through Operations

Throughout its history, colostomy has been considered a disabling procedure. Few attempts have been made to correct imperforate anus at a later date. In the year 1798, Martin de Lyon suggested the use of a colostomy as an aid in a rectal

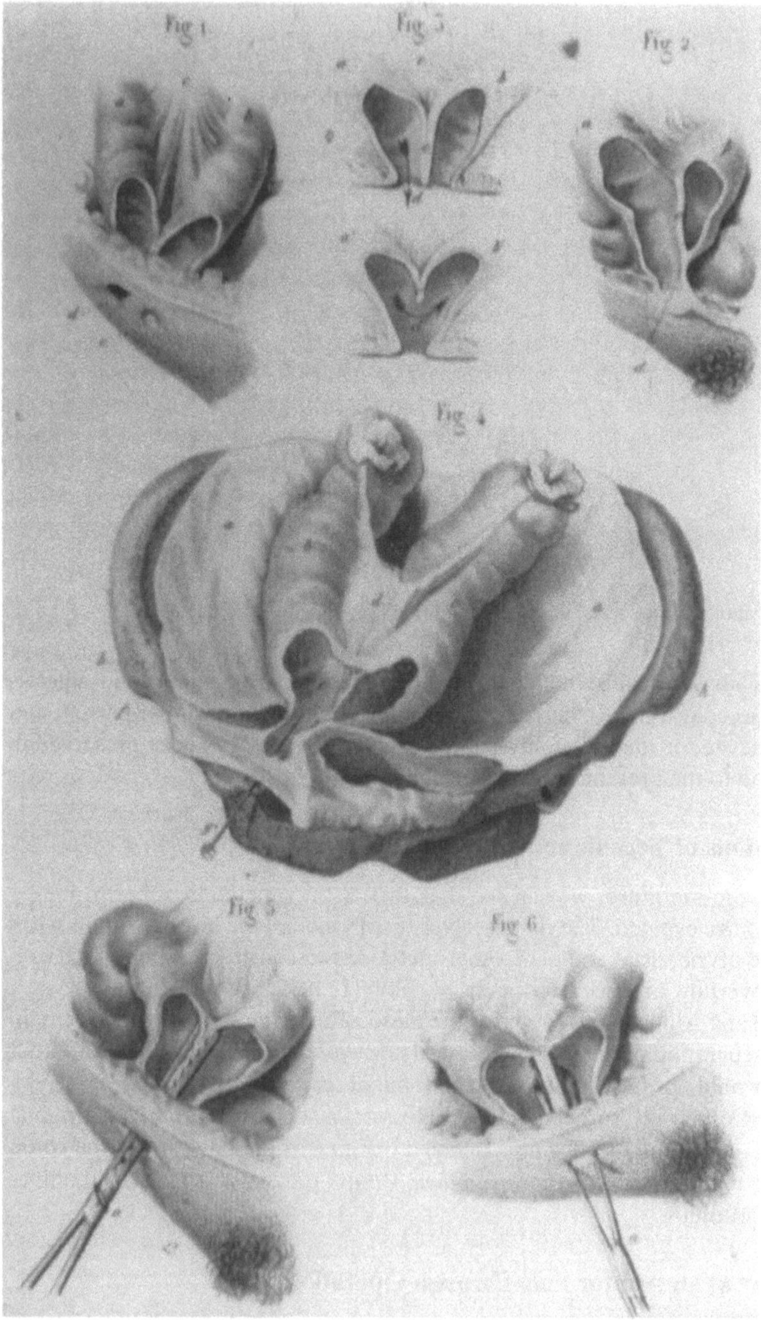

Fig. 8. Various types of colostomy with or without spur preservation and with operative spur resection are illustrated in Bernard's atlas of operation surgery [9a]

pull-through [28]. In February 1856, Chassaignac was the first to use this procedure successfully. However, by the beginning of the twentieth century, this technique had been employed only seven times.

In 1863, Demarquay [13], a French surgeon in Paris, suggested introducing a pointed, threaded probe into the distal stoma of an inguinal colostomy. This probe could be pulled out through the center of the anal dimple and the blind rectal pouch then brought close to the anal skin by means of a leaden ball. The dissection could then be carried out in the direction of the terminal rectum, enabling the rectal pull-through to be achieved. It is not known whether this brillant idea has ever been put into practice.

After an unsuccessful perineal operation for rectoanal atresia, Krönlein [26] performed an inguinal colostomy (Fig. 9). Seven months later, he was able to bring the rectum down to the perineal wound by pushing it down with the index finger. The enterostomy could then be closed.

Opponents of Colostomy

Opinions regarding colostomy were not unanimous, especially as far as newborn infants were concerned. Foucart [20] wanted to perform this operation only when he was compelled to by the parents. He expressed the wish that no surgeon would opt for it in order to uphold the honor of the profession. Some surgeons of this period opposed the operation with vehemence. For example, Bushe worte, "It is to be hoped that no surgeon at the present time would be so cruel as to subject an infant to this operation" [8]. In the opinion of Bigelow, "It is better that a child born with those imperfections would die without operation" (Fig. 10). Gross [22] wrote, "I cannot appreciate the benevolence which prompts a surgeon to form an

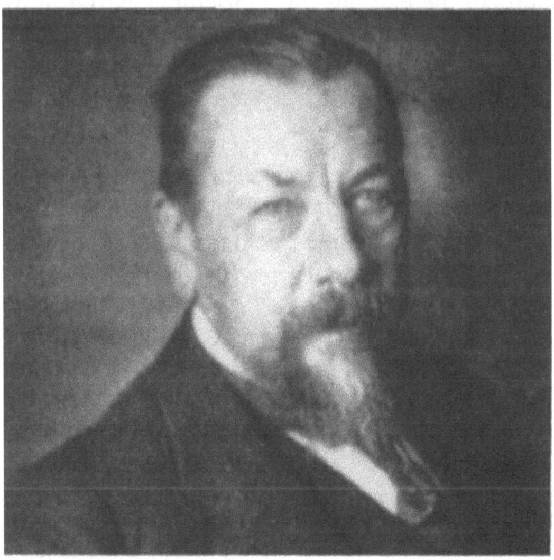

Fig. 9. Rudolf Krönlein (1847–1910) did a pull-through operation as a "staged procedure" in a child with rectal atresia [26]

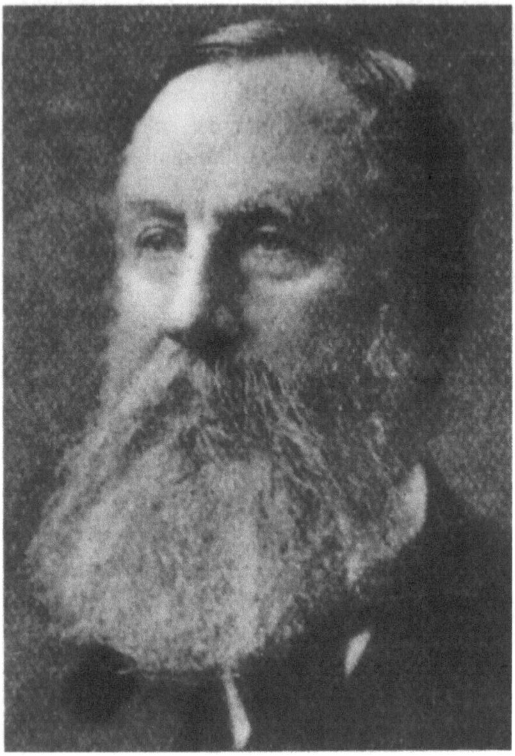

Fig. 10. Bigelow (1828–1890) was one of the strongest opponents of any kind of colostomy [5]

artificial outlet of faeces. Would the surgeon not rather see the child die without an attempt of relief, than to undertake the eke out for a miserable existence by such a pitiful and disgusting operation."

Epicrisis

Little attention was paid to this critical outery. As surgical experience increased toward the end of the nineteenth century, the laparocolostomy had an important place in the treatment of patients with imperforate anus, colonic obstructions, and rectal carcinoma. Despite all the more recent variations currently used, undiminished credit goes to those men who conceived of the colostomy – Littré and Callisen – and to those who had the courage to implement it – Pillore, Dumas, Duret, Amussat, and many others.

Summary

The idea of performing a colostomy in a child was first brought up by Littré in 1710. It lasted, however, 50 years until the first successful operation was published.

Especially in the 19th century various ways to approach the colon have been practized with frequently disappointing results (lumbar, inguinal approach). Only at the end of the century, colostomy was used as a guide for a pull-through operation.

With improved surgical and anaesthesiological techniques, colostomy has gained more importance as a temporary measure in order to postpone definitive surgery. Various new techniques have been developed within the same time. In our days, colostomy is a safe procedure and has a more defined place in handling children with imperforate anus and Hirschsprung's disease.

Résumé

En 1710, Littré était déjà d'avis qu'il était possible de pratiquer une colostomie et pourtant ce n'est que 50 ans plus tard que la première intervention fut couronnée de succès.

Au XIXe siècle on essaya plusieurs méthodes d'accès au colon (voie lombaire ou inguinale). Ce n'est qu'à la fin du siècle que l'on pratiqua une colostomie.

Avec les progrès des techniques chirurgicales et de l'anesthésie, la colostomie prit de plus en plus d'importance. Aujourd'hui il s'agit d'une intervention ne présentant pratiquement aucun risque et elle joue un rôle très important dans le traitement des imperforations et de la maladie de Hirschsprung.

Zusammenfassung

1710 hielt Littré als erster die Kolostomie für durchführbar. Es vergingen jedoch 50 Jahre, bis die erste erfolgreiche Operation stattfand.

Besonders im 19. Jahrhundert versuchte man auf die verschiedenste Art und Weise, einen Zugang zum Dickdarm zu finden (durch die Lende oder durch die Leiste).

Erst am Ende des Jahrhunderts wurde die Kolostomie im Zusammenhang mit einer Durchzugsoperation durchgeführt.

Mit dem Fortschritt der chirurgischen Methoden und der Anästhesie hat die Kolostomie als Übergangsmaßnahme, bis ein endgültiger Eingriff vorgenommen werden kann, an Bedeutung gewonnen. Heute ist sie ein risikoloser Eingriff, der bei der Behandlung der Imperforation und der Hirschsprung-Krankheit einen festen Platz einnimmt.

References

1. Allingham W (1873) Diseases of the rectum. London
2. Amussat JZ (1839) Mémoire sur la possibilité d'établir un anus artificiel dans la région lombaire sans pénétrer le peritoine. Lu à l'Académie Royale de Médicine, 1 Oct 1839
3. Amussat JZ (1841) Deuxième mémoire d'établir un anus artificiel dans les régions lombaires sans ouvrir le peritoine. Lu à l'Académie Royale de Médécine, 6 Sept 1841

4. Ball CB (1887) The rectum and anus. Lea, Philadelphia
5. Bigelow HJ (1857) Boston Med Surg J 57:240
6. Book of Judges 3:19–22
7. Bougon P (1828) Imperforation de l'anus. Lancette française 1:78
8. Bushe G (1837) A treatise on the malformations, injuries and diseases of the rectum and anus. New York, chap 3, p 37
9. Callisen H (1800) Systema chirurgiae hodiernae, in usum publicum et privatum adornatum. Copenhagen (Hafniae), vol 2, p 688
9a. Bernard C, Huette C (1858) Atlas der chirurgischen Operationslehre. Hoffmann, Leipzig
10. Cripps H (1892) The treatment of imperforate anus. Br Med J 1:1197
11. Curling TB (1876) Observations on the diseases of the rectum. Lindsay and Blakiston, Philadelphia
12. Davies-Colley (1885) Lapare colostomy. Trans Clin Soc XVIII:204
13. Demarquay M (1863) Operation de Littré, pratiquée sur un enfant né avec unanus imperforé. Gaz Hôpitaux (Paris) 129:450 (3 Nov 1863)
14. Desault PJ (1792) Imperforation de l'anus. J Chir 4:248
15. Dinnick T (1934) The origins and evolution of colostomy. Br J Surg 22:142
16. Dubois A (1783) Recueil Périodique Soc Méd Paris 3:125
17. Dupuytren M (1818) Leçons orales clin chirur 3:663
18. Duret C (1798) Observation sur un enfant sans anus. Recueil Périodique Soc Méd Paris 4:45
19. Erichsen J (1850) Imperforate rectum. Lancet 1:235
20. Foucart (1857) Imperation de l'anus. Gaz Hôpitaux (Paris) 21:86
21. Friedberg H (1857) Recherches cliniques et critiques sur l'anus artificiel. Arch Gen Med (Paris) IX:565, 701
22. Gross SD (1859) A system of surgery. Hoffmann, Philadelphia, vol 2, chap 13, p 763
23. Heister L (1718) Wundartzney. Nuremberg
24. Fabricius Guilhelmus Hildanus (Wilhelm Fabry) (1606) Observationum et curationum chirurgicarum centuria. Centur I Obs 74, Basel
25. Knie A (1885) Zur Technik der Kolostomie. Zentralbl Chir 25:433, 18:188, 313
26. Krönlein RU (1879) Casuistische Beiträge zur operativen Chirurgie des Digestionstractus. Berl Klin Wochenschr 16:505, 526
27. Littré A (1710) Diverses observations anatomiques. In: Histoire de l'Académie des Sciences Paris, p 36
28. Martin J (1798) Rapport sur une observation d'imperation d'anus. Rec Act Soc Sante de Lyon 1:180
29. Maydl K (1888) Zur Technik der Kolostomie. Zentralbl Chir 24:433
30. Miriel PL (1835) Vices congenitaux de confirmation de l'extremite inférieure du tube digestif. Dissertation, Paris
31. Pillore H (1797) Operation d'anus artificiel par la methode de Littré. Actes de la Société de Lyon 189
32. Reeves HA (1892) Inguinal colotomy. Br Med J 1:66
33. Schlagintweit WAJ (1826) La thèse inaugurale de Ottinger sur les imperforations de l'anus. Munich

Hirschsprung's Disease: An Historical Review

D. Cass[1]

The history of Hirschsprung's disease (congenital megacolon) is a fascinating progression from early, astute observations of an uncommon condition to the present-day more detailed understanding. This progress was not one of steady building on previous careful work, but one of forgotten, dismissed or fallacious theories, ignored isolated observations, and then an almost synchronous appearance of clinical understanding, histological demonstration of the defect and animal experiments leading to effective surgical treatment. In recent years there has been extensive investigation of the underlying pathology in both animals and humans, indicating that our knowledge is incomplete and that treatment needs further refinement.

The first observation of congenital megacolon is attributed to Frederick Ruysch in 1691 (cited by [1]). In a postmortem examination of a 5-year-old girl, the colon proximal to the upper rectum was grossly dilated. Over the next 200 years there were numerous sporadic reports of congenital megacolon, but these were inadequate in detail, and may have included other diseases [2–5]. Hirschsprung in 1886 provided the classical description, presenting two patients with clinical and postmortem features that established the presence of a distinct congenital disease [6]. However, while he noted that "the rectum was not enlarged, but actually somewhat narrowed", it was Hirschsprung's emphasis on the dilated, hypertrophied proximal colon that was to continue as the predominant focus of attention for the next 60 years [6–8]. He and most others felt the disease must be a congenital disorder, since megacolon was noted so soon after birth.

While the concept of congenital dilatation of the colon was the most widely accepted view, there were many other theories. In 1893 Walker and Griffith suggested, in the absence of any obstructing agent, a chronic colitis with much gas being produced, resulting in a distended gut with poor peristalsis. Interestingly, this postmortem report contained a histological section of the bowel, but it was the transverse colon and thus showed the changes produced by colitis. The rectum was macroscopically normal and the pathological report was that its muscular walls were thicker than normal [9]. In 1895 Marfan implicated a congenital long redundant sigmoid, with resultant increased water resorption producing drier than normal faeces, which caused obstruction followed by dilatation and hypertrophy of the more proximal colon [10]. The passage of a rectal tube 8–10 inches from the anus often led to drainage of faeces and gas, and this observation led

[1] Paediatric Surgery Unit, Weastmead Centre, Sydney 2145, Australia

Progress in Pediatric Surgery, Vol. 20
Ed. by P. P. Rickham

Roser and others [11] to suggest "valve formation", "folding" and "kinking" as the underlying mechanism. There was, however, no postmortem evidence to support these "anatomical factors", and these theories lost influence [11].

A congenital neuropathic origin was mentioned by many early workers, but the affected region of colon and the nature of the disorders were not defined. Terms such as "spasm", "contraction" and "mechanical obstruction" often confused the discussion and have led some reviewers to suggest these authors were discussing other mechanisms [12]. However, several physicians at the end of the last century were very close to the truth: firstly, in supposing a neurogenic cause; secondly, in suggesting that the lower rectum and colon were the primary cause, with proximal dilatation being a consequence; and thirdly in presenting an effective surgical approach. In 1880, Hilton Fagge diagnosed "spasm of rectum" in a 12-month-old child suffering from constipation and abdominal distension since birth [11]. When the child died 3 years later, Gee [13] performed a postmortem which revealed a dilated pelvic colon, below which "the rectum and perhaps the lower end of the pelvic colon, showed a spastic contraction, but not a very tight stricture, easily admitting the index finger". In 1893 Osler [14] described two cases (one treated successfully by colostomy, the other by irrigation and the passage of a flatus tube) in which he thought there appeared to be some defect in the innervation of the colon and in the contracting power of the muscles, but he was not specific as to which segment of bowel was abnormal. In 1900 Fenwick [15] provided a logical argument for dismissing "congenital dilation of the colon", as well as kinks and congenital narrowing. Instead he suggested spasm of the sphincter ani as the congenital prime cause, with proximal dilatation and hypertrophy developing secondarily after birth. In 1907 Hawkins [11] reiterated this view and spoke of a

> neuromuscular defect, through which a section of the colon, though it oppose no obstacle, is yet incapable of forwarding its contents. ... One cannot doubt that the hypertrophy is a secondary compensatory development. In cases in which life is prolonged for many years, no doubt this hypertrophy is for a time sufficient to counterbalance the paretic or spastic section of the bowel below, but a relative insufficiency must set in sooner or later.

Within this conceptual framework, operative procedures were performed. In 1898 Sir Frederick Treves reported an abdominal perineal resection of the distal colon and rectum with cure of the obstructive symptoms [16]. His paper reviews the literature and concludes

> I venture to think that there is strong evidence to support the suggestion that all cases of 'idiopathic' dilatation of the colon in young children are due to congenital defects in the terminal part of the bowel, that there is in these cases an actual mechanical obstruction and that the dilatation of the bowel is not idiopathic.

His patient was a 6-year-old girl, who at 2 days of age had developed distension, vomiting and constipation. Her bowels never acted naturally and relief of obstruction was obtained only by passing a rigid tube some 10 in. beyond the anus and then administering an enema. At operation in 1897, the distal 8 or 9 in. of the bowel was "a straight solid-looking tube about the size of an adult fore-finger" with hypertrophied ascending and transverse parts of the colon. Initially a colostomy was performed, and 9 months later Treves reoperated. On this occasion the colon was less distended. He excised part of the transverse, descending and sigmoid colon along with the rectum in a combined abdominoperineal approach, effecting a transverse colo-anal anastomosis. Postoperatively the child did well and had no further obstructive episodes, although at the time of the report she was still incontinent. Treves in his paper, was clear as to *where* the primary pathology was – the rectum; but it is not clear *what* he considered the pathology to be. He spoke of "congenital narrowing", but then noted that this narrowed part exhibited "no structural change and there was no mechanical obstruction nor disesae of the mucous or muscular coats". The use of the words "narrowing" and "mechanical obstruction" early in the paper have led some reviewers [12, 17] to suggest Treves held an anatomical (stenotic) concept of Hirschsprung's disease. His ideas and operation, however, fitted in with the current neuropathic theories. Hawkins in 1907 quoted Treves' work to support his well-stated neuropathic theory [11]. The specimen from this first abdomino-perineal resection was placed in the Museum of the Royal College of Surgeons of England, and it would be of interest to know if microscopic examination confirmed Hirschsprung's disesae. There was some improvement, but symptoms remained.

This neuropathic concept, very similar to our modern understanding, failed to gain acceptance because there was no definite proof in the face of more popular theories. Even when a lack of ganglion cells was later noted [18], which should have given new life to this theory, the evidence was dismissed, as others had found normal ganglion cells in the dilated proximal colon and in the "lower bowel" [19]. The essential problems impeding progress were therefore a plethora of theories for a rare disease; a popular concept that the abnormality lay in the proximal dilated colon, with the histological examination often restricted to this area; and probably a "mixed" collection of patients, only some of whom had aganglionosis.

With increased knowledge of the autonomic nervous system, a disorder in its function was implicated by many, with some suggesting parasympathetic underactivity [20] or sympathetic overactivity [21, 22]. Others were of the opinion that, while there was no imbalance of the system in Hirschsprung's disease, the stimulation of the parasympathetic or inhibition of the sympathetic system would improve the clinical situation. The theory of gut function was that the parasympathetic outflow was tonic to the bowel and relaxant to the sphincter, while the sympathetic outflow was relaxant to the bowel and tonic to the sphincter.

Ishikawa (1923) demonstrated an absence of parasympathetic nerves to the pelvic colon in a 4-year-old girl with Hirschsprung's disease, and found that he could induce megacolon in animals after division of the parasympathetic nerves [23]. Frazer (1926) spoke of the "hypertrophies of infancy", in which he discovered an imbalance of the neuronal elements that led to insufficient relaxation of the associated sphincters. This "imbalance theory" was used to explain, among other disorders, pyloric stenosis and Hirschsprung's disease, where the problem allegedly lay at O'Beirne's sphincter (the junction of the rectum and sigmoid colon) [21, 22]. It is interesting how such a simplified view of gut function arose, as early physiological investigations had revealed a complex system with variable responses under differing experimental conditions, and marked differences existed between species, especially at the level of the sphincters [24, 25].

In the human, Rankin and Learmonth (1930) stimulated the peripheral end of the cut presacral nerve in a young anaesthetised woman. A surgical assistant, whose finger was in the rectum, described "strong clonic contractions of the sphincter followed by several weaker clonic contractions". No manometric recordings were made [26]. This single observation and work in the dog formed the experimental basis of resection of the presacral nerve along with the lumbar sympathetics [27, 28]. More recent observations have not confirmed this physiological situation in the human. Using manometric measurements, Shepard and Wright (1968) found that stimulation of the presacral (pelvic) nerve in humans and primates resulted in relaxation of the internal anal sphincter. Interestingly, this relaxation of the internal sphincter after presacral nerve stimulation also occurred in patients with Hirschsprung's disease [29]. Pharmacological studies on the internal anal sphincter of the monkey have revealed a complex situation with cholinergic inhibition and adrenergic excitation and inhibition, along with nonadrenergic noncholinergic inhibition [30].

Nevertheless, the simplified idea of autonomic function led to the use of sympathectomy in the treatment of Hirschsprung's disease. Royle (1927) reported success in relieving the peripheral motor aspects of spastic paresis by sympathectomy, attributing the role of control of plastic and postural tone to the sympathetic nerves [31]. Wade (1927), linking Frazer's ideas of an autonomic imbalance in Hirschsprung's disease to Royle's operative success in relieving sympathetic overdrive in spastic paresis, performed a sympathectomy in a patient with Hirschsprung's disease which led to clinical and radiological improvement [31]. There were many subsequent sympathectomies, some extensive [32, 33] and others localized [26]. Success was generally reported, with a decrease in the abdominal distension and more frequent bowel actions. However, follow-up was short – 6 weeks and 7 months [26] – and later reports noted a return of obstructive symptoms and a significant incidence of late complications [34].

Other forms of treatment consisted of enemas and the passage of rectal tubes [11, 14]. Often washouts were performed with tap water, with resultant electrolyte problems [35]. Electrical stimulation [36], anal sphincter dilatation [37], rectosigmoid myotomy [38] and parasympathomimetic [39] or anticholinergic [40] drugs were all suggested, but not generally accepted. Spinal anaesthesia was reported to give good long-term results even after one or two instillations [41], but this was disputed by other authors [34]. Operative techniques included the single abdomino-perineal resection [16] and sympathectomies [26, 31–33] previously mentioned, but most often involved colostomies alone or in combination with later resections of the dilated colon [34]. Attempts to close colostomies often resulted in the return of obstructive symptoms or fistulas. Assessment of the operative results was difficult, as those patients said to have Hirschsprung's disease were a mixture of cases; moreover, the obstruction could vary between individuals and with time in the same person. Judd and Adson (1928), reviewing 26 cases from the Mayo Clinic treated by ileosigmoidectomy, Mikulicz procedure, total colectomy or anterior partial resection, reported that "61.5% were cured or improved" [32]. A later review from the same institution in 1943 reported 29 patients treated by colectomy with 7 deaths. Among the 16 long-term follow-ups, results were described as excellent in 13 and good in 3 [34]. Even today, objective follow-up and comparison of different treatment methods is difficult.

After 60 years of confusion, the solution came remarkably quickly. Classical papers bearing on clinical, histological and surgical aspects of Hirschsprung's disease appeared in rapid succession and formed the basis of modern treatment. The clinical features were described in detail in 1946 by Ehrenpreis [42], with a clear description of neonatal signs and symptoms. Using radiological methods, he demonstrated that the cause of the problem was a failure by the terminal colon to allow the passage of faeces. The histological demonstration of aganglionosis was firmly established by Whitehouse and Kernohan [43] and Zueler and Wilson [44] in 1948. These papers with their extensive literature reviews, the number of cases (11 and 6), and detailed histology, clearly established aganglionosis as the underlying pathological cause.

The first histological report on ganglion cells in Hirschsprung's disease was by Tittel [45] in 1901. The intrinsic plexus was sparsely developed throughout the colon, but was normal in the ileum. In 1904 Brentano [46] reported similar findings. Total absence of ganglion cells was described by Dalla Valla (1920, 1924), Cameron (1928), Robertson and Kernohan (1938), and Tiffin et al. (1940) [18, 47–50]. But these were isolated reports and, as mentioned previously, other workers had reported normal histological findings [19, 51, 52]. Aganglionosis had therefore been thought to represent a rare secondary event. The 1948 papers [43, 44] left no doubt that the ganglion cells were absent. In addition, they described increased numbers of nerve trunks in the distal colon (often in association with blood vessels). The transition zone was variable in its extent, and had occasional isolated ganglion cells with few nerve trunks. In some cases there appeared to be a very long transition zone with variability in the number of ganglion cells (zones) or hyperganglionosis [43].

Appropriate surgical treatment was first reported by Swenson and Bill in 1948 [53]. Radiographic and balloon manometry demonstrated an area of spasm and lack of peristalsis in the terminal colon. Experimental surgery was then performed using dogs and a surgical procedure was developed, whereby the entire rectum (and appropriate lengths of proximal bowel) could be removed with subsequent retention of continence. This anal pull-through technique was then applied successfully in a patient [53]. At this stage Swenson and Bill were unaware of the aganglionosis reports, and had based their work on clinical observation. The final classic paper that helped establish the modern treatment of Hirschsprung's disease was that of Bodian et al. in 1949 [54]. A review of 73 patients with megacolon revealed 39 with characteristic clinical and radiological features of what we now accept as Hirschsprung's disease. In 15 out of 15 specimens examined, aganglionosis was found. The second group of patients had a milder clinical course and it was safe to pursue non-operative methods of treatment. Many of this group had previously been considered to have had Hirschsprung's disease and eight had in fact had operations on the sympathetic nervous system. Today we consider this second group as "idiopathic", although many such patients will probably be found to have subtle neuropathic lesions as the cause of their megacolon. In an overview, Hiatt (1951) again identified the distal colon as the pathological site by manometric studies and showed this to be spastic contracted bowel incapable of ongoing peristalsis, but capable of mass contraction [55]. There was a lack of the normal reflex relaxation of the internal sphincter. Hiatt described patients with very short segments of aganglionosis involving only the distal half or third of the rectum. After inadequate resection of the aganglionic bowel the initial result was often excellent, but with time the obstruction tended to return [55].

In recent years much has been learned about normal physiology of the bowel [56] and the pathophysiology of Hirschsprung's disease [11, 57, 58]. There are still gaps in this knowledge and areas of controversy. The three basic components of intestinal motility are the smooth muscle itself, the intrinsic nervous system and the extrinsic nerves.

Smooth muscle has considerable autonomy. The membrane potential and depolarization depend on Ca^{++} and K^{+} channels. In uterine muscle, hormones can influence these channels and so modify the response to stimulation. The contraction is not an all-or-nothing response, but can be graded. In the gut, the smooth-muscle cells act as syncytial units and the muscle itself can respond to stretch [59]. Normally, smooth muscle has a predominantly inhibitory neural input, so the natural state of denervated muscle is a tendency towards contraction. Bayliss and Starling first demonstrated this in 1901 [24]. In 1922 Alvarez [60] reiterated this, and even proposed denervation as a cause of Hirschsprung's disease, long before aganglionosis was definitely established as the cause. In Hirschsprung's disease, some workers have reported a contracted spastic distal colon capable only of mass contraction [11, 55], while others have found that in vitro the basal tension of resected tissue is normal [61]. Denervation hypersensitivity has been suggested [11, 62], but others have found decreased [63] or normal [61] sensitivity. Detailed analysis in the mouse model has revealed no excess of receptors, nor any evidence of denervation hypersensitivity [64]. Electrophysiological studies have shown that the muscle cells have normal resting membrane potentials and respond normally to field stimulation [65, 66]. Smooth muscle is a difficult tissue to study, with many variables such as initial tension and stretch affecting the results. Conclusions from this work suggests that in Hirschsprung's disease the smooth muscle is eletrophysiologically normal, but that if deprived of its innervation, the tendency of smooth muscle is towards a contracted state. However, the degree of contraction may weell depend on hormones and ion channels.

The intrinsic neural network of ganglia is absent in Hirschsprung's disease. Normally, this complex neural system coordinates the peristaltic reflex and has a marked inhibitory effect on smooth muscle (especially the inner circular layer) by way of an non-adrenergic inhibitory substance as yet to be conclusively identified [56]. Electrophysiological recording in Hirschsprung's disease reveals an electrically quiescent tissue with no inhibitory junction potential or relaxation on stimulation [65, 66]. This lack of the peristaltic mechanism is the prime reason for the functional obstruction in Hirschsprung's disease. In addition, the lack of the non-adrenergic inhibitory neurons results in a tendency to contract.

Histological, histochemical and ultrastructural studies have shown that the extrinsic nerves are greatly increased in the aganglionic segment [67]. These nerve trunks represent sympathetic and parasympathetic nerves that enter the bowel with blood vessels and then grow aimlessly through the muscle in the absence of their normal target cells. The increase is not uniform over the whole area of ganglionosis; it is more pronounced distally, and varies between individuals. This variability has been suggested as the reason for the different clinical presentations between patients with similar lengths of aganglionosis [68]. While it is accepted that there are an increased number of nerve trunks, increased tissue content and increased turnover [69], it is not certain how functionally significant these nerve bundles are. When isolated strips of human aganglionic bowel are perfused with atropine, propanolol and pentolamine, the normal decrease in tone or tension does not occur. This would suggest that the extrinsic nerve trunks are not contributing to an increase in tone. Conversely, field stimulation results in excitatory junction potentials and contraction, suggesting that these nerve fibres can release transmitters and contribute to a contraction of the aganglionic bowel [65]. In addition, spinal anaesthesia can result in slight dilatation of contracted bowel, as seen on barium enema [54] or as visualised by proctoscopy [42], suggesting that the extrinsic innervation does contribute to the tonic state of aganglionic bowel.

Therefore, the predominant cellular pathophysiology in Hirschsprung's disease is a lack of the intrinsic ganglion cells, with resultant aperistaltic obstruction. The muscle cells, lacking their normal neural input, tend to lapse into a state of contraction, and the extrinsic nerve trunks in the rectosigmoid can elicit further contraction. These effects are particularly pronounced at the level of the internal anal sphincter, where there is a failure to relax in reaction to the local stimulus of more proximal distension, and a tendency to tonic contraction. However, even in patients with Hirschsprung's disease the internal anal sphincter will relax when the pelvic nerves are electrically stimulated [29], suggesting that the extrinsic neural arch to the sphincter can function normally. The gut has a complex nervous system, and improved understanding of normal function and peristalsis are required before a clear understanding of the cellular pathophysiology of Hirschsprung's disease is possible. In addition, there are probably many functional disorders, such as pseudo-Hirschsprung's disease and pseudo-obstruction, that are related to subtle disorders of the intrinsic gut nervous system [42, 58].

The embryology of Hirschsprung's disease is unknown. Environmental factors are involved, as evidenced by the occurrence of Hirschsprung's disease in only one of monozygotic twins [70]. Genetic influences also play a part [71], especially in some families [72], where there may be associated defects such as the congenital deafness and streaks of white hair of cephalosyndactylia (Waardenburg's syndrome).

The failure of the distal bowel to be normally innervated could be due to a migratory defect of the neural crest cells, a defect in the local microenvironment (such that primitive neuroblasts lack trophic support), or later anoxic destruction of established ganglion cells.

Okamoto and Ueda [73], using silver stains in human embryos, demonstrated a single wave of vagal innervation that was at the stomach at 6 weeks, the transverse colon at 8 weeks, and complete by 12 weeks, of gestation. They suggested a migratory defect as the most satisfactory explanation of a disease that always affects the lower rectum and a variable proximal segment of bowel.

In embryonic studies in strains of mice that develop aganglionosis as an autosomal recessive disorder, Webster [74] showed that the normal migration times are slowed, to such a degree that the aganglionic cells never reach the lower bowel. This supports the concept of a migratory defect. Other workers have suggested anoxic damage to established ganglion cells [75–78]. Ganglion cells can be selectively destroyed by local infusion of chemicals [75, 76] or anoxia [78], with a resultant aperistaltic obstruction. These results have been disputed by other work, with the implication that ganglion cells are quite resistant to anoxia [79]. In addition, the anoxia theory does not adequately explain the universal distal to proximal distribution of aganglionosis, nor does it allow explanation of the actual mechanism of ganglion cell damage. An abnormality in the local microenvironment has been postulated in tissue culture experiments using the lethal spotted mouse model [80].

It is difficult to study the embryogenesis of Hirschsprung's disease, as the experimental production of aganglionosis may not reflect intrauterine events, and in animal models the disorder differs in several important respects from that in humans [81].

The clinical features are well known. Most infants present with bile-stained vomiting, abdominal distension and delayed passage of meconium [12, 58]. Older children present with severe constipation and in this group, even in the 1980s, there is often delay in diagnosis. Of 30 patients presenting at the Royal Children's Hospital in Melbourne between 1980 and 1983, 8 had an average delay of 4 years from the onset of symptoms to diagnosis. Of equal concern is the number of patients with Hirschsprung's disease (17%) who present undiagnosed at an encopresis clinic [82].

A barium enema in an unprepared colon excludes other causes of neonatal bowel obstruction and usually allows the demonstration of the narrowed segment [12, 53]. Rectal suction biopsy is a reliable method of diagnosing Hirschsprung's disease [83, 84], especially when the absence of ganglion cells is combined with histochemical staining for excess acetylcholinesterase that is associated with the increased number of nerve trunks [85]. Balloon manometry aids diagnosis by showing an absence of the normal recto-anal reflex [55, 86–88]. Normally, distension of the lower rectum leads to a reflex relaxation of the internal anal sphincter in some full-term infants and in all normal infants by 12 days of age [88]. More recent studies using a semiconductor manometer and smaller probes have demonstrated a normal recto-anal reflex even in premature infants, suggesting that previous negative recordings may have been due to technical difficulties rather than a "maturation" of the reflex after birth [89]. Therefore, manometry should be of diagnostic use regardless of gestation and birth weight. Electrical recording has also been shown to be of assistance in the diagnosis of Hirschsprung's disease [90, 91], but has not been widely used because of technical difficulties, especially in documenting the length of aganglionosis [58].

The classic surgical treatment consists of a defunctionalizing colostomy and a subsequent rectosigmoidectomy with abdomino-perineal resection and pull-through. The *Swenson* procedure was the first described and although there have been modifications, none has conclusively proved to be superior [58, 92]. Swenson's original description was of a horizontal anal anastomosis 2–3 cm above the mucocutaneous line [53]. Modifications were made to achieve improved sterility [93, 94] – delayed anastomosis [95, 96] or partial sphincterotomy [94, 97]. *Duhamel* originally described a colorectal end-to-side anastomosis just above the internal sphincter with crushing of the septum using V-shaped Kocher clamps [98]. This was done to leave some sensitive rectal mucosa anteriorly, and to decrease injury to pelvic nerves. Modifications included minimization of the anterior rectal pouch [99–101], the use of staples instead of clamps [102], and performing the anastomosis at a lower level so as to include part of the internal anal sphincter [103, 104]. *Soave's* procedure involved a submucosal dissection starting 8 cm above the peritoneal reflection and descending to 1 cm above the mucocutaneous line. The everted mucosa was excised and the pull-through bowel left for 12 days, so that adhesions developed, after which the prolapsed bowel was amputated [105]. The advantages were technical ease and minimization of pelvic dissection. The principal modifications were a primary anastomosis [106, 107] and longitudinal splitting of the aganglionic muscular cuff with a higher anastomosis [108]. The *Rehbein* technique involved an anterior resection and abdomino-rectal anastomosis 4–7 cm above the mucocutaneous line [109, 110]. The procedure was combined with dilatation of the internal anal sphincter, to overcome the obstructive tendency of the remaining aganglionic bowel.

The results of these procedures are similar, with some surgeons reporting poor results and others good ones. Each procedure, however, has characteristic problems: an anastomotic leak with Swenson's, dilatation of the rectal pouch with Duhamel's, cuff stenosis and incontinence with Soave's, and obstruction in Rehbein's [58, 92]. However, in all procedures, the principal complications relate to the internal anal sphincter. If too much sphincter is damaged then incontinence results, if too much remains, obstructive symptoms can return and fatal enterocolitis can ensue, even years after the operative procedure [12].

In a recent review, each of the operative techniques is described in detail by its originator, followed by reports of other surgeons' experience using these techniques and finally by a large independent multicentre follow-up comparing the results [58]. The final conclusion is that no procedure is clearly superior. Even the basic question remains of whether it is better to leave a short terminal segment with intact sphincters or to totally remove the rectum and partially weaken the internal anal sphincter. This inconclusive result and the variability of experience is of concern especially since many forms of treatment, such as cholinergics, anticholinergics, spinal anaesthesia, and sympathectomy and colectomy of the megacolonic segment, have all been reported by various authors as having provided excellent results. The gastrointestinal tract has a complex physiological structure that is influenced by many as yet unknown factors. More needs to be known before a completely adequate operation can be devised. However, at the moment it is possible to state the aims of operative repair and to extrapolate from recent physiological discoveries.

The ideal operative procedure would remove the aganglionic bowel, lead to the restoration of the recto-anal relaxation reflex, and permit normal central control of defaecation. All the current procedures remove most of the aganglionic bowel, leaving at most only a few centimetres. The restoration of the ano-rectal reflex would depend on reinnervation of the sphincter with inhibitory fibres from ganglia above [58]. Normally, the ganglion cells end several centimeters above the anal valves and send their processes down to the sphincteric muscle [111]. In resections and anastomoses in the small bowel, the intrinsic axons degenerate for about 2 cm distal to an incision, but then regenerate [112]. It is theoretically possible that a similar reinnervation could occur at the colo-anal anastomosis. An end-to-end anastomosis, as well as the absence of infection and excessive scar formation, would be a theoretical advantage [58]. The extent of central control would depend on intact neural pathways and their normal functioning. Stimulation nof the distal ends of the pelvic nerves results in relaxation of the internal anal sphincter in patients with Hirschsprung's disease, demonstrating the neural pathway to be intact [29]. Central awareness of rectal stimulation has been shown to develop normally at about 3–4 months of age [113]. In infants with imperforate anus and who have undergone a pull-through procedure at 1 year of age, the anal cortical evoked potential is absent [114]. However, early pull-through operations result in the normal development of an anal evoked potential [115].

As with the development of vision, it is probably important that an infant receive some normal anal stimuli for this awareness of rectal fullness and function to develop, with the resultant development of continence. This therefore constitutes a theoretical advantage of early definitive surgery, which was traditionally avoided because of the stress of a major operation in a neonate and the anatomical difficulties in operating in the small infant pelvis. It was felt safest to perform a defunctionalizing colostomy and defer the definitive operation until 1 year of age. In a large series, Swenson showed an increased mortality in infants operated on under 6 months of age [116]. But more recently, definitive operations for Hirschsprung's disease have been performed in the neonatal period with no mortality and minimal morbidity [117]. The follow-up periods were unfortunately short. It would have been of interest to know whether physiological measurements and the attainment of continence were normal in these patients. A further recent series of definitive operations in the first few months of life showed that a higher percentage of infants had a normal post-operative ano-rectal reflex [118] (suggesting perhaps intrinsic reinnervation, but also the functional action of higher neural pathways) and the early attainment of continence. With improved peri-operative support and technique, early corrective surgery is possible with minimal risk and a theoretical advantage.

In summary, the history of Hirschsprung's disease represents a fascinating unravelling of a congenital disorder, leading to adequate treatment for what was frequently a fatal disease. However, much remains to be learnt. An exact knowledge of the cause of Hirschsprung's disease would contribute to the understanding of normal mechanisms of embryogenesis, and would perhaps aid diagnosis and treatment. An improved knowledge of the normal and pathological physiology may explain the perplexing variability between patients and help to determine the optimal surgical technique and the timing of operation. The aim of treatment should be to ensure normal colo-anal function.

Summary

A historical review of Hirschsprung's disease is of relevance for several reasons. The historical events are revealing as to how clinical diseases are often slowly unravelled. In addition, many unsolved problems are highlighted. *Firstly* the exact cause is unknown. There is obviously an interaction between genetic and environmental factors, the nature of which is of interest to basic scientists as well as clinicians. *Secondly* the pathophysiological explanation for the functional obstruction, and especially its variability, is still incomplete. Much more needs to be known about normal gastrointestinal physiology before this question can be fully answered. *Thirdly* the technique and timing of operative correction remains inconclusive. Despite extensive postoperative assessment there is no one operation that is clear superior. Each have characteristic problems, but all share the main problem; the abnormal internal sphincter. It remains uncertain how much (if any) of the sphincter should be bypassed. As well the optimal timing of operation is uncertain, with some theoretical advantages being suggested for earlier operation. However, these advantages need to be balanced against possible technical problems. Nevertheless the aim of surgical correction should be the full attainment of normal faecal continence.

Résumé

L'histoire de la maladie de Hirschsprung est intéressante à plus d'un point de vue. Elle montre d'abord qu'il faut souvent un temps considérable pour arriver à percer le mystère de manifestations cliniques. Elle souligne aussi qu'un nombre considérable de problèmes attendent toujours une solution. *Premièrement:* la cause exacte n'est pas encore connue. Il s'agit probablement d'un concours de facteurs congénitaux et du milieu ambiant qui présentent un très grand intérêt tant pour la recherche fondamentale que pour la clinique. *Deuxièmement:* l'explication physiopathologique de l'occlusion est encore incomplète. Il faudra attendre d'en savoir plus sur la physiologie gastro-intestinale normale. *Troisièmement:*

comment et quand pratiquer l'intervention? On en discute encore. Il existe déjà un grand nombre de contrôles post-opératoires mais aucune méthode ne s'est révélée nettement supérieure. Elles présentent toutes leurs problèmes propres en plus de celui qu'elles ont en commun: le sphincter anormal. On ne sait pas encore si le pontage doit l'inclure et dans quelle proportion. On ne sait pas non plus quand exactement pratiquer l'intervention bien qu'il semble utile qu'elle ait lieu tôt. Une opération précoce, par contre, peut présenter des problèmes techniques. Quoi qu'il en soit, le but est partout et toujours de rétablir un contrôle complet.

Zusammenfassung

Die Geschichte der Hirschsprung-Krankheit ist aus vielen Gründen sehr aufschlußreich. Die geschichtliche Entwicklung zeigt, wie langsam in vielen Fällen klinische Krankheitsbilder enträtselt werden. Sie zeigt auch, wie viele Probleme noch ungelöst sind. 1) Die genaue Ursache ist noch unbekannt. Es handelt sich vermutlich um ein Zusammentreffen von genetischen und Umweltfaktoren, die sowohl für die Grundlagenforschung als auch für die Klinik von großem Interesse sind. 2) Die pathophysiologische Erklärung des funktionellen Verschlusses ist noch unvollständig. Es bleibt noch viel über die normale gastrointestinale Physiologie zu erfahren, bevor diese Frage zufriedenstellend beantwortet werden kann. 3) Technik und Zeitpunkt der Operation sind noch umstritten. Obwohl viele postoperative Untersuchungsergebnisse vorliegen, kann man noch nicht eine Methode als eindeutig überlegen ansehen. Alle haben ihre eigenen Probleme, aber *ein* Problem haben sie alle gemeinsam: den abnormalen inneren Schließmuskel. Es ist noch unklar, wieviel von dem Schließmuskel (oder ob überhaupt) von dem Bypass erfaßt werden soll. Der günstigste Zeitpunkt für die Operation steht auch immer noch nicht eindeutig fest, obwohl theoretisch vieles für eine frühe Operation spricht. Dem Vorteil einer frühen Operation stehen jedoch eventuelle technische Probleme entgegen. Das Ziel jedoch bleibt in allen Fällen die Wiederherstellung einer funktionierenden Peristaltik.

References

1. Leenders E, Sieber WK (1970) Congenital megacolon, observation by Frederick Ruysch 1691. J Pediatr Surg 5:1–3
2. Bristowe JS (1985) Clinical lecture on the consequences of long continued constipation. Br Med J I:1085–1088
3. Finney JMT (1908) Congenital idiopathic dilatation of the colon. Surg Gynecol Obstet 6: 624–643
4. Schneiderholn O (1915) Die Therapie der Hirschsprungschen Krankheit. Z Kinderth 12:321
5. Jayle F (1909) La dilatation congenitale idiopathique du colon. Presse Med 17:803
6. Hirschsprung H (1981) Stuhlträgheit Neugeborener infolge von Dilatation und Hypertrophie des Colons. Dis Colon Rectum 24:408–410
7. Hirschsprung H (1904) Dilatation congenitale du colon. In: Grancher, Comby (eds) Traité des maladies de l'enfance, 2nd edn. Paris

8. Hirschsprung H (1905) 107 Fälle von Darminvagination bei Kindern, behandelt in Königin Louises Kinderhospital in Kopenhagen während der Jahre 1871–1904. Mitt Grenzgeb Med Chir 14:555
9. Walker TJ, Griffith J (1893) Congenital dilatation and hypertrophy of the colon fatal at age of 11 years. Br Med J 2:230–231
10. Marfan A (1895) De la constipation des nourrissons et en particular de la constipation d'origine congénitale. Rev Mens Mal De Lenf 13:153
11. Hawkins HP (1907) Remarks on idiopathic dilatation of the colon. Br Med J I:477–483
12. Ehrenpreis T (1970) Hirschsprung's disease. Yearbook Medical, Chicago
13. Gee (1884) St Barth Hosp Rep
14. Osler W (1893) Cases of dilatation of the colon in young children. John Hopkins Hosp Bull 30:41–43
15. Fenwick WS (1900) Hypertrophy and dilatations of the colon in infancy. Br Med J ii: 564–567
16. Treves F (1898) Idiopathic dilatation of the colon. Lancet i:276–279
17. Swenson O, Rheinlander HF, Diamond I (1949) Hirschsprung's disease: a new concept of the etiology. N Engl J Med 241:551–556
18. Cameron JAM (1928) On the etiology of Hirschsprung's disease. Arch Dis Child 3:210–211
19. Adamson WAD, Aird I (1932) Megacolon: evidence in favour of a neurogenic origin. Br J Surg 20:220–233
20. Hurst AF (1934) Anal achalasia and megacolon (Hirschsprung's disease: idiopathic dilatation of the colon). Guys Hosp Rep 84:317–350
21. Frazer J (1926) Surgical aspects of certain disturbances of involuntary nervous system met within alimentary tract. Br Med J i:359–364
22. Frazer J (1927) The involuntary nervous system in relation to abdominal disease. Surg Gynecol Obstet 44:289–300
23. Ishikawa N (1923) Experimentelle und klinische Untersuchungen über die Pathogenese und das Wesen des Megacolons. Mitt Med Fak Kaiserl Kyushu Univ 7:339
24. Bayliss WM, Starling EH (1900) The movements and the innervation of the large intestine. J Physiol (Lond) 26:107–118
25. Langley JN, Anderson HK (1895) On the innervation of the pelvic and adjoining viscera. I. The lower portion of the intestine. J Physiol (Lond) 18:67–105
26. Rankin EW, Learmonth JR (1930) Section of the sympathetic nerves of the distal part of the colon and the rectum in the treatment of Hirschsprung's disease and certain types of constipation. Ann Surg 92:710–720
27. Learmonth JR, Markowitz J (1929) Studies on the function of the lumbar sympathetic outflow to the Sphincter ani internus. Am J Physiol 89:686–691
28. Learmonth JR, Markowitz J (1930) Studies on the innervation of the large bowel. II. The influence of the lumbar colonic nerve on the distal part of the colon. Am J Physiol 94: 501–504
29. Shephard JJ, Wright PG (1968) The response of the anal sphincter in man to stimulation of the presacral nerve. Am J Dig Dis 13:421–427
30. Rayner V (1970) Observations on the functional internal and sphincter of the vervet monkey. Proc Physiol Soc:27–28
31. Wade R, Royle ND (1927) The operative treatment of Hirschsprung's disease, new method; with explanation of the technique and results of operation. Med J Aust 1:137–141
32. Judd E, Adson AW, Lumber (1928) Sympathetic ganglionectomy and ramisectomy for congenital idiopathic dilatation of the colon. Ann Surg 88:479–498
33. Adson AW (1937) Hirschsprung's disease; indications for and results obtained by sympathectomy. Surgery I:859–877
34. Whitehouse F, Bargen JA, Dixon CF (1943) Congenital megacolon: favourable end results of treatment by resection. Gastroenterology I:922–937
35. Steinbach HL, Rosenberg RH, Grossman M, Nelson TL (1955) The potential hazard of enemas in patients with Hirschsprung's disease. Radiology 64:45–50
36. Lennander KG (1900) Fall av medfodd? Dilatation och hypertrofi av flexura sigmoidea hos ett barn (Maladie de Hirschsprung). Nord Med Ark II:1

37. Wilms M (1918) Dauerspasmus an Pylorus, Cardia, Sphincter der Blase und des Mastdarmes. Dtsch Z Chir 144:68
38. Martin E, Burden VG (1927) The surgical significance of the rectosigmoid sphincter. Ann Surg 86:86–91
39. Law JL (1940) Treatment of megacolon with acetylbetametylcholine bromide. Am J Dis Child 60:262–282
40. Klingman WO (1938) The treatment of neurogenic megacolon with selective drugs. J Pediatr 13:805
41. Hawksley M (1944–45) Spinal anaesthesia in the treatment of Hirschsprung's disease – with reports of twelve cases. Br J Surg 31:245–252
42. Ehrenpreis TL (1946) Megacolon in the newborn. A clinical and roentgenological study with special regard to the pathogenesis. Acta Chir Scand [Suppl] 94:112
43. Whitehouse FR, Kernohan JW (1948) Myenteric plexus in congenital megacolon. Arch Intern Med 82:75–111
44. Zueler WW, Wilson JL (1948) Functional intestinal obstruction on congenital neurogenic basis in infancy. Am J Dis Child 75:40–64
45. Tittel K (1901) Über eine angeborene Mißbildung des Dickdarmes. Wien Klin Wochenschr 14:903–907
46. Brentano A (1904) Über einen Fall von Hirschsprungscher Krankheit. Verh Dtsch Ges Chir I:265–268
47. Dalla Valla A (1920) Richerche istologiche su di un caso di megacolon congenito. Pediatria 28:740–752
48. Dalla Valla A (1924) Contributo alla conoscenza della forme famigliare del megacolon congenito. Pediatria 32:569–599
49. Robertson HE, Kernohan JW (1938) The myenteric plexus in congenital megacolon. Proc Staff Meet Mayo Clinic 13:123–125
50. Tiffin ME, Chandler LR, Faber HK (1940) Localised absence of the ganglion cells of the myenteric plexus in congenital megacolon. Am J Dis Child 59:1071–1082
51. Schmidt JE (1909) Über Hirschsprungsche Krankheit, insbesondere ihre chirurgische Behandlung. Klin Chir 61:682
52. Hurst A (1934) Anal achalasia and megacolon. Guys Hosp Rep 84:317
53. Swenson O, Bill AH Jr (1948) Resection of rectum and rectosigmoid with preservation of the sphincter for benign spastic lesions producing megacolon. Surgery 24:212–220
54. Bodian M, Stephens FD, Ward BCH (1949) Hirschsprung's disease and idiopathic megacolon. Lancet i:6–11
55. Hiatt RB (1951) The pathological physiology of congenital megacolon. Ann Surg 133:313–320
56. Hirst GDS (1979) Mechanics of peristalsis. Br Med Bull 35:263–268
57. Nixon HH (1964) Review article. Hirschsprung's disease. Arch Dis Child 39:109–115
58. Holschneider AM (ed) (1982) Hirschsprung's disease. Hippokrates, Stuttgart
59. Bulbring E, Brading AF, Johes AW, Tomita T (eds) (1981) Smooth muscle: an assessment of current knowledge. Arnold, Leeds
60. Alvarez WC (1949) A simple explanation for cardiospasm and Hirschsprung's disease. Gastroeneterology 13:422–429
61. Penninck FM, Kerremans RP (1975) Evolution of anorectal motility and rectoan reflex in Hirschsprung's disease and functional constipation. Acta Paediatr Scand 64:148–149
62. McElhannon FM (1959) Experimental production of megacolon resembling Hirschsprung's disease. Surg Forum 10:218–221
63. Weinberg AG (1970) The anorectal myenteric plexus: its relation to hypoganglionosis of the colon. Am J Clin Pathol 54:637–642
64. Seidal ER, Woods J, Elkenberg BA, Johnson LR (1983) Muscarinic cholinergic receptors in piebald mouse model for Hirschsprung's disease. Gastroenterology 85:335–338
65. Kubota M, Ito Y, Ikeda K (1983) Membrane properties and innervation of smooth muscle cells in Hirschsprung's disease. Am J Physiol 244:G406–415
66. Taylor G, Bywater B: Unpublished observations

67. Howard ER, Garrett JR (1970) Histochemistry and electron microscopy of rectum and colon in Hirschsprung's disease. Proc Roy Soc Med 63:1264–1266
68. Garrett JR, Howard ER, Nixon HH (1969) Autonomic nerves in rectum and colon in Hirschsprung's disease. A cholinesterase and catecholamine histochemical study. Arch Dis Child 44:406–417
69. Frigo GM, Del Tacca M, Lecchini S, Crema A (1973) Some observations on the intrinsic nervous mechanism in Hirschsprung's disease. Gut 14:35–40
70. Moore TC, Landers DB, Lachman RS, Ament ME (1979) Hirschsprung's disease in discordant monozygotic twins: a study of possible environmental factors in production of colonic aganglionosis. J Pediatr Surg 14:158–161
71. Passarge E (1967) The genetics of Hirschsprung's disease. Evidence for heterogeneous etiology and a study of sixty-three families. N Engl J Med 276:138–143
72. Cohen IT, Gadd MA (1982) Hirschsprung's disease in a kindred: a possible clue to the genetics of the disease. J Pediatr Surg 17:632–634
73. Okamoto E, Ueda T (1967) Embryogenesis of intraneural ganglia of the gut and its relation to Hirschsprung's disease. J Pediatr Surg 2:437–443
74. Webster W (1973) Embryogenesis of the enteric ganglia in normal mice and mice that develop congenital aganglionic megacolon. J Embryol Exp Morphol 30:573–585
75. Hukuhara T, Kotani S, Sato G (1961) Effects of destruction of intraneural ganglion cells on colon motility: possible genesis of congenital megacolon. Jpn J Physiol II:635–641
76. Okamoto E, Iwasaki T, Kakutani T, Ueda T (1967) Selective destruction of the myenteric plexus: its relation to Hirschsprung's disease, achalasia of the oesophagus and hypertrophic pyloric stenosis. J Pediatr Surg 2:444–454
77. Bolande RP, Towler WF (1972) Ultrastructural and histochemical studies of murine mega colon. Am J Pathol 69:139–152
78. Earlam RJ (1972) A vascular cause for aganglionic bowel: a new hypothesis. Dig Dis Sci 17:255–261
79. De Villiers DR (1966) Ischaemia of the colon: an experimental study. Br J Surg 53:497–503
80. Rothman TP, Gershon MD (1982) Colonization of the bowel by neuronal precursors in normal and aganglionic (1^s1^s) mutant mice. Anat Rec 202:161–162
81. Boley SJ (1975) Pathophysiology of Hirschsprung's disease. J Pediatr Surg 10:861–863
82. Orr JD, Scobie WG (1983) Presentation and incidence of Hirschsprung's disease. Br Med J 287:1671
83. Dobbins WO, Bill AH (1965) Diagnosis of Hirschsprung's disease excluded by rectal section biopsy. N Engl J Med 272:990–993
84. Campbell PE, Noblett HR (1969) Experience with rectal suction biopsy in the diagnosis of Hirschsprung's disease. J Pediatr Surg 4:410–415
85. Meier-Ruge W, Morger R (1968) Neue Gesichtspunkte zur Pathogenese und Klinik des Morbus Hirschsprung. Schweiz Med Wochenschr 98:20
86. Lawson JON, Nixon NH (1967) Anal canal pressure in the diagnosis of Hirschsprung's disease. J Pediatr Surg 2:544–552
87. Shafie H, Suzuki H, Schnaufer L, Haller JA Jr, White JJ (1972) A simplified method of anorectal manometry for wider clinical application. J Pediatr Surg 7:230–235
88. Holschneider AM, Kellner E, Streibl P, Sippell WG (1976) The development of anorectal continence and its significance in the diagnosis of Hirschsprung's disease. J Pediatr Surg II:151–156
89. Tamate S et al (1984) Manometric diagnosis of Hirschsprung's disease in the neonatal period. J Pediatr Surg 19:285–288
90. Marin AM, Riarola A, Garcia H (1976) Electromyography of the rectum and colon in Hirschsprung's disease. J Pediatr Surg II:457–552
91. Sharma LK, Marya RK, Chandran AP (1981) A clinical evaluation of anorectal electromyography in the diagnosis of Hirschsprung's disease. Acta Paediatr Scand 70:865–867
92. Rowe MI (1984) Hirschsprung's disease: is the Boley procedure better? International congress of paediatric surgery, Perth, Australia, 7–9 March 1984
93. Ehrenpreis TL (1951) Rectosigmoidectomy for Hirschsprung's disease. Acta Chir Scand 102:251–259

94. Grob M (1952) Zur Technik der Rectosigmoidektomie bei Megacolon congenitum (Hirschsprung). Helv Chir Acta 19:336
95. Toupet A (1950) Technique de resection du rectum abdominotransanale par retournement sans anus prévalable avec abaissement systématique du colon transverse. J Chir 66:37
96. Cutiat DE (1965) Technique of rectosigmoidectomy for megacolon. Dis Colon Rectum 8:107–114
97. Swenson O (1964) Partial internal sphincterectomy in the treatment of Hirschsprung's disease. Ann Surg 160:540–550
98. Duhamel B (1960) A new operation for the treatment of Hirschsprung's disease. Arch Dis Child 35:38–39
99. Grob M (1960) Intestinal obstruction in the newborn infant. Arch Dis Child 35:40–50
100. Louw JH (1961) The Duhamel operation for Hirschsprung's disease. S Afr Med J 35:1033–1036
101. Martin LW, Altemeier WA (1962) Clinical experience with a new operation (modified Duhamel procedure) for Hirschsprung's disease. Ann Surg 156:678–681
102. Steichen SM, Talbert JL, Ravitch MM (1968) Primary side-to-side colo-rectal anastomosis in the Duhamel's operation for Hirschsprung's disease. Surgery 64:475–483
103. Grob M, Genton N, Vontobel V (1959) Erfahrungen in der Behandlung des Megacolon congenitum und Vorschlag einer neuen Operationstechnik. Zentralbl Chir 84:1781
104. Duhamel B (1964) Retrorectal and transanal pull-through procedure for the treatment of Hirschsprung's disease Dis Colon Rectum 7:455–458
105. Soave F (1964) Hirschsprung's disease: a new surgical technique. Arch Dis Child 39:116–124
106. Boley SJ (1964) New modification of the surgical treatment of Hirschsprung's disease. Surgery 56:1015–1017
107. Boley SJ et al (1968) Endorectal pull-through procedure for Hirschsprung's disease with and without primary anastomosis. J Pediatr Surg 3:258–262
108. Kasai M, Suzuki H, Watanabe K (1971) Rectal myotomy with colectomy: a new radical operation for Hirschsprung's disease. J Pediatr Surg 6:36–41
109. Rehbein F, Von S, Zimmermann H (1960) Results with abdominal resection in Hirschsprung's disease. Arch Dis Child 35:29–37
110. Rehbein F, Morger R, Kundert JG, Meier-Ruge W (1966) Surgical problems in congenital megacolon. J Pediatr Surg I:526–533
111. Stephens FD (1980) Anorectal continence and idiopathic constipation. In: Holder TM, Ashcraft KW (eds) Pediatric surgery. Saunders, Philadelphia, p 421
112. Costa M, Furness JB (1982) Neuronal peptides in the intestine. Br Med Bull 38:247–252
113. Freeman NV, Burge DM, Soar JS, Sedgewick EM (1980) The normal development of cortical evoked potentials in response to anal stimulation. Z Kinderchir 31:22–30
114. Freeman NV, Cass DT (1981) Unpublished observations
115. Freeman NV (1984) Personal communication
116. Swenson O, Sherman JO, Fisher JH, Cohen E (1975) The treatment and post-operation complications of congenital megacolon: A 25-year follow-up. Ann Surg 182:266–273
117. So HB, Schwartz DL, Becker JM, Daum F, Schneider KM (1980) Endorectal "pull-through" without preliminary colostomy in neonates with Hirschsprung's disease. J Pediatr Surg 15:470–471
118. Carcassonne M (1984) The definitive operation: which, when, why, and how. International congress of paediatric surgery, symposium on management of Hirschsprung's disease, Perth, Australia, 7–9 March 1984

Club-foot Through the Centuries

E. H. STRACH[1]

The early history of club-foot is the history of the lame and crippled child. Throughout the ages the fate of a deformed child depended on the attitude of the society.

Ancient man led a nomadic life, hence a lame or sickly child was a burden to the family in the struggle for existence – it did not survive long.

The Spartans 'laid out' their deformed children for different reasons: the elimination furthered their ideal of aesthetic supremacy and was carried out scientifically and without sentiment. The future Orthodox Church was unmoved by such ideals – after all a deformity was considered to be a 'curse of God'. This attitude is undoubtedly based on the Levitican laws of the Old Testament:

> Whosoever has any blemish, let him not approach to offer the bread of his God... a blind man or a lame, or he that has a flat nose or anything superfluous, or a man that is brokenfooted or brokenhanded, or crookbackt, or a dwarf...

Ancient Indian Society considered the cripple and the dwarf an outcast, and it is significant that the Sanscrit word for dwarf (dhvaros) is translated as "the evil one".

Smith and Warren [58] in their studies of Egyptian Mummies found that Pharaoh Siptah of the XIX Dynasty was afflicted with talipes, or "club-foot" (Fig. 1). He lived around 1210 B.C.; to judge from the Elliot Smith drawing of the foot this was a case of extreme equinus deformity, possibly from poliomyelitis or cerebral palsy rather than congenital club-foot. Many authorities describe any foot deformity as talipes or club-foot.

In Greek mythology Hephaestus, the blacksmith of Olympus, was lame from birth, his feet were twisted. His stumbling gait aroused "unquenchable laughter of the Immortals". There is little doubt that he had bilateral club-feet and this was represented by several ancient Greek artists: an example is the small amphora painted in the 6th century B.C. and found in Corinth (Fig. 2), at present in the National Archaeological Museum in Athens.

In view of the negative attitude of society towards the deformed, very little attention was paid to cure or alleviate the suffering cripple or the lame afflicted by foot deformities. There are exceptions. The old Indian Literature, the Ajur-Veda, way back in the tenth century B.C. contains the first known description of club-foot and advises massage.

[1] Consultant Orthopaedic Surgeon, Liverpool, United Kingdom

Progress in Pediatric Surgery, Vol. 20
Ed. by P. P. Rickham

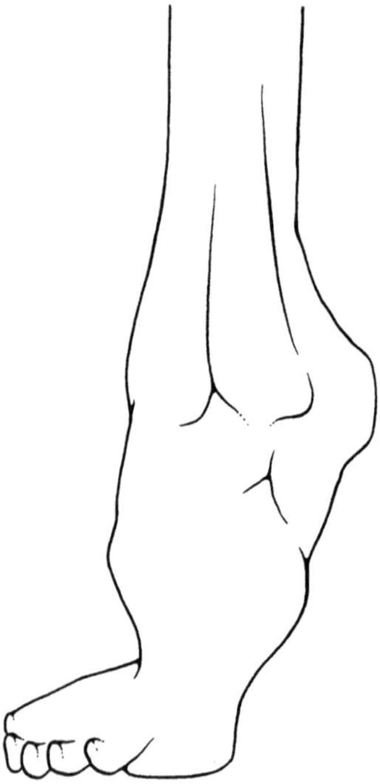

Fig. 1. Tracing of Elliot Smith drawing of the talipes of the Pharaoh Siptah [58]

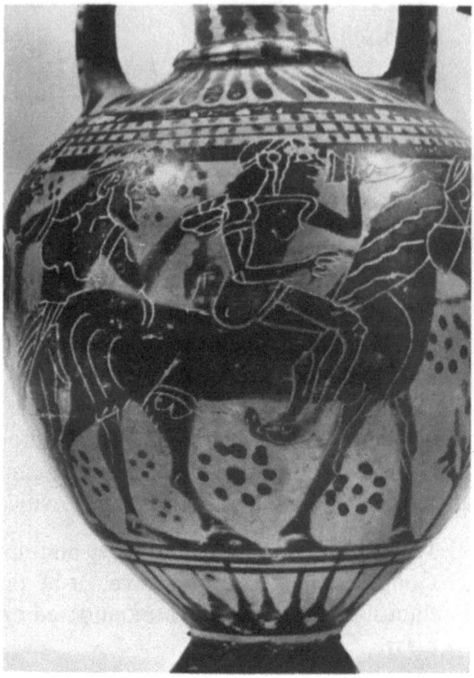

Fig. 2. Small Amphora showing the club-foot Hephaestus riding a horse. By courtesy of the National Archaeological Museum, Athens

In ancient Graeco-Roman civilisation the cult of Asklepios (Aesculapius) flourished. Aesculap was the son of Apollo and became the God of Medicine. Temples were erected (Aesclopeiae), which though primarily religious became centres of medical service. The great establishments of Cos and Epidauros can be considered as the forerunners of Hospitals. In these mountain retreats the cripples and disabled were cared for.

Hippocrates was born about 460 B.C. of an Aesclepiad family on the island of Cos. He was thought to be a descendant of Aesculapius and Hercules. He gave Greek medicine its scientific spirit and its ethical ideals. Amongst the great volumes of writings which were continued over the next four centuries and collected as the monumental 'Corpus Hippocrates' are descriptions of spinal deformities, congenital dislocation of the hip and club-foot [33]. He recognised that some club-feet are congenital, while some are acquired in early infancy. He believed mechanical pressure in utero to be the cause of congenital club-foot, a theory which has been upheld by Galen and by modern workers [16, 50] and is still valid today at least for the milder type of club-feet. Hippocrates defined the principles of treatment of club-foot, urging that treatment should start as soon as possible after birth. He recommended repeated manipulation and fixation by strong bandages which should be maintained for a long time, aiming at over-correction. These principles of treatment are as valid today as they were 2300 years ago. His teaching has been passed on over the centuries, but his plea for treatment to be commenced soon after birth has been forgotten.

No further written account of club-foot appeared for the next 2000 years. These were the dark ages in the history of orthopaedic surgery during which the Hippocratic teaching faded. There were exceptions, notably Galen (second century A.D.), whose greatest contribution to orthopaedic surgery was the study of muscles, nerves and blood vessels and also the treatment of deformities. Anthyllus (third century A.D.) was the first to recommend tenotomy in the treatment of contracted joints.

The Middle Ages (Fifth–Fifteenth Centuries)

The Middle Ages added little to the progress of surgery and the light of Hippocrates was extinguished or at the best burned but dimly in hidden places. Medicine and surgery were influenced by mysticism arising in Asia Minor and by Arabic culture with its antipathy towards dissection. Throughout the centuries a deformity represented a mark of divine discipline and the victims were scorned without pity or at the best were subject for derision. Devils were pictured as hunchbacks with crooked limbs and deformed feet. The derision led to the fashion of cripples as court jesters. This became widespread and led to the deliberate maiming of children.

Footbinding in China was done for different reasons: a small and delicate foot was a symbol of feminine beauty; the footwear required a raised heel (Fig. 3) and caused a slow and graceful gait. The resulting foot (Fig. 4) and shoe (Fig. 5) resemble the shape of a lotus flower (Fig. 6), hence the name of lotus feet. The custom may have started about 1000 years ago amongst the dancers and court women

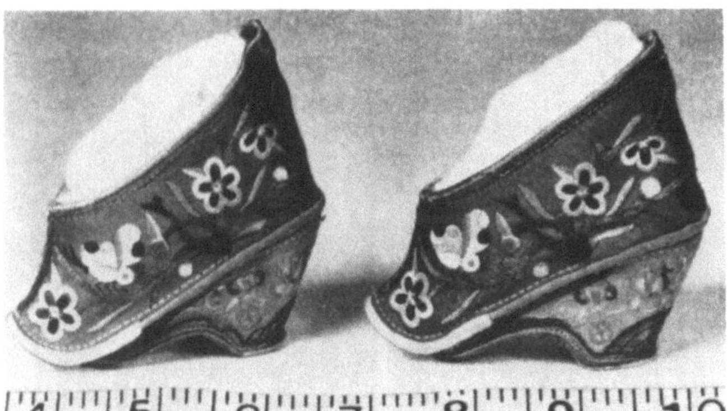

Fig. 3. Shoes to fit bound feet. Note the raised heel. (From [27]). Measurement in inches

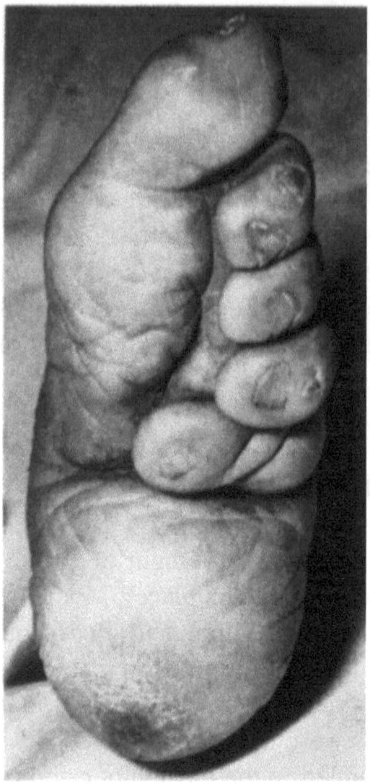

Fig. 4. Bound foot. (From [27])

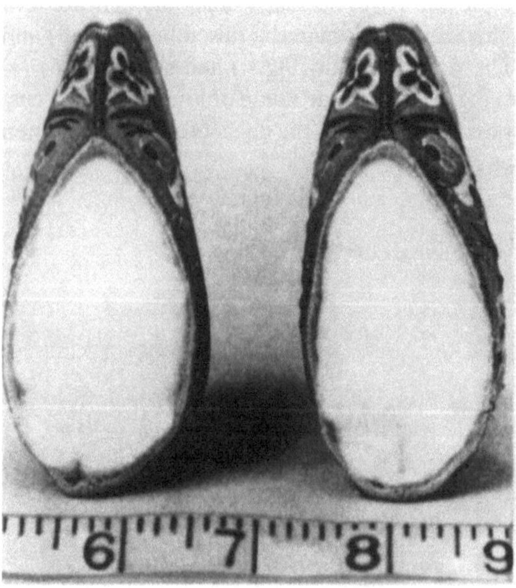

Fig. 5. Bound feet shoes showing resemblance to lotus flower. (From [27]). Measurement in inches

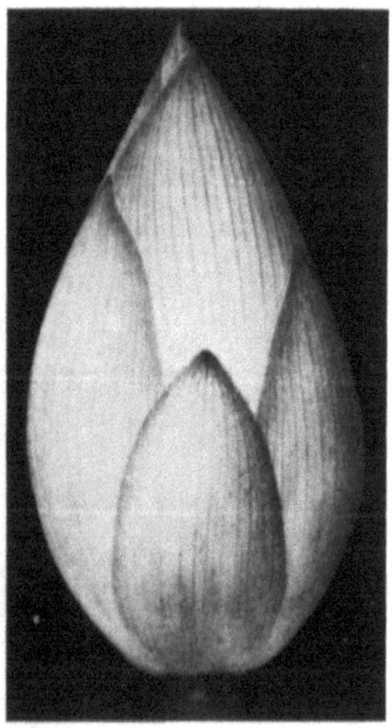

Fig. 6. Lotus flower bud. (From [27])

and eventually spread like any fashion and became a symbol of social standing. Footbinding was started at the age of two to six among the rich, but at a later age in poorer families; starting later produced a less disabling foot which would not prevent the girls from working in adult life. The method of producing the deformity closely resembles the method used to treat club-feet; repeated moulding and strapping and bandaging is effective in producing or correcting a deformity. The custom of footbinding was resisted in the late nineteenth century and became illegal in the first half of the twentieth century.

The fourteenth and fifteenth centuries saw a great awakening of medical sciences with the birth of the great universities of western civilisation.

The Renaissance (Fifteenth–Sixteenth Centuries)

The Renaissance brought widespread acceptance of scientific methods, including anatomical studies. Leonardo da Vinci studied the human framework, notably muscles and their function. Vesalius added physiology. Ambroise Paré described spinal deformities as well as club-foot (1575) [49]. He advised treatment by manipulation, bandaging and special boots.

Dr. O. Bohne [11] reported on the orthopaedic treatment of club-foot in the sixteenth century. He relates the case of the infant Duke of Braunschweig who was taken to many countries for consultation; no one was found who could help the little Prince, not even Ambroise Paré. Finally Dr. Haerdael of Holland undertook his treatment. He and his sons took the Prince in a huge carriage, packed with instruments and medicaments, out of town where no one could see or hear them. The Prince was placed in an instrument which did not allow him to move at all: then additional instruments were applied to his feet; the screws were turned every hour, increasing the Prince's discomfort; this was relieved to some extent by "essences" and "strong waters" [probably alcohol]. The procedure was carried out six times in one day and eventually the feet were restored to an almost normal position, allowing him to walk far better than before.

The Seventeenth Century

The seventeenth century augured well for progress of orthopaedic surgery as society became more considerate towards its crippled and maimed, who were shunned no longer. The Poor Relief Act of 1601 included the care of the crippled, and derision gave way to sympathy. This attitude became also manifest in art. Velasquez painted sympathetic portraits of dwarfs. Ribera's picture of the boy with club-foot betrays the commiseration felt by the artist for his model (Fig. 7). The artist captured the boy's sad smile which expresses a suspicion of hidden suffering, the deformed foot not being a prominent feature. Such facial expressions can be found even today in children undergoing long term treatment in orthopaedic wards.

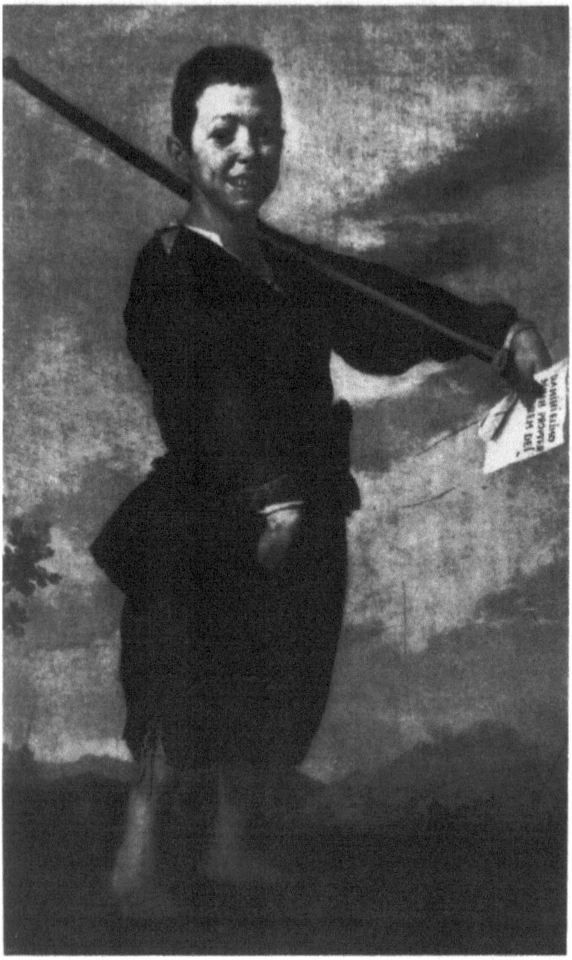

Fig. 7. 'Boy with club-foot'. Painting by José Ribera (1589–c. 1656). Musée du Louvre, Paris. This young vagabond is carrying his crutch with the proud air of an hildago bearing arms. His smile seems to be making game of his own infirmity; he is also careful to inform us by means of a scrap of writing he holds, that he is dumb as well as crippled, because he appeals to charity with a card which bears the inscription: "Da mihi elimosinam propter amorem Dei". J. Ruhrah [52] suggests that this boy is suffering from right-sided hemiplegia and has a speech defect

At that time the first description of club-foot appeared since Hippocrates: Arcaeus in 1658 [4] described club-foot and devised a mechanical contraption for its correction.

William Fabrig or Fabry of Hilden (Fabricius Hildanus) [26] described an apparatus which included a turnbuckle for gradual correction of the "Pes distortus".

The Dutch surgeon Isacius Minnius established the principle of dividing tight tendons to correct deformity and he performed the first tenotomy for wry neck in 1685 (cited by [62]).

The Eighteenth Century

Orthopaedic surgery became established in the eighteenth century as a result of two events: the appearance of the first book specially devoted to orthopaedics and the creation of the first orthopaedic hospital.

Nicholas André produced his treatise in 1741 at the ripe age of 83. His whole life had been a struggle: in his youth against poverty, in his manhood he was involved in polemics against other writers. He studied theology and turned to medicine later, qualifying in Reims and later in Paris. His inaugural thesis was: "What part in the care of disease have cheerfulness in the doctor and obedience in the patient?" He eventually became professor of medicine. His famous treatise is entitled 'Orthopaedia' and he explains how he coined the word: "As to the title, I have formed it of Greek words, viz. ορθός [orthos] which specifies streight [sic], free from deformity, and παις [pais], a child. Out of these two words I have compounded that of Orthopaedia, to express in one term the design I propose which is to teach the different methods of preventing and correcting deformities in children." André died in 1742. In 1743 the English translation appeared with the authors's name spelled Andry [3].

He described "Bolt feet" as such "as resemble those of a horse and they are called Pedes Equinae". He laid great stress on the role of muscle balance in the creation of deformities. He described how to manage feet "when the heel does not touch the ground easily. ... Children are sometimes born with the defect, and sometimes come by it afterwards. ... It may be cured by such remedies as are proper to relax tendons and muscles, and by great motions of the leg and foot ... to rub the leg with the Oil of Worms ... to bathe the leg in a bucket full of Trip-Broth. ... He then describes passive and active exercises in detail and recommends frequent climbing up some sloping ascents, thus stretching the tendon of the leg so that the heel must fall lower. He also recommends a heel of lead to the shoe instead of timber.

"If the feet of a young child are turned inwards the Nurse ought to turn the feet gently to that position which is natural to those parts." In long-standing deformities of the older child he recommends remedies which soften the ligaments such as formations followed by manual manipulation and splinting on a strong pasteboard, wood or a small plate of iron, held on carefully with a bandage.

He mentions that "it is reckoned a beauty amongst the ladies of China to have the feet less than the natural size" and describes the foot-binding of girls after the third year. The women feel the effect all their life and can scarcely walk. Yet, they suffer the inconvenience with pleasure, as nothing is more esteemed amongst them than exceedingly small feet.

The effect of moulding and bandaging is exemplified in his treatment of knock knees and bow legs of young children. His method of "recovering the shape of the leg is the same as is used for making streight [sic] the crooked trunk of a young tree". He illustrates this with a drawing of a crooked tree tied to a straight pole (Fig. 8). This has remained the symbol of orthopaedic surgery up to the present day. As orthopaedic surgery developed over the years it outgrew the original meaning proposed by André. It can now be interpreted as 'to educate' (παιδέτω) 'to grow straight' (ορθός).

The idea of an orthopaedic hospital was conceived by Jean André Venel [64], a physician in Geneva and the first of these institutions was inaugurated in Orbe in 1780. Venel treated curvatures of the spine by prolonged recumbency and he developed several types of braces for club-feet, notably the club-foot shoe.

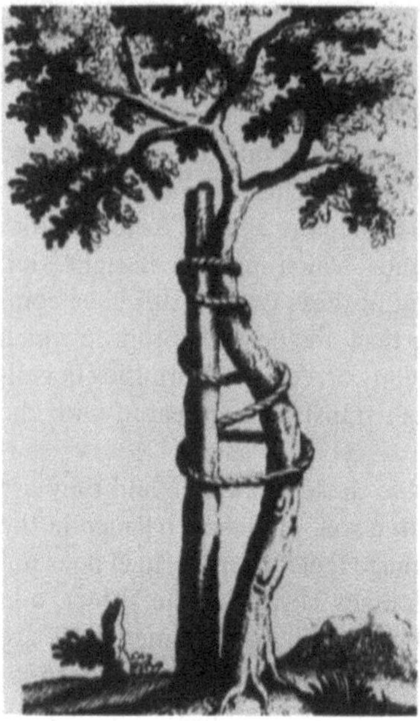

Fig. 8. The crooked trunk of a young tree tied to a straight pole has become the symbol of orthopaedic surgery. (From [3])

Eighteenth century medicine relegated surgery to the barber – anaesthesia was unknown, antisepsis had not survived antiquity, the genius of Pasteur was unborn – the scene was set for the golden age for the bone-setter.

In England, William Chesledon, surgeon and anatomist, became interested in talipes in the first half of the eighteenth century. Not knowing how to cure club-foot he referred such cases to Mr. Presgrove, a professional bone-setter and studied his method; this was by holding the foot as near the natural position as he could and then rolling it up with straps of sticking plaster. This procedure was repeated until the foot was restored to its natural position. There were some imperfections of this method: the bandages caused wasting of the legs and swelling of the top of the feet. Chesledon modified the method: he remembered the method of treatment for his own fracture of the cubit when a boy. The fracture was set by Mr. Cowper, bone-setter at Leicester; he wrapped the arm in rags dipped in whites of eggs mixed with a little flour. Whilst drying, the rags grew stiff, thus keeping the limb in good position. He applied the same method to the treatment of club-feet. Nine years later a description of his method appeared in the textbook *Operations in Surgery* by the Paris surgeon Le Dran together with illustrations (Fig. 9). Chesledon used this method for 40 years with great success.

There were isolated attempts at surgical treatment: Lorenz in Frankfurt performed the first section of the Achilles tendon for club-foot in 1782 following a suggestion by the physician Thilemus (cited by [28]).

Bruckner's monograph on club-foot appeared in 1796 [18] and generated renewed interest in the subject in the German-speaking world. He was the first to

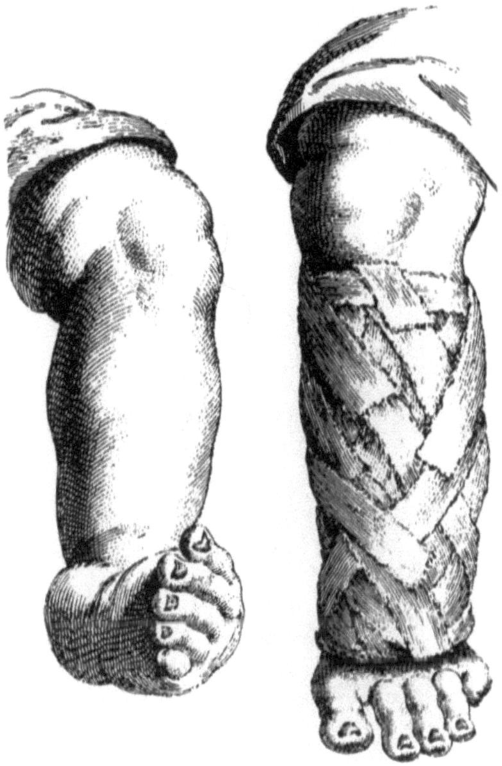

Fig. 9. Cheselden's method of correction of club-foot using egg and flour bandages. (From [42, p. 11])

recommend forcible manipulation followed by corrective footwear. John Hunter's experimental work on tendon healing laid the foundation for future tendon surgery.

The Nineteenth Century

The turn of the century saw the gradual development of modern orthopaedic surgery; conservative and manipulative treatment of club-foot was supplemented by surgical interventions.

It is significant that hitherto club-foot was mostly managed by bone setters and instrument makers. Timothy Sheldrake, trussmaker to Westminster Hospital, was a staunch defender of conservative treatment of club-foot and published his "Essay on Club-Foot" in 1798 (cited by Little [42]). He showed considerable knowledge of anatomy and pathology and attributed foot deformities to defective muscle action. He never fully described his method. Although his writings were abundant, he had a veritable gift for hiding his meaning in a cloud of words. But it is known that his appliance provided a spring to replace defective muscle action. He claimed great success but admits to the occurrence of relapses. One of his not-

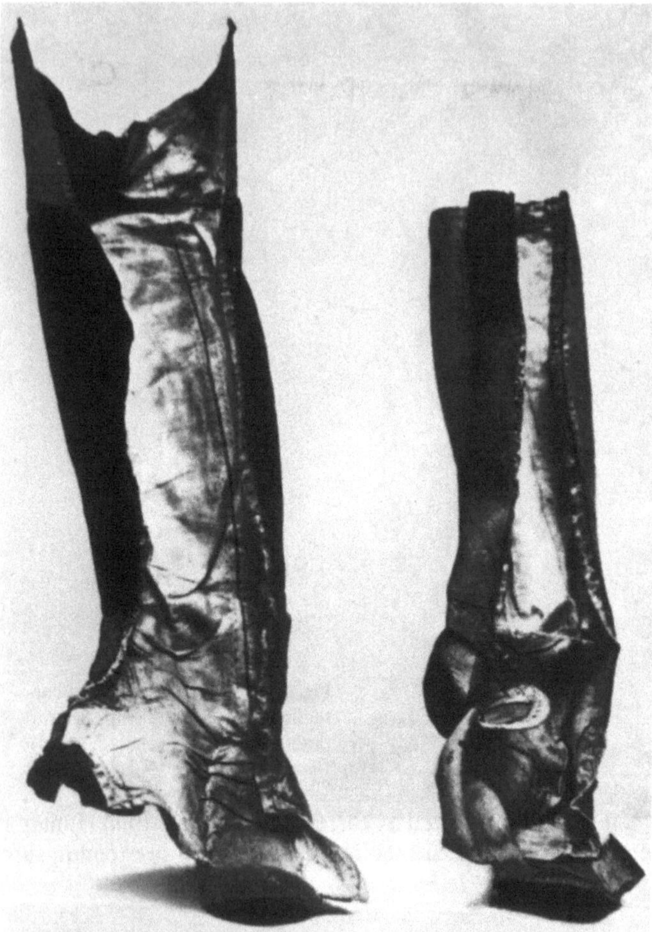

Fig. 10. Byron's walking instruments. (From [42, p. 24])

able failures was the case of Lord Byron. But he explains that Byron, whilst at school at Dulwich, had his club-foot treated by William Sheldrake, his younger brother and unfair competitor who also made a mess of his case! Later on he complained that he was unable to cure Lord Byron's lameness "from unwillingness of the noble patient to submit to restraint and confinement." Fortunately he was successful in constructing a sort of shoe which in some degree alleviated the inconvenience (Fig. 10).

Sheldrake strongly opposed tenotomy but he could not halt the progress of surgical treatment which was based on the studies of John Hunter and on the description of the pathological anatomy of the club-foot by Antonio Scarpa, the Italian anatomist who published his work in 1803 [55]. Scarpa thought that the talus was normal in club-foot but that the soft tissues were deranged by an inward

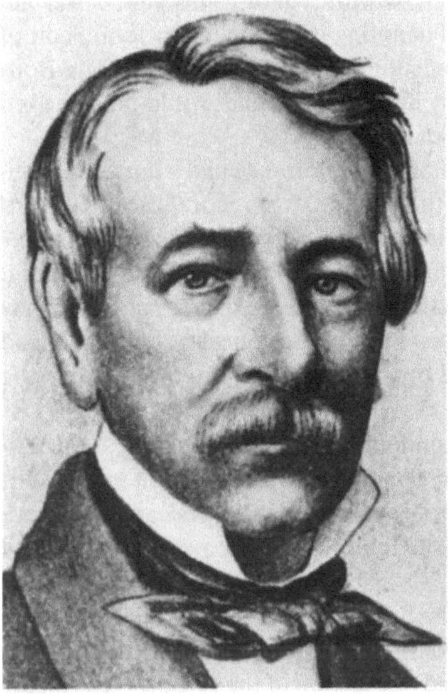

Fig. 11. G. F. L. Stromeyer. (From [38])

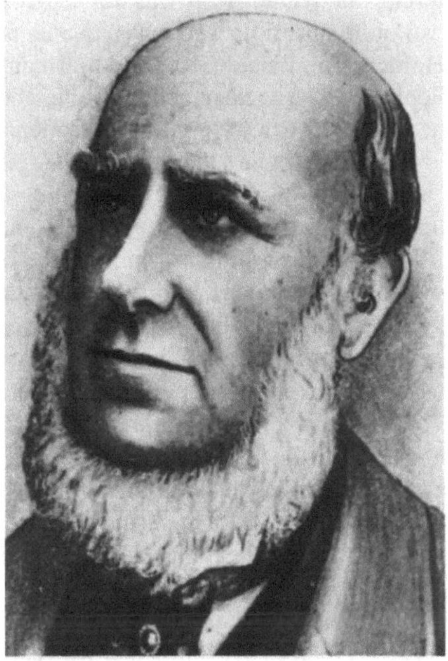

Fig. 12. W. J. Little. (From [38])

dislocation of the forefoot; the bone changes were secondary. His book marked a turning point in interest on this subject. Many studies followed, especially in France and England, but were chiefly therapeutic rather than descriptive. Adams [1], some 60 years later, agreed that the essential changes in idiopathic club-foot were in the tarsus and that all soft tissue abnormalities were secondary. However, he disagreed on the nature of the osseous changes; he was convinced that the principal deformity was in the head and neck of the talus.

Tendon surgery was revived and tenotomy was rediscovered: Delpech of Montpellier [22] used it for several cases but the infection rate was high.

George Friedrich Louis Stromeyer [60] (Fig. 11) of Hanover had the ingenious idea of cutting the contracted Achilles tendon subcutaneously so as to avoid infection. He did the first subcutaneous tenotomy on a 14-year-old schoolboy in 1831, whom he had treated for the previous 18 months without success. The tenotomy corrected the equinus so well that Stromeyer became enthusiastic about his method; he perfected it and it was quickly adopted by other surgeons. By 1833 some 400 cases were reported. He now came to consider deformed feet as a reproach to surgeons. He saw in the streets of great cities people with club-feet, the healing of which no one even thought of and which could have been helped.

Two of the greatest poets, Lord Byron and Sir Walter Scott and the greatest diplomat of his time, Prince Talleyrand, suffered from club-feet and were not cured. The psychological reaction of the two poets to their lameness was quite different. Sir Walter Scott was not self-conscious with regard to his gait. After all, two of his ancestors were given nicknames denoting their lameness: John Scott of Harden, The Lammiter, in the fourteenth century and his son William The Bolt-Foot. Byron was extremely sensitive about his deformity and would have moved heaven and earth to suppress all evidence of it.

Stromeyer found the theory of congenitalism a hindrance and a curse to surgical progress. "Congenital" was a shibboleth used to cover ignorance; it does not imply that a condition is not curable, and left to nature it will only get worse.

In spite of his enthusiasm he had a balanced view and he made no claim that sectioning of tendons, aponeurosis and muscles displaced existing methods, they merely offer a valuable help in difficult cases. Purely mechanical orthopaedics and operative orthopaedics must be cultivated together and both methods should be followed and perfected by the same man.

Stromeyer's most famous patient was undoubtedly W. J. Little (Fig. 12). William John Little was born in the east end of London in 1810; a fever in infancy left him with a palsied and deformed foot and as he grew up his heel became inverted. He began the study of medicine with the fixed intention of discovering what could be done for the relief of his deformed foot. At that time, club-foot was outside the domaine of legitimate surgery and was in the hands of bone setters, sprain rubbers and instrument makers. He studied the French literature and heard of the French surgeon Delpech of Montpellier who carried out section of the Achilles tendon for club-foot. He approached Delpech who advised against surgery because of fear of infection.

Little studied comparative anatomy and at the age of 22 he became a Member of the Royal College of Surgeons. He started a practice and also lectured in comparative anatomy at the London Hospital. He was unsuccessful in obtaining a surgical position at that hospital, as a result of which he became a physician, a fact which changed his life and caused him to become a pioneer of orthopaedic surgery. He was seconded to work at the University of Berlin under Johannes Muller. This was a great medical centre where he met Schwann, Henle and other famous workers. He was able to continue his dissections of deformed feet. He found that the soft tissues, especially muscles and tendons were the cause of deformed feed, and he postulated that they should be amenable to surgical treatment and Muller agreed. Little had heard of Stromeyer and went out to Hanover to see him. He underwent the operation which proved to be a great success. He stayed on in Hanover, perfected himself in the technique of the operation. When he returned to Berlin he was convinced that a new era had dawned for the deformed. Muller and Dieffenbach were amazed by the result. Dieffenbach immediately adopted the operation and within 12 months operated on 140 club-feet. Little read his doctor's thesis of the University of Berlin on "The Nature and Treatment of Club-Foot".

He returned to London and started his practice specially for the treatment of club-foot. On the 20th February 1837 he performed the first tenotomy for club-foot in England; he also devided the tibialis posterior and the flexor hallucis longus tendons. The reaction of his British collegues were divided; some were interested, some sceptical, some were opposed. In 1838 he founded the Orthopaedic Institution with the help of friends and relatives and this became later the Royal Orthopaedic Hospital, the first public charity institution for the relief of the maimed and deformed poor. Here his third son, Louis Stromeyer Little performed the first subcutaneous osteotomy for knock-knee in 1865. His son Muirhead Little became senior surgeon at the Royal Orthopaedic Hospital.

W. J. Little published his *Treatise on the Nature of Club-Foot and Analogous Distortions* in 1839 [43]. In it he distinguished the various types of club-feet and recognised pes cavus as a different entity. He gave lectures and published his course of lectures; he became a pioneer of subcutaneous tenotomy and of orthopaedic surgery. Yet, his real aim was to become a physician. He was appointed assistant physician to the London Hospital, but his surgical endeavours prevented his election to the Fellowship until he was 67 years of age. He continued his work on deformities and muscle action and he described that curious form of infantile spastic paralysis known as "Little's disease".

In later life he became disillusioned with the results of tenotomy. Like any new method it gave poor results if used indiscriminately. Like Stromeyer, he concluded that tenotomy as a sole treatment can lead to disastrous results; it must be combined with conservative treatment to be effective.

In the United States D. L. Rogers of New York performed the first tenotomy for club-foot, assisted by Lewis Sayre in 1885 (cited in [54]).

Subcutaneous section of the Achilles tendon was often unsuccessful in correcting club-foot because other soft tissues were maintaining the deformity. With the introduction of antiseptic and aseptic methods in surgery by Lister in 1862, operative treatment of club-foot became more adventurous: Streckeisen (cited in [7]) described the medial release operation in 1867 to correct the varus element of the deformity. This soft tissue operation was extended by Phelps in 1884 [51] to include elongation of the tibialis posterior and flexor hallucis longus tendons and the division of the medial ligament of the ankle.

Even more radical were operations on the bones, probably for the more resistant forms of club-feet. In 1875 Solly (cited in [40]), at the suggestion of Little, removed the cuboid bone, but the operation failed to correct the foot. In 1872 Lund of Manchester excised the talus, and in 1875 Davies Colley removed a bone wedge from the outer side of the foot. Pughe of Liverpool resected the head of the talus in 1883, and Phelps extended his soft tissue release operation to include osteotomy of the neck of the talus and wedge resection of the calcaneum.

There were many opponents to radical treatment, and conservative management received an impetus by a new type of plaster bandage which was used to splint the corrected club-foot. It was first developed by Guerin in 1836 [32], but it took 20 years for plaster of Paris to be used in these cases.

There were advocates for treatment to begin as early after birth as possible, as first recommended by Hippocrates. Yet until the end of the nineteenth century treatment was deliberately delayed until early childhood. Even Little started treatment of club-foot when the child was old enough to walk; but Dieffenbach and William Adams recommended that the treatment start as early as possible. This was a great step forward, and considerable resistance had to be overcome.

Fundamental research was done in the dissecting room by Little and Adams and led to the concept of the role of muscle action in causing the deformity. Gradually the various types of club-feet were recognised; the neurogenic type (poliomyelitis, cerebral palsy) was distinguished from the congenital type. The old Hippocratic theory of mechanical pressure in utero, also upheld by Paré and Scarpa, was revived by the work of Parker and Shattock of 1884 [50]. They believed, like Tubby (1896, cited in [9]), that the foetal feet are inverted in early pregnancy; the increased intra-uterine pressure leads to muscle damage and to club-foot. Bessel-Hagen [8] studied the human foetus and came to the same conclusion.

At the Robert Jones Clinic in Liverpool manual correction as a daily routine was considered sufficient in many cases. At the Hospital for the Ruptured and Crippled in New York, manual overcorrection was used as a weakly routine and the corrected foot was immobilised in plaster of Paris or by strapping.

Even manipulative treatment became more radical, and Hugh Owen Thomas (Fig. 13), the great protagonist of manipulation, devised a wrench "to aid in the treatment of club-feet of every variety" (Fig. 14). He maintains that "the foot becomes instantly more pliable after stretching..., the use of the wrench very materially shortens the period of treatment..." [61].

His method was adopted by Grattan of Cork, Bradford of Boston and by Lorenz of Vienna. Lorenz later made use of a padded pyramid over whose apex he 'broke' the deformity.

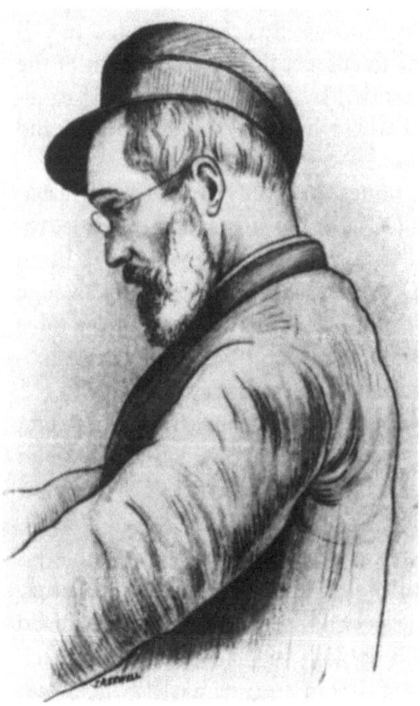

Fig. 13. Hugh Owen Thomas. 1834–1891. (From [38].) 'Frail in body, strong in mind, with a brusque manner and a big heart, he was an independent thinker, a careful yet bold surgeon and an expert mechanician' [48]

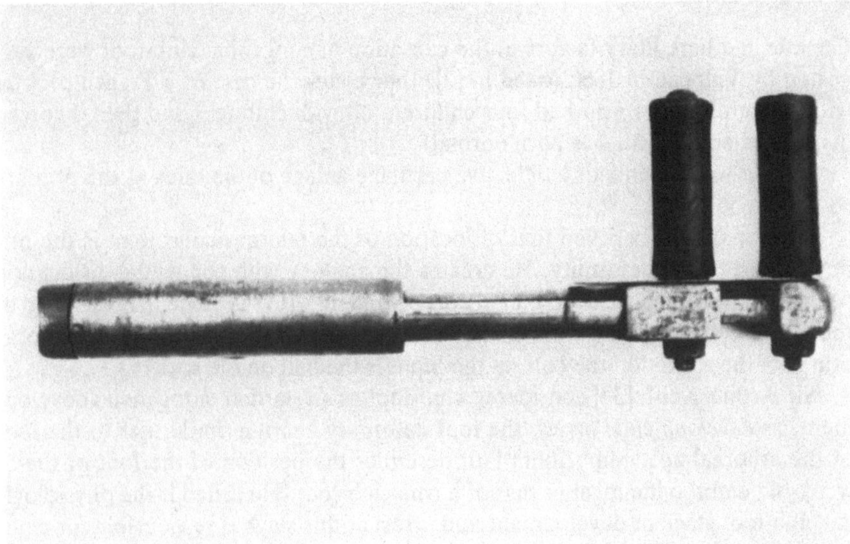

Fig. 14. The original Thomas' wrench. (From the collection of surgical instruments, held by the Liverpool Medical Institution)

Such treatment would be considered cruel today. Flaubert in his Madame Bovary [29] vividly describes the attempted forceful correction of a mature club-foot with its tragic consequences. It is not surprising that surgeons like Taylor and Freiburg in the United States advocated correction by prolonged and gradual leverage.

The Twentieth Century

Although the writings of the twentieth century are plentiful, no fundamental advance was made in the study of aetiology, pathology or treatment of club-foot. Club-foot was and still is one of the commonest congenital deformities of the skeletal system. Its high incidence alone has exercised the enquiring mind of many workers. All published work is based on previous writings, but enlarged by modern facilities.

Incidence

Modern society facilitated epidemiological studies and the overall incidence of the deformities has been reported to vary from 1 to 4 per 1000 live births. In some races the incidence is as low as 0.6 per 1000, in others as high as 6.8 per 1000 (Polynesia) indicating an hereditary factor in its causation. All workers agree that there is a higher incidence in males (2 to 2½:1), but occurring as often bilaterally as on one side only.

Primary Causes

Genetic and hereditary factors in the causation of congenital club-foot were suggested by Velpeau in 1860 (cited in [2]): he relates the case of a French cobbler with bilateral talipes who had four children, all with club-feet and then divorced his wife when the fifth was born normal!

Recent work points to a defective cartilage anlage of the talus as the primary cause [35, 56].

Brockman [15] believed that dislocation of the talo-navicular joint is the primary cause of the deformity. He creates the analogy with congenital dislocation of the hip, the defective acetabulum corresponding with the navicular, the head of the femur corresponding with the head of the talus. But in club-foot the dislocation is of the socket on the ball, in the hip it is the ball on the socket.

Sir Arthur Keith [39] considered club-foot as a retarded ontogenetic development, as *developmental arrest,* the foot deformity bearing similarities to the foot of the arboreal ape. Max Böhm [10] describes the position of the foot of the 5-week-old embryo identical to that of a true club-foot. He called it the physiological club-foot stage of development and arrest at this stage is responsible for club-foot.

Secondary Causes

Mechanical Factors. The old Hippocratic idea of intra-uterine compression causing club-foot found new support in the twentieth century, notably by Denis Browne [16], who demonstrated mechanical pressure of the foetal foot against the uterine wall as a potent cause of the deformity. Oligo-hydramnios causes similar deformities in lambs and calves but is a doubtful factor in humans.

Soft Tissue Causes. It remains debatable whether the soft tissue abnormalities are primary and causing the deformity or are the result of adaptive changes. Dittrich (cited in [66]) maintains that the soft tissues determine the position of the foot. Middleton (cited in [66]), Wiley [66] and others emphasize the importance of muscles in determining the deformity. Others believe that a neurological defect is the cause of congenital club-foot. This paralytic theory was proposed by Little [43] probably because his own club-foot was of paralytic origin and at that time there was no clear distinction between the congenital club-foot and the acquired deformity caused by infantile paralysis and other neurological conditions. Stewart [59] found that the Achilles tendon is inserted more medially in the calcaneum, and he deduced that abnormal tendon insertions determine the club-foot position.

Classification

The greatest advance in the understanding of club-foot was made by the recognition of the various types of club-feet and the realisation that some respond better to treatment than others. If we speak of club-foot generally we usually mean the congenital type, which bears the full name of 'congenital talipes equino-varus'. Coleman [21] rightly points out that the term 'talipes' [talus = ankle, pes = foot] simply implies a non-specific deformity of the ankle and foot and is therefore superfluous. He prefers to speak of 'equino-varus congenita'. By definition it is present at birth but the causation may be developmental or antenatal.

Broadly speaking there are three types of congenital club-foot:

1. The postural type of congenital club-foot. This is probably the type which is produced by excess intra-uterine pressure on the developing foot. It responds readily to treatment, which mostly results in a normal foot.
2. The idiopathic congenital club-foot. This is the commonest and most important type. It is a developmental abnormality, at times associated with other congenital defects. There is a wide variation of the rigidity of the deformity and its reponse to treatment. Excellent results can be obtained but the foot will never be completely normal.
3. The teratological club-foot. This is a very severe deformity often associated with arthrogryposis and most resistant to treatment. Maud Forrester-Brown [31] aptly called it "the intrinsically vicious club-foot".

Earlier writers made no distinction between congenital and acquired club-feet. Such differentiation is important from the treatment point of view. Little's club-foot was of paralytic origin and therefore responded well to tenotomy of the Achilles tendon. Quite understandably Little became disillusioned in later life when he applied the operation to congenital club-feet. Infantile paralysis, cerebral palsy, myelo-meningocele, muscular dystrophy and trauma may give rise to deformities similar to club-foot but may require quite different management.

Treatment

All twentieth century workers agree that treatment should be started as soon as possible after birth. At the turn of the century forcible correction of the deformity was in vogue as taught by Hugh Owen Thomas [61]. It was practiced in modified forms by Elmslie [24], who insisted that the forefoot adduction and varus should be corrected first and only after that has been achieved should the equinus be corrected. Denis Browne [16] popularised his splint and also practised forceful correction.

Kite [40] realised the harmful effects of forcible manipulation, leading to damage of articular cartilage and to joint stiffness. He therefore recommended repeated gentle manipulations and serial plaster casts. It was generally realized that the soft tissues of a child's foot are more resistant to pressure than the bones. A forcible manipulation would not achieve stretching of the joint capsule and ligaments but would cause damage to the articular cartilage and crushing of the bones.

This concept led to the soft tissue operation; the division of the tight capsule and ligaments by the scalpel is much less damaging than the pressure on articular cartilage and bone by forcible manipulation. The simple elongation of the Achilles tendon is insufficient to correct the congenital equino-varus deformity. Zadek and Barnett [69] added the posterior capsular release of the ankle. Codivilla [20] recommended elongation of the tibialis posterior, flexor digitorum longus, flexor hallucis longus and elongation of the Achilles tendon. Ober [47] divides the deltoid ligament to correct the varus element. Other additions to the soft tissue operation were made by Brockman [15] and Turco [63].

Amongst the more conservative bone operations ranks the procedure developed by Dillwyn Evans [25]; he combines the soft tissue release operation with calcaneo-cuboid fusion to "shorten the outer pillar of the foot". F. C. Dwyer [23] advocates calcaneal osteotomy to correct persistant hindfoot varus. The great advantage of this procedure is that it does not involve any of the foot joints and therefore does not lead to rigidity.

More drastic bone operations have been evolved for persistent deformities of older children such as triple arthrodesis, crescentic wedge tarsectomy and astragalectomy. These are clearly salvage operations.

Historical, Aphorisms

"What is so exasperating in the treatment of club-foot is that the growth force is continuously at work undoing the labour of the orthopaedic surgeon."

Maud Forrester-Brown, 1935 [31]

"The literature of the treatment of club-foot is, as a rule, that of unvarying success. It is often as brilliant as an advertising sheet, and yet in practice there is no lack of half-cured or relapsed cases, sufficient evidence that methods of cure are not universally understood."

Bradford, 1892 [14]

"Different methods are capable of producing the same results in different ways."

Robert Jones, 1895 [36]

"The foot with congenital talipes is not cured until the patient can voluntarily place it in the position of valgus."

Robert Jones, 1894 [36]

"I have been told that there is no relapse of club-foot; there is reappearance of uncorrected club-foot. If correction includes active eversion the foot will not relapse."

T. P. McMurray, 1920 [45]

"Nature cannot cure club-foot, it can only make it worse."

Louis Stromeyer, cited in [43]

Summary

This is a study of the history of club-foot from ancient times up to the present. It embraces not only the clinical aspects of the deformity but also its social implications, particularly of its early history when the attitude of society towards the lame and crippled in general and to foot deformities in particular is discussed.

Relevant references from Greek mythology and also from the Old Testament are quoted. A close study is made of the old Chinese custom of foot-binding which produced club-foot like deformities which became a symbol of social standing.

Inevitably, like most other medical conditions, club-foot has been well described by Hippocrates and it is a sobering thought that his concepts of causation and his principles of treatment are as valid today as they were 2300 years ago.

This paper also briefly describes club-foot in history and art. Encouraged by society's compassionate approach towards the cripple, famous painters of the 17th century produced sympathetic portraits of the deformed and the club-footed. Well-known personalities who suffered from club-foot, such as Lord Byron and Sir Walter Scott, are mentioned and it is shown how the deformity affected them.

The saga of the physician and surgeon W. J. Little, himself afflicted by club-foot, is unfolded. His life was dedicated to the study and relief of his own deformity and later he devoted his efforts towards the cure of his fellow sufferers. W. J. Little has done so much for the advancement of orthopaedic surgery that Sir Robert Jones called him the father of orthopaedic surgery; yet at heart W. J. Little was a physician!

Another physician, Nicholas André, deserves the title of father of orthopaedic surgery. He coined the word 'orthopaedia' and laid down the principles of preventing and correcting deformities and he detailed the conservative management of club-foot. The treatment of the deformity came into the hands of bone setters and instrument makers and it was almost beneath the dignity of a surgeon to treat it.

Yet, with the advent of tenotomy, popularised by Little, surgical treatment of the condition increased, aided by the development of antiseptic and aseptic technique and anaesthesia.

It is shown how both conservative and operative methods developed side by side to reach their present standing.

Fundamental research into aetiology, pathology and epidemiology is described leading to the present concepts of a condition which is still ill-understood, controversial and fascinating.

Résumé

L'auteur fait l'historique du pied-bot de l'Antiquité à nos jours. Il insiste surtout sur les répercussions sociales de cette malformation et sur l'attitude des sociétés d'autrefois envers les handicapés en général et les personnes présentant des malformations du pied en particulier.

Il cite des exemples de la mythologie grecque et de l'ancien testament. it traite en détail de la coutume chinoise du bandage des pieds qui provoquait une déformation ressemblant au pied-bot et qui était le symbole de la classe aristocratique.

Hippocrate a bien sûr traité aussi de ce problème médical et sa théorie tant sur les causes que sur le remèdes est aussi valable aujourd'hui qu'il y a 2300 ans.

Ce chapitre évoque aussi les œuvres d'art représentant des pieds-bots (surtout au XVIIe siècle) et les personnages historiques présentant cettee malformation, tels que les écrivains Lord Byron et Sir Walter Scott.

Suit la biographie de W. J. Little qui avait lui-même un pied-bot et qui consacra toute son énergie et sa vie entière à l'étude et au traitement de cette malformation et qui a tant fait progresser la chirurgie orthopédique que Sir Robert Jones disait de lui qu'il était le père de la chirurgie orthopédique.

C'est à un autre médecin, Nicholas André, que l'on devrait conférer le titre de père de la chirurgie orthopédique. Il a créé le terme "orthopédie" et a avancé les principes fondamentaux de la prévention et du traitement des malformations ainsi que du traitement non-chirurgical du pied-bot, traitement qui fut par la suite uniquement le fait des guérisseurs et des cordonniers orthopédiques, les chirurgiens n'éprouvant que mépris pour ce genre de traitement.

Toutefois, après que Little eût introduit la ténotomie, le traitement chirurgical a pris de plus en plus d'importance. Parallèlement, les mesures antiseptiques, les méthodes aseptiques et l'anesthésie faisaient de grands progrès.

Le traitement non-chirurgical et le traitement chirurgical ont donc évolué simultanément.

Le chapitre traite aussi de la recherche fondamentale à l'heure actuelle – étiologie, pathologie et épidémiologie – qui est la base de ce que nous savons de cette malformation encore mal comprise.

Zusammenfassung

Der Beitrag gibt einen Überblick über die Geschichte des Klumpfußes von der Antike bis zur Gegenwart. Es werden nicht nur die klinischen Aspekte der Mißbildung beleuchtet, sondern auch ihre sozialen Implikationen, besonders das gesellschaftliche Verhalten gegenüber Behinderten jeder Art und besonders gegenüber Fußmißbildungen in früheren Zeiten.

Neben der Anführung von Beispielen aus der griechischen Mythologie und aus dem Alten Testament wird besonders auf die alt-chinesische Sitte des Fußeinbindens eingegangen, die eine klumpfußähnliche Mißbildung hervorrief und Symbol einer höheren gesellschaftlichen Stellung war.

Wie so viele andere wurde auch diese medizinische Frage von Hippokrates behandelt, und es ist ernüchternd festzustellen, daß seine Theorie über die Ursache und seine Behandlungsgrundsätze heute noch genausoviel Gültigkeit haben wie vor 2300 Jahren.

Der Beitrag befaßt sich auch mit der Darstellung des Klumpfußes in Geschichte und Kunst. Ermutigt durch das Mitgefühl in der Gesellschaft ihrer Zeit haben viele Maler aus dem 17. Jahrhundert Bilder von behinderten und klumpfüßigen Menschen gemalt. Es werden auch berühmte Persönlichkeiten angeführt, die einen Klumpfuß hatten, wie Lord Byron und Sir Walter Scott, und es wird gezeigt, wie sehr diese Mißbildung sie prägte.

Aus dem Leben und Wirken von W. J. Little, der selbst einen Klumpfuß hatte, werden Einzelheiten mitgeteilt. Little widmete sich sein Leben lang dem Studium und der Behandlung dieser Mißbildung; er hat so viel zum Fortschritt der orthopädischen Chirurgie beigetragen, daß Sir Robert Jones ihn als den Vater der orthopädischen Chirurgie bezeichnete. Jedoch war Little am liebsten nur Arzt.

Ein anderer Arzt, Nicolas André (engl. auch: Andry), verdiente eher den Titel des Vaters der orthopädischen Chirurgie. Er hat das Wort „Orthopädie" geprägt und die Grundprinzipien der Vorsorge und der Behandlung von Mißbildungen aufgestellt sowie die konservative Behandlung des Klumpfußes eingeleitet. Diese Behandlung wurde dann gänzlich den Heilpraktikern und den orthopädischen Werkstätten überlassen, und es war fast unter der Würde eines Chirurgen, sich damit zu beschäftigen.

Jedoch nachdem Little die Tenotomie eingeführt hatte und diese zunehmende Bedeutung erlangte, trat die chirurgische Behandlung immer mehr in den Vordergrund. Gleichzeitig machten antiseptische Maßnahmen, aseptische Methoden und die Anästhesie entsprechende Fortschritte.

Es wird also gezeigt, daß die konservative und die chirurgische Behandlungsmethode sich gleichzeitig entwickelten.

Der Beitrag schließt mit Bemerkungen zur heutigen Grundlagenforschung (Ätiologie, Pathologie und Epidemiologie), die zum derzeitigen Verständnis dieser immer noch schlecht verstandenen kontroversen und faszinierenden Frage geführt hat.

Acknowledgements. I am indebted to the staff of the Liverpool Medical Institution for providing books and journals, to the Department of Medical Illustrations of the University of Liverpool for the photographs and to Mr. Athanasios Kontossi for obtaining the photograph of the amphora from the National Archaelogical Museum in Athens, and last but not least to my wife for helpful suggestions and patient proof-reading.

References

1. Adams W (1866) Club-foot: its causes, pathology and treatment. Churchill, London
2. Almond HGA (1947) Congenital talipes equino varus. Thesis, Liverpool
3. André N (1743) Orthopaedia, or the art of preventing and correcting deformities in children. London
4. Arcaeus F (1658) De curandis vulneribus
5. Attenborough CG (1966) Severe congenital talipes equinovarus. J Bone Joint Surg 48B:31
6. Bartsocas C (1972) Hephaestus and club-foot. J Hist Med 27:450
7. Baumgartner R, Taillard W (1963) Treatment of congenital club-foot at the Kinderspital Basel. Ann Paediatr (Basel) 200:363
8. Bessel-Hagen (1889) Die Pathologie und Therapie des Klumpfußes. Heidelberg
9. Bick EM (1948) Source book of orthopaedics. Williams and Wilkins, Baltimore
10. Böhm M (1929) The embryological origin of club-foot. J Bone Joint Surg 11:229

11. Bohne O (1938) Orthopaedic treatment of club-foot in the 16th century. Z Krüppel Fürsorge 31:104
12. Bose K (1971) A clinical review of the treatment of congenital talipes equinovarus. Thesis, Liverpool
13. Bracken BC (1958) Perspectives of congenital club-foot. Thesis, Liverpool
14. Bradford EH (1892) Operative treatment of resistant club-feet. Trans Am Orthop Assoc 5:182
15. Brockman EP (1930) Congenital club-foot. Marshall, London
16. Browne D (1934) Talipes equinovarus. Lancet II:969
17. Bruce-Chwatt R (1983) The lure of the lotus. World Med 18(19):40–41
18. Bruckner (1796) Über die Natur, Ursachen und Behandlung der einwärts gekrümmten Füsse oder der sogenannten Klumpfüsse. Gotha
19. Cheng WN (1969) Congenital club-foot – incidence and aetiology. Thesis, Liverpool
20. Codivilla A (1976) The classic. Tendon transplant in orthopaedic practice. Clin Orthop 118: 2–6
21. Coleman SS (1983) Complex foot deformities in children. Lea and Febiger, Philadelphia
22. Delpech JM (1823) Tenotomie du tendon d'Achille. Chir Clin Montepellier 1:184
23. Dwyer FC (1963) The treatment of relapsed club-foot by the insertion of a wedge into the calcaneum. J Bone Joint Surg 45B:67
24. Elmslie RC (1920) The principles of treatment of congenital talipes equinovarus. J Orthop Surg 2:669
25. Evans D (1961) Relapsed club-foot. J Bone Joint Surg 43B:722
26. Fabricius Hildanus (1641) Observationum et curationum medico-chirurgarum centurae sex. Lugduni
27. Fang HS (1960) Footbinding in Chinese women. Can J Surg 3:195
28. Fergusson WA (1843) A system of practical surgery. Lea and Blanckard, Philadelphia, p 350
29. Flaubert G (1950) Madame Bovary. Penguin, Harmandsworth
30. Flinchum D (1952) Pathological anatomy in talipes equinovarus. J Bone Joint Surg 35A:111
31. Forrester-Brown M (1935) The treatment of congenital equinovarus. J Bone Joint Surg 17:661
32. Guérin JR (1838) Memoire sur l'étiologie génerale de pieds bots congénitaux. Paris
33. Hippocrates (1939) The genuine works of Hippocrates. Williams and Wilkins, Baltimore
34. Hirsch C (1960) Observations on early operative treatment of congenital club-foot. Bull Hosp Joint Dis 21:173
35. Irani RN, Sherman MS (1963) The pathological anatomy of club-foot. J Bone Joint Surg 45A:45
36. Jones R (1895) Discussion on the treatment of intractable talipes equinovarus. Trans Br Orthop Soc 1:20
37. Jones R (1923) The treatment of club-foot in the newly born. Lancet 1:713–714
38. Keith A (1919) Menders of the maimed. Oxford Medical Publications, Oxford
39. Keith A (1929) History of the human foot. J Bone Joint Surg 11:10
40. Kite JH (1932) The treatment of congenital clubfeet. JAMA 99:1156
41. Larousse encyclopedia of mythology. Batchworth, London, pp 139, 148
42. Little EM (1928) Orthopaedics before Stromeyer. The Robert Jones birthday volume. Oxford Medical Publications, Oxford
43. Little WJ (1839) A treatise on the nature of club-foot and analogous distorsions. Jeffs, London
44. McCauley JC (1966) Clubfoot. Clin Orthop 44:51
45. McMurray TP (1920) Discussions. J Orthop Surg 2:683
46. Mottram ME, Pyle IR (1973) Mandarin feet. Am J Roentgenol 118:318
47. Ober FR (1920) An operation for the relief of congenital equinovarus deformity. J Orthop Surg 2:558
48. Osgood RB (1925) The evolution of orthopaedic surgery. Mosby, St. Louis
49. Pare A (1642) Collected works. London
50. Parker RW, Shattock SG (1884) The pathology and etiology of congenital club-foot. Trans Pathol Soc Lond 35:423

51. Phelps AM (1884) International Congress of Medical Science, Copenhagen
52. Ruhrah J (1933) Paediatrics in art. Am J Dis Child 46:1397
53. Salz M (1961) Congenital club-foot. Med Press June:535
54. Sayre LA (1885) Orthopaedic surgery. Appleton, New York
55. Scarpa A (1818) A memoir on the congenital club-foot of children and the mode of correcting that deformity. Constable, Edinburgh
56. Settle GW (1963) The anatomy of congenital talipes equino varus. J Bone Joint Surg 45A:45
57. Sheldrake T (1806) Distorsions of the legs and feet of children. London
58. Smith EG, Warren RD (1924) Egyptian mummies. Allen and Unwin, London, p 100
59. Stewart SF (1951) Club-foot; its incidence, cause and treatment. An anatomical-physiological study. J Bone Joint Surg 33A:557
60. Stromeyer L (1973) The classic contributions to operative orthopaedics or experiences with subcutaneous section of shortenend muscles and their tendons. Clin Orthop 97:2–4
61. Thomas HO (1886) A new wrench for club-foot. Provincial Med J 5:286
62. Tulpius N (1685) Observationes medicae. Amsterdam
63. Turco VJ (1979) Resistant congenital club-foot. J Bone Joint Surg 61A:805
64. Venel JA (1789) Mémoires de la Societé des sciences physiques de Lausanne, vol 2, pp 66, 197
65. Watson F (1930) Civilization and the cripple. Bale Sons and Danielson, London
66. Wiley AM (1959) Club-foot, an anatomical and experimental study of muscle growth. J Bone Joint Surg 41B:821
67. Wishart JH (1818) Memoir on congenital club-foot in children. Edinburgh
68. Wynn-Davies R (1946) Family studies and the cause of congenital club-foot. J Bone Joint Surg 46B:445
69. Zadek I, Barnett E (1917) The importance of the ligaments of the ankle in correction of congenital clubfoot. JAMA 69:1057

The History of Treatment of Cleft Lip and Palate

M. Perko[1]

The first report of an operation for a cleft lip was by Boo Chai [5], in which an unnamed surgeon successfully closed a cleft lip in 390 B.C.

No operations for clefts were carried out in ancient Egypt, but a mummy with a cleft palate has been found. In the great epoch of Greek and Roman medicine, no cleft operations were described, although operations were performed in the mouth and on the uvula.

In Europe, Saxon surgeons described an operation for cleft lip in the *Leech-Book of Bald* in 950 A.D.: "For harelip, pound mastic very small, add the white of an egg and mingle as thou dost vermilion, cut with a knife the false edges of the lip, sew fast with silk, then smear without and within with the salve ere the silk rot. If it draw together, arrange it with the hand; anoint again soon."

The first exact description of a cleft lip operation was given by Johan Yperman (1325–1351) (Fig. 1). This author was the first to perform a two-layer operation with waxed, twisted thread that was additionally secured by stitches inserted at a distance from the cleft [3]. He warned that lateral incisions to relieve tension should not be made, as they would cause malformations of the lip later on. The first description of a cleft palate was by Franco in 1556 [2]. Syphilitic perforations of the palate were, however, frequently encountered in those times, so that surgeons believed that cleft palates were the result of syphilis. For this reason, operations for cleft palates were not advised. Ambroise Paré [40] and Amatus Lusitanus [29] introduced the use of an obturator. Gaspare Tagliacozzi described a cleft lip oper-

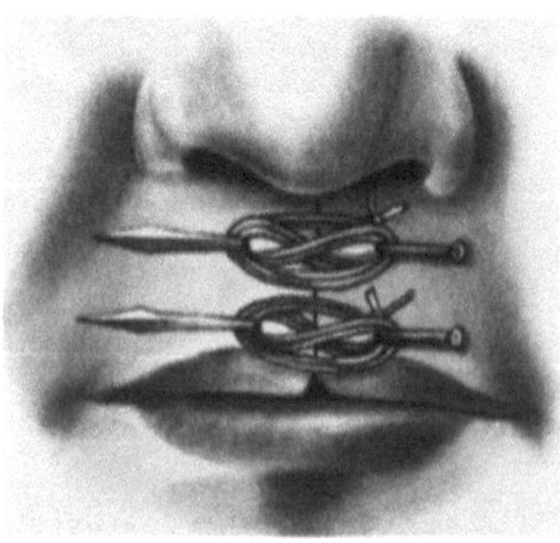

Fig. 1. Lip repair by Pancoast (1844) similar to the method used by Yperman [36]

[1] Children's University Hospital, Department of Surgery, Steinwiesstr. 75, CH-8032 Zürich, Switzerland

Progress in Pediatric Surgery, Vol. 20
Ed. by P. P. Rickham

ation in 1579 [55]. There were no reports of cleft palate operations in the sixteenth and seventeenth centuries, probably because surgeons were frightened of the copious bleeding and the severe pain caused by the operation [3].

It is interesting to note that Hendrik van Roonhuyze (1622–1672) advised that cleft lips should be operated upon between 3 and 4 months of age [59]. In his opinion, if they were operated earlier, the results would not be favorable. James Cook of Warwick (1614–1688) was the first to warn that the premaxilla should not be removed because of the danger of interfering with subsequent growth [9]. Pierre Fauchard (1678–1761) in his book "Le Chirurgien Dentiste" described several different obturators to close the cleft palate defect (Fig. 2) [18].

In the United States, Matthew Wilson (1736–1790) was the first to publish an account of a cleft lip operation (Fig. 3) [3]. In 1766, Le Monnier [47a] described a cleft palate operation in which for the first time the margins of the gap were freshened. This caused an inflammation which the author thought would stimulate healing. Eustache is said to have closed the soft palate as early as 1779, but this

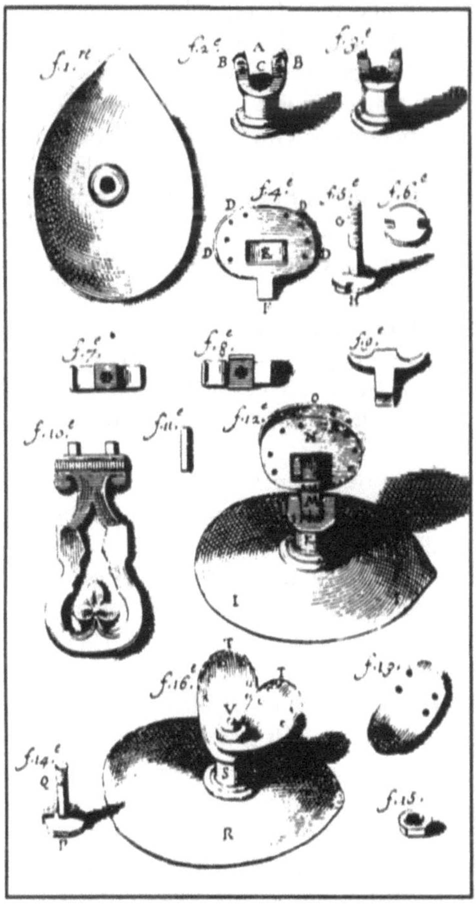

Fig. 2. Obturators for palatal defects [18]

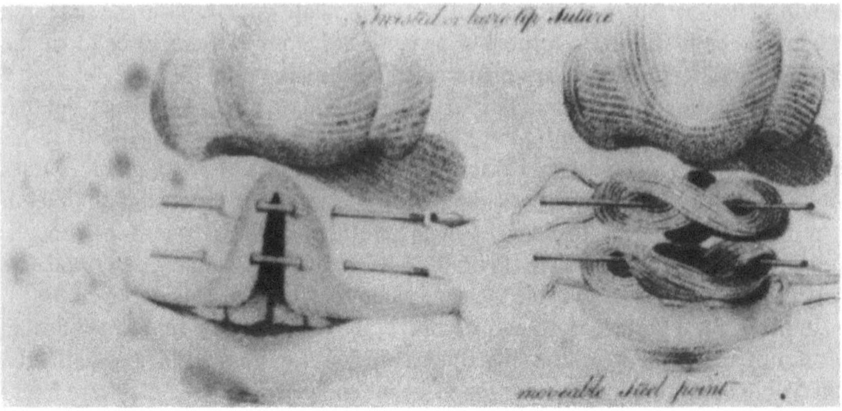

Fig. 3. Probably the first illustration of cleft lip repair in the USA [15a]

has not been proven [15]. In 1798, Desault and Bichat [12] published an article stressing the importance of approximation of the margins of the cleft palate. The same author also practiced repositioning of the premaxilla with an extraoral fraction mechanism (Fig. 4). The literature recognizes Graefe [20a] and Roux [49] as the first authors of a proper cleft palate operation. Graefe first cauterized the margins and then sewed them together. After failure to achieve healing, he freshened the wound margins and fixed the stitches to the cheeks, so that they could not rip out.

Roux's operation is well known because the first patient to undergo this procedure, the medical student John Stephenson [54a] wrote a thesis about it to complete his degree in medicine (Fig. 5). Since then, surgery for cleft palates has made rapid progress, but the results have not been very good. In 1820, Warren was the first American surgeon to close a palate successfully. He developed special instruments for the operation but did not know about the operative technique devised by Roux [64, 65].

Dorrance [15] described the development of cleft palate surgery. He was of the opinion that the frequent failures of the various operative techniques employed were due to premature removal of the stitches. For instance, Alcock [1] removed the stitches on the 4th day and Mayo [32] on the 3rd day after operation. In 1826, Dieffenbach [14] of Berlin recommended the dissection of the mucosa from the hard palate, combined with lateral incisions to relieve tension. This operation was first carried out in 1828. Velpeau [63] thought that the first to introduce lateral incisions to relieve tension was Krimer of Aix La Chapelle in 1827 [26]. In 1828, Warren [64] reported a successful closure of the soft palate which he had carried out in 1820. Warren, Desault and Bichat [12], and, 150 years later, Schweckendiek [51] noticed that the gap in the hard palate decreased in size following the operation. Thus, the advisability of the two-stage closure of the palate was discovered. Warren [65] and Cathrall [6a] were the first to advise extraoral bandages in order to compress the gap in a bilateral cleft lip and palate. They are therefore

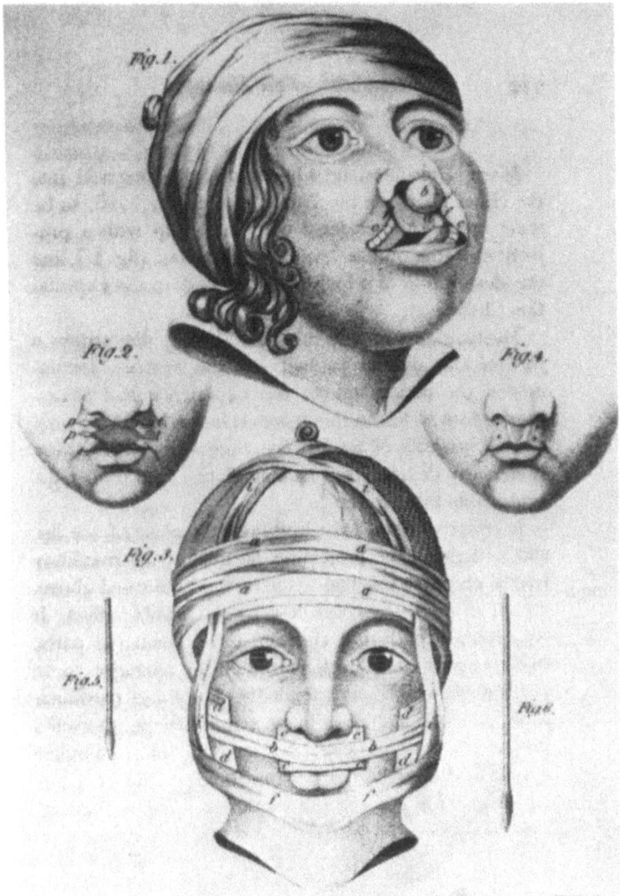

Fig. 4. Desault's repositioning of the premaxilla [12]

throught to be the pioneers of preoperative orthopedic treatment of the maxilla. Hofmann had previously described a skullcap with elastic compression as early as 1686 [23]. Chronologically, the names of Nathan Smith [54], Georg Bushe [6], James Deane [11], and John P. Mettauer [33] should be mentioned, as they all introduced a number of improvements in cleft surgery. In 1843, John Pancoast described the necessity of joining the muscles when doing palate surgery [39], and Fergusson [19] advised relieving the muscle tension by using relaxing incisions with scissors in the neighborhood of the eustachian tube. Considering the year of this report, the results described are remarkable.

During this period, the surgical treatment of cleft lip also improved. In 1843, Malgaigné [31] advised the use of a flap for closing the lip, and in 1844, Mirault [37] removed a skin flap in order to improve the symmetry of the lip (Fig. 6). Since then, different skin flaps have been used, which are described at length by Washio [66].

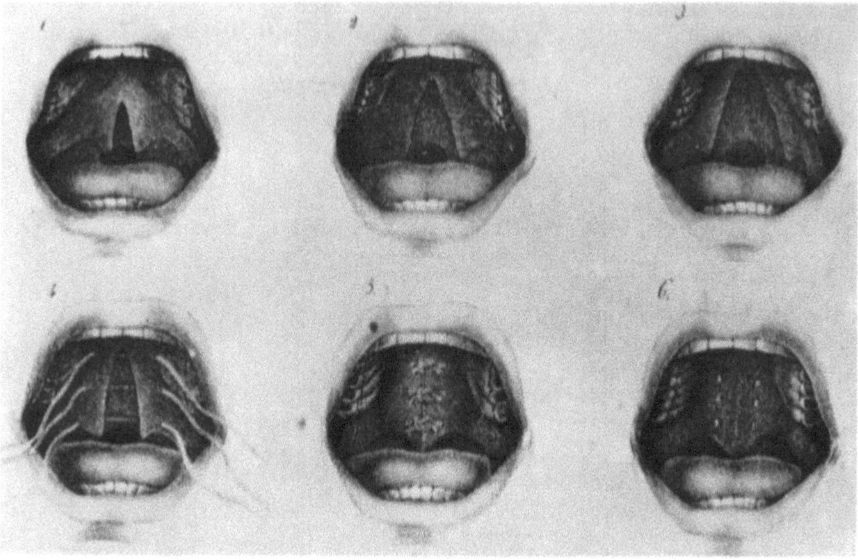

Fig. 5. Roux's method of closing a cleft of the soft palate [49]

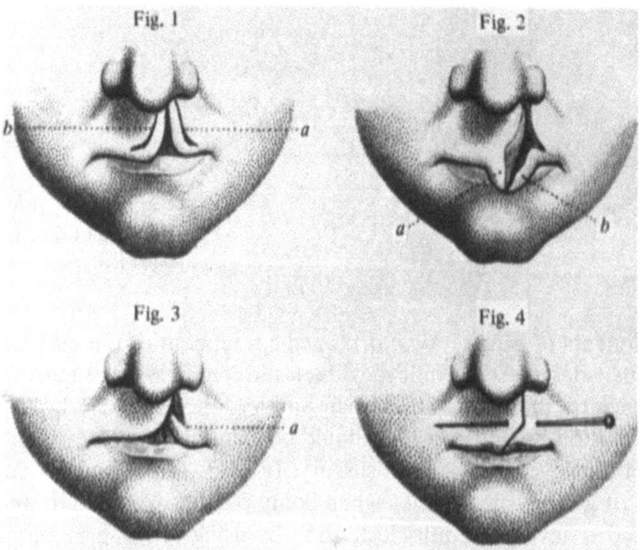

Fig. 6. Malgaigné's harelip operation [31]

The great advance in cleft palate surgery was due to Langenbeck [26a], who was the first to use a mucoperiosteal flap, which was separated from the hard palate. This method is still used today in many places (Fig. 7). The introduction of chloroform as an anesthetic was of course of enormous importance. Cleft palate surgery thus became much easier, especially in children.

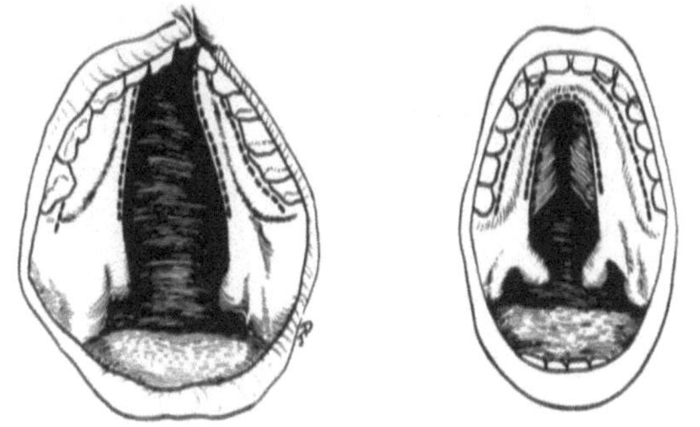

A. One palate plate horizontal, one vertical. B. Both plates horizontal.

Fig. 7. Langenbeck's cleft palate operation [26a]

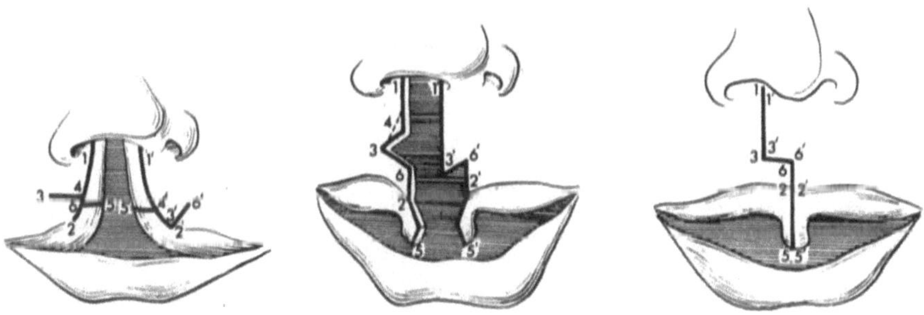

Fig. 8. Hagedorn's quadrangular lip repair [21]

In 1868, Collis [8] was the first to close the floor of the nose with a nasal mucosal flap. A drawback of this operation was that the red mucosa was often visible in the nasal floor. The first surgeons recognized that a straight closure of the lip often shortened it. Thompson [57] introduced the use of a pair of compasses to measure the length of the lip. His method did not however produce satisfactory results.

The real pioneers of cleft lip surgery were Hagedorn [21] who used a quadrangular flap to increase the thickness of the medial part of the lip (Fig. 8) and Blair and Brown [4], who attempted to correct the anterior nares by shifting the tissues towards the middle line. Veau [60] was impressed by this procedure, and his method is very similar (Fig. 9). Le Mesurier reintroduced Hagedorn's method and published his experience extending over a period of 13 years in 1948 [27]. Many surgeons followed his lead. Unfortunately, subsequent results often revealed that the lip became too long. Today, the method of Tennison [56] for closure of the unilateral cleft with a triangular flap is often used (Figs. 10, 11). The method is relatively simple and esthetically satisfactory; it was modified by Randall in 1959 [46] and Hagerty in 1958 [22]. Trauner [58] and Skoog [52] (Fig. 12) introduced an additional triangular flap at the base of the alae nasi. In 1967, Millard [35] reported the "rotation advancement principle" using an exchange flap in the

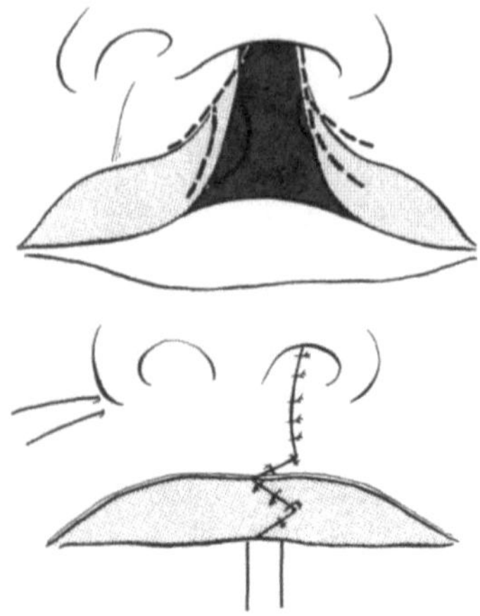

Fig. 9. Veau's lip closure [60]

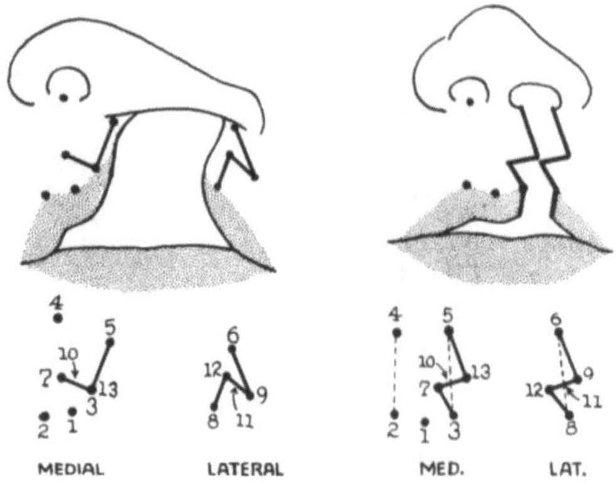

Fig. 10. Tennison's triangular flap [56]

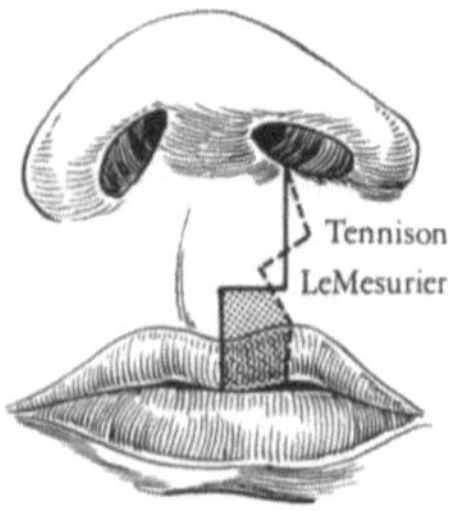

Fig. 11. Tennison's triangular and the Le Mesurier-Hagedorn quadrangular incisions. ---, Tennison; ——, Le Mesurier. [21, 27, 56]

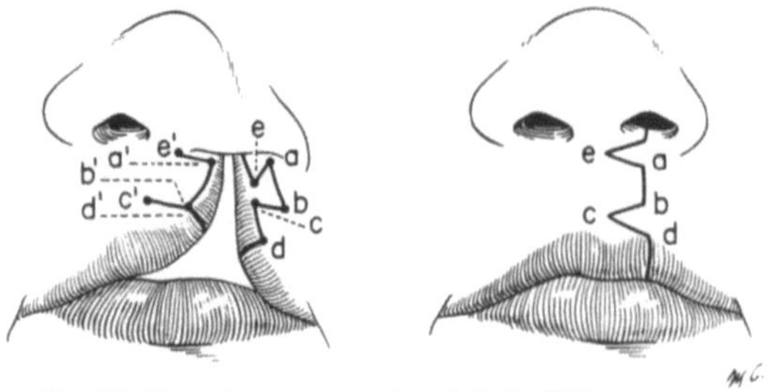

Fig. 12. Skoog's operation for cleft lip [52]

region of the anterior nares. This method has also been modified several times. The advantage of the procedure is improved nasal form and better anatomical joining of the musculature compared with that achieved by the Tennison operation.

Another original operative method is the so-called wave-shaped incision of Pfeifer [43]. It is said that this method joins the musculature better than any other. However, only a few surgeons outside Germany have used this technique.

The operative techniques for unilateral clefts of the lip are now satisfactory, with the exception of the primary nasal cleft, but the plastic closure of bilateral clefts is still a great problem because the anatomical situation is difficult, especially when compounded by the often unfortunate position of the premaxilla. The short columella and the absence of muscles in the prolabium are further problems.

Many authors have tried to use the technique which has been so successful in unilateral clefts for bilateral clefts. We agree with Millard [36] that this is unsatisfactory. As early as 1790, Desault [13] advised that the cleft lip should be operated on one side only after the premaxilla is repositioned by external bandages before the operation. Veau [60], during his life time a leading figure in cleft surgery, advised that bilateral lips should be closed in two to three stages, depending on the width of the gap.

Surgeons like Franco [2], van Roonhuyze [47b], and de la Faye [18a] excised the premaxilla in order to be able to suture the gap in the lip. Excision was also practiced by Dupuytren [16] and Rose and Sims [48], who valued the advantages of excision without realizing the damage done to maxillary growth through this operation. Elastic traction was introduced by von Bardeleben [1a] and von Esmarch and Kowalzig [17]. This technique is still practiced today. In addition to traction, McNeil [34] introduced treatment with maxillary plates, which represented a milestone for the modern orthopedic treatment of the maxilla. Hotz [25] stopped using elastic repositioning of the premaxilla after the operative technique of Celesnik [7] was introduced in Zürich (Fig. 13a, b). This method has been called "lip adhesion" by Millard; however, it consists of joining the upper lip musculature beneath the prolabium in the upper part of bilateral clefts [41] and not in an adhesion of the lip. Hotz comments that this method stimulates the lateral segments of the premaxilla to grow instead of forcing the premaxilla to move backwards. Many authors have described surgical repositioning of the premaxilla. Gensoul [20] used a forced fracture of the premaxilla, von Bardeleben [1a] a subperiosteal resection, while Pichler [45] employed osteotomy of the overlapping vomer in combination with his vomer flap technique. Veau and Ruppe [61] followed up 208 cases, commenting that *"Le malheur de cette chirurgie est que nous ne pouvons tirer un enseignement de notre opération que plusieurs années après l'avoir pratiquée."*

Impaired growth following osteotomy of the premaxilla in infancy has now been generally recognized, even if this operation is combined with a bone transplantation, as advised by Pfeifer in 1962 [44]. The unsatisfactory long-term results, especially the impaired growth, have persuaded many surgeons to look for other techniques. Several authors, such as Schmid [50], Nordin and Johanson [38], and others believe that bone transplantation in the alveolar cleft performed simultaneously with rotation of the lip will enhance bone growth. However, experience has shown that these primary plastic bone operations do not stimulate growth, and the method has therefore been abandoned by most surgeons.

Skoog [53] bridged the alveolar gap by periosteal flaps in the hope that subperiosteal bone would form and close the gap (Fig. 14). Rintala et al. [47] introduced the free periosteal flap taken from the tibia with the idea that this would stimulate osseous growth. The long-term results were not very satisfactory. Schweckendiek [51] introduced staged closure in order to avoid growth impairment. In this method, the soft palate is closed early, but the hard palate is not closed until the patient is 13 years old. The results are good as far as growth is concerned, but the disadvantage is the late development of proper speech (Fig. 15a, b). Perko [42] has

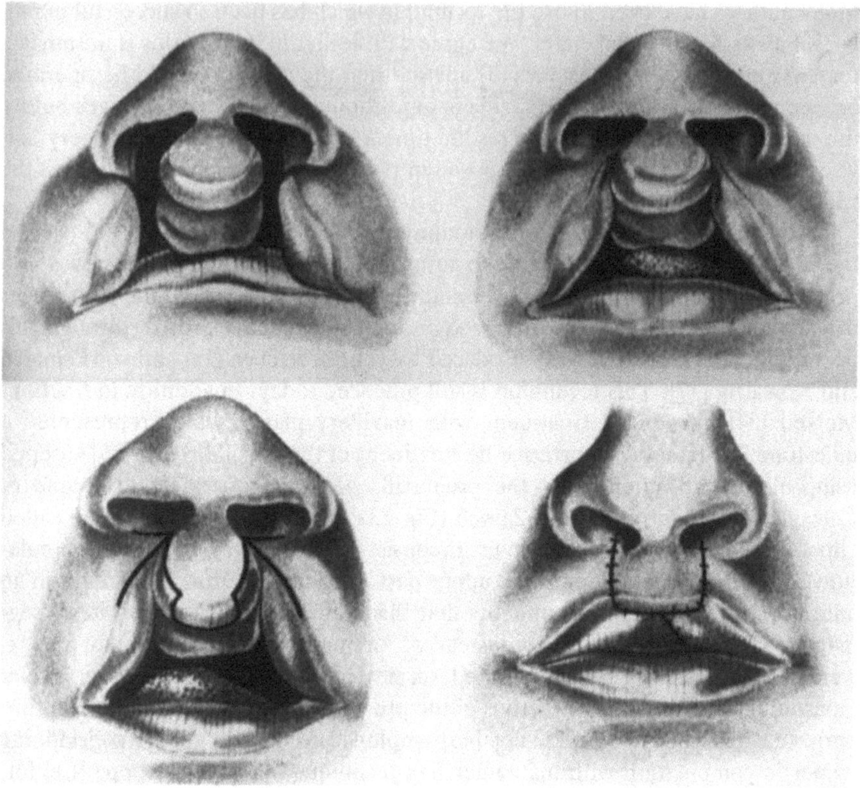

a

b

Fig. 13a, b. Celesnik's method for two-step closure of bilateral cleft lip and palate [7]

followed this principle, advising anatomical reconstruction of the soft palate at 18 months of age and closure of the hard palate at 5 years. This has the advantage of minimizing growth impairment and allows children to attend a regular school and learn to speak normally.

In the last few years, there has been a tendency again to close clefts very early in life. Malek [30] closes the total lip and palatal cleft at the age of 6–8 months. Follow-up has as yet been too brief to be able to draw relevant long-term conclusions.

Modern cleft management has shown that the range of problems, which involve maxillary growth, speech, hearing, and esthetics, can only be solved by a "team approach." In spite of great advances, no one method of treatment has as yet been universally accepted. Whether one specific method of treatment is better than another can only be judged by the same team using the same method for many years. Unfortunately, at least 20 years are required to evaluate results. It is probably a mistake to change the method of treatment again and again, although at times one would like to do so. It is questionable whether the recent tendency to

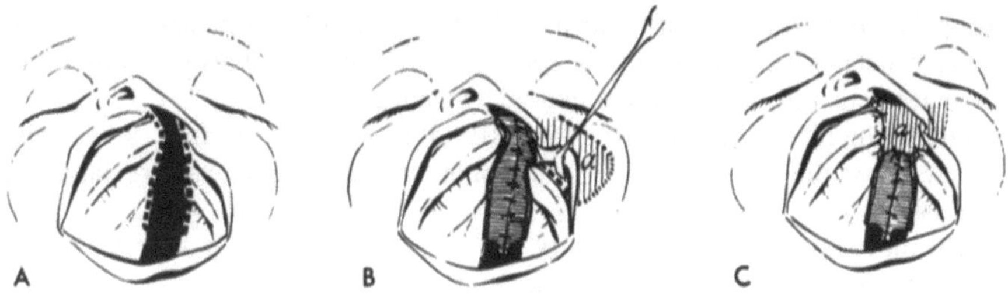

Fig. 14. Skoog's periostoplasty [53]

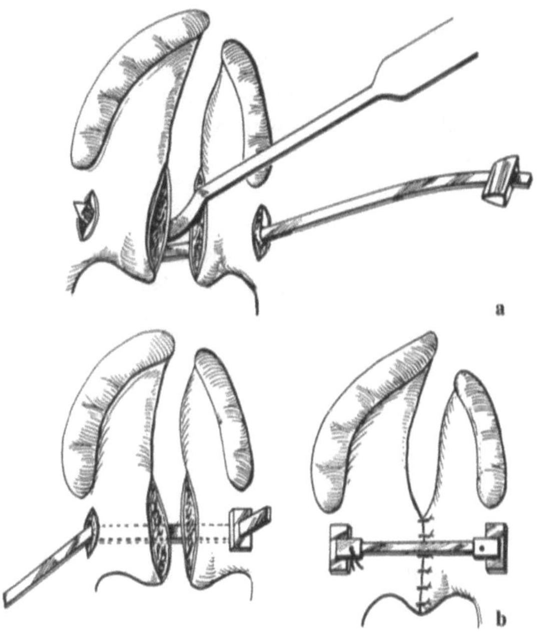

Fig. 15a, b. Schweckendiek's soft palate closure [51]

return to early operations on the assumption that damage in later years will not be incurred is well advised. One wonders whether the old masters were not right to reject early operations for clefts. Only time will tell.

Summary

The history of surgery of cleft lip and palates reaches as far backwards as the pre-christian era to 390 B.C. when for the first time a cleft lip was closed successfully in China. Although Egyptian and Greek medicines developed to a remarkable degree, no descriptions of cleft operations have survived. In the middle ages operations on cleft lip have been several times described. A successful operation on a cleft palate did however not occur until 1816. This can be explained by the fact that cleft palates were thought to be secondary to syphilis, but also because without anaesthetic this operation was extremely painful and difficult.

Graefe in 1816 [20a] and Roux in 1819 [49] published the first satisfactory results. After the introduction of chlorophorm cleft surgery made remarkable progress.

The development of cleft surgery has been chronologically described and finally the present state of affairs is discussed.

Résumé

L'histoire du traitement chirurgical des fentes labiopalatines remonte à 390 avant. J.C., date à laquelle une intervention a été couronnée de succès en Chine. Bien que la médecine égyptienne et grecque aient été très évoluées, il n'était pas question du traitement des fentes labiopalatines. Au Moyen-Age, ces fentes sont décrites fréquemment mais ce n'est qu'en 1816 que la première opération a été pratiquée avec succès. Cela est dû d'une part au fait que l'on croyait qu'il s'agissait d'une manifestation secondaire de la syphilis et que d'autre part, cette opération était extrêmement délicate et douloureuse sans anesthésie suffisante.

Graefe en 1816 et Roux en 1819 ont publié les premiers résultats. Quand l'usage du chloroforme fut devenu courant, le traitement chirurgical fit des progrès rapides.

Le chapitre se termine par une historique de l'intervention et une discussion des méthodes d'intervention de nos jours.

Zusammenfassung

Die Geschichte der chirurgischen Behandlung der Gaumenspalte und der Lippenspalte reicht bis in die Zeit um 390 vor Christus zurück, als zum ersten Mal in China eine Lippenspalte erfolgreich geschlossen wurde. Obwohl die ägyptische und die griechische Medizin einen hohen Entwicklungsstand erreichten, wird nichts über Spaltoperationen berichtet. Im Mittelalter dagegen werden sie mehrmals beschrieben. Jedoch fand erst 1816 die erste erfolgreiche Gaumenspaltenoperation statt. Dies erklärt sich dadurch, daß man annahm, daß Gaumenspalten sekundäre Erscheinungen der Syphilis waren, aber auch dadurch, daß ohne Anästhetika diese Operation äußerst schmerzhaft und schwierig war.

Graefe (1816) und Roux (1819) haben die ersten Erfolgsmeldungen veröffentlicht. Nach Einführung des Chloroforms machte die chirurgische Behandlung von Spalten beachtliche Fortschritte.

Es wird eine chronologische Darstellung der Entwicklung der Spaltenoperationen angeschlossen sowie eine Diskussion über den heutigen Stand der Behandlung.

References

1. Alcock T (1823) Case of congenital division of the palate in which union of the divided parts was effected. Trans Assoc Apothec Surg Apothec Engl Wales 1:377
1a. Bardeleben A von (1865) Lehrbuch der Chirurgie und Operationslehre, 4th edn. Reimer, Berlin
2. Barsky AJ (1964) Pierre Franco, father of cleft lip surgery – his life and times. Br J Plast Surg 17:335
3. Blair OR (1971) History of cleft lip and palate treatment. In: Grab et al (eds) Cleft lip and palate. Little, Brown and Co, Boston
4. Blair VP, Brown JB (1930) Mirault operation for single harelip. Surg Gynecol Obstet 51:81
5. Boo Chai K (1966) An ancient Chinese text on a cleft lip. Plast Reconstr Surg 38:89
6. Bushe G (1835) An essay on the operation for cleft palate. Jackson, New York
6a. Cathrall I (1819) A case of double hair-lip. Med Recorder 2:372
7. Celesnik F (1962) Notre procédé de traitement chirurgical du bec-de-lièvre bilatéral totale. Rev Stomatol 63:386
8. Collis MH (1868) The esthetic treatment of harelip. Dublin J Med Sci 45:392
9. Cooke J (1693) Mellificium chirurgiae or the marrow of chirurgery. With the anatomy of human bodies, 4th edn, p 195
10. Deleted in production
11. Deane J (1837) Congenital fissures of the palate. Boston Med Surg J 16:333
12. Desault PJ, Bichat X (1798) Sur l'opération du bec-de-lièvre. In: Oeuvres chirurgicales ou exposé de la doctrine et de la pratique. Méquignon, Paris, vol 2
13. Desault PJ, Bichat X (1798) Sur l'opération du bec-de-lièvre. In: Oeuvres chirurgicales ou exposé de la doctrine et de la pratique. Méquignon, Paris, vol 2
14. Dieffenbach JF (1928) Beiträge zur Gaumennaht. Ann Heilkd 10:322
15. Dorrance GM (1933) The operative story of cleft palate. Saunders, Philadelphia, vol 3
15a. Dorsey JS (1813) Elements of surgery for the use of students. Parker, Kimber and Conrad, Philadelphia
16. Dupuytren G (1832–34) Leçons orales de clinique chirurgicale faite à l'Hôtel-Dieu de Paris. Baillière, Paris, vol 1
17. Esmarch F von, Kowalzig E (1901) Plastic operations for congenital fissure formations of the oral region: surgical technique. In: Sims N (ed) A textbook on operative surgery. McMillan, New York
18. Fauchard P (1728) Le chirurgien dentiste ou traité des dents. Mariette, Paris, vol II, p 285
18a. Faye G de la (1743) Mémoires de l-Académie Royale de Chirurgie, vol 1, p 605
19. Fergusson W (1844–45) Observations on cleft palate and on staphylorraphy. Med Times 2:256
20. Gensoul J (1833) J Hébd Med Chir Pratique 29
20a. Graefe C von (1820) Die Gaumennaht – ein neu entdecktes Mittel gegen angeborene Fehler der Sprache. J Chir Augenheilkd 1:1
21. Hagedorn (1884) Über eine Modifikation der Hasenschartenoperation. Zentralbl Chir 11:756
22. Hagerty R (1958) Unilateral cleft lip repair. Surg Gynecol Obstet 106:119
23. Hofmann JP (1686) De labiis leporinis: von Hasenscharten. Bergmann, Heidelberg
24. Hollerii (Stempani) I (1623) Omnio opera pratica. De morbis internis. Singulares aliquot Hollerii observationes, quai ad consilia curandi pertinent. In: Excudebat Iacobus Stoer, Coloniae Allobrogum, Observation IV. Stoer, Geneva, vol I, p 573
25. Hotz M, Perko M (1974) Koordinierte kieferorthopädisch-chirurgische Behandlung von Lippen-Kiefer-Gaumen-Spalten. Schweiz Med Wochenschr 104/20:718–723
26. Krimer W (1827) Heilung eines beträchtlichen Wolfrachens. Chir Augenheilkd 10:625
26a. Langenbeck B von (1861) Operation der angeborenen totalen Spaltung des harten Gaumens nach einer neuen Methode. Dtsch Klin 8:231
27. Le Mesurier AB (1949) A method of cutting and suturing the lip in the treatment of complete unilateral clefts. J Plast Reconstr Surg 4:1

28. Deleted in production
29. Lusitanus A (1566) Curationum medicinalium... Tomus secundus, continens enturias tres, quintam videlicet. Venetiis: Apud Vincentium Valgrisium, curatio 14, 39
30. Malek R, Psaume J (1979) Results of first and early closure of cleft palate with cleft lip. 3. Internationales Symposium für Lippen-Kiefer-Gaumen-Spalten, Hamburg, 1st Sep 1979
31. Malgaigné JF (1843) Manuel de médecine opératoire, 4th edn. Baillière, Paris
32. Mayo H (1927) Fissure of the soft palate. Med Physiol J (Lond) 57:119
33. Mettauer JP (1837) On staphylorraphy. Am J Med Sci 21:309
34. McNeil CK (1950) Orthodontic procedures in the treatment of congenital cleft palate. Dent Rec 79:126
35. Millard DR (1967) Rotation advancement in wide cleft lips. 4th International congress of plastic surgery, Rome 1967
36. Millard DR (1977) Cleft craft. Little, Brown and Co, Boston
37. Mirault (1844) Lettre sur le bec-de-lièvre. J Chir 2:257
38. Nordin KE, Johanson B (1955) Freie Knochentransplantation bei Defekten im Alveolarkamm nach kieferorthopädischer Einstellung der Maxilla bei Lippen-Kiefer-Gaumen-Spalten. In: Schuchardt K, Wassmund M (eds) Fortschritte der Kiefer- und Gesichtschirurgie. Thieme, Stuttgart, vol I, pp 168–171
39. Pancoast JA (1843) On staphylorraphy. Am J Med Sci 66
40. Paré A (1564) Dix livres de la chirurgie. Jean le Royer, Paris, p 211
41. Perko M (1973) Vorteile und Ergebnisse der Operation. Fortschritte Kiefer- und Gesichtschirurgie XVI:77
42. Perko M (1974) Primary closure of the cleft palate using a palatal mucosal flap: An attempt to prevent growth impairment. J Maxillofac Surg 2:40–43
43. Pfeifer G (1970) Über ein entwicklungsgeschichtlich begründetes Verfahren des Verschlusses von Lippenspalten. Dtsch Zahn Mund Kieferkl 54:69
44. Pfeifer G (1966) Die sekundäre osteoplastische Stabilisierung des beweglichen Zwischenkiefers bei frisch operierten, doppelseitigen Kieferspalten. Chir Plast Reconstr 2:96
45. Pichler H (1926) Zur Operation der doppelten Lippen-Gaumen-Spalten. Dtsch Z Chir 195:104
46. Randall PA (1959) A triangular flap operation for the primary repair of unilateral clefts of the lip. J Plast Reconstr Surg 23:331
47. Rintala A, Soivio A, Ranta R, Oikari T, Haataja J (1974) On the bone-forming capacity of periosteal flap in surgery for cleft lip and palate. Scand J Plast Reconstr Surg 8:58–61
47a. Robert (1766) Traité des principaux objets de médecine avec un sommaire de la plupart des thèses soutenues aux écoles de Paris, depuio 1762 jusqu'à 1746. Lacombe, Paris, vol 1, p 8
47b. Roonhuyze H van (1674) Historische Heil-Curen in zwey Theile verfasste Anmerckungen... Endtern, Nürnberg, p 26
48. Rose W, Sims N (1891) Harelip and cleft palate. Lewis, London
49. Roux PJ (1819) Observation sur une division congénitale du voile du palais et de la luette, guérie au moyen d'une opération analogue à celle du bec-de-lièvre. J Univ Sci Med 15:356
50. Schmid E (1955) Die Annäherung der Kieferstümpfe bei Lippen-Kiefer-Gaumen-Spalten; ihre schädlichen Folgen und Vermeidung. In: Schuchardt K, Wassmund M (eds) Fortschritte der Kiefer- und Gesichtschirurgie. Thieme, Stuttgart, vol I, pp 37–39
51. Schweckendiek H (1951) Zur Frage der Früh- und Spätoperationen der angeborenen Lippen-Kiefer-Gaumen-Spalten. Z Laryngol Rhinol 30:51
52. Skoog T (1958) A design for the repair of unilateral cleft lips. Am J Surg 95:223
53. Skoog T (1967) The use of periosteum and surgical for bone restoration in congenital clefts of the maxilla. Scand J Plast Reconstr Surg 1:113–130
54. Smith N (1826) Suture of the palate. Med Physiol J (NY) 5:525
54a. Stephenson J (1820)
55. Tagliacozzi G (1597) De curtorum chirurgia per ifitionem. Bindonus, Venice
56. Tennison CW (1952) The repair of unilateral cleft lip by the stencil method. J Plast Reconstr Surg 9:115

57. Thompson JE (1912) An artistic and mathematically accurate method of repairing the defect in cases of harelip. Surg Gynecol Obstet 14:498
58. Trauner R (1955) Die Operation der Lippenspalte. Fortschr Kiefer Gesichtschir 1:16
59. Deleted in production
60. Veau V (1938) Bec-de-lièvre. Masson, Paris
61. Veau V, Ruppe C (1922) Les résultats anatomiques et fonctionnels de la staphylorrhaphie par les procédés classiques. Rev Chir 60:81–89
62. Veau V (1926) Le rôle tubercle médian dans la constitution de la face. Ann Anat Pathol (Paris) 3:305–348
63. Velpeau AALM (1845) New elements of operative surgery. Langley, New York, vol I, pp 652
64. Warren JC (1828) On an operation for the cure of natural fissure of the soft palate. Am J Med Sci 1:1
65. Warren JC (1828) Double harelip with fissure through the hard and soft palate. Boston Med Surg J 1:140
66. Washio H (1968) History of cleft lip surgery. In: Stark RB (ed) Cleft palate – a multidiscipline approach. Harper and Row, New York, vol 1

Professor Bochdalek and His Hernia: Then and Now

J. A. Haller, Jr.[1]

Vincent Alexander Bochdalek was born in 1801 of a Czech father who was a gamekeeper and a Slovak mother who lived in the village of Skripov in northern Moravia. Before his death in 1883, he became one of the most outstanding university anatomists and pathologists of his era. He studied in Opava and Vienna and graduated with a degree in medicine from the Carolinum in Prague in 1833. The dissertation he submitted for his graduate degree, entitled "Instruction to Practical Autopsy of the Human Brain with Special Attention to the Cerebellum," was published as a monograph containing 19 defended theses that clearly indicate Bochdalek's lively interest in the broad problems of medicine of his time. Bochdalek spent his entire career in the Prague dissecting rooms and was appointed to the faculty of the Carolinum, where he became a much respected senior academician. He was also very active in the general infirmary, where he introduced the keeping of post mortem records and reported a few microscopic examinations of autopsied material even before his more famous successor, J. E. Purkyne. Following an extensive trip to Scandinavia, he brought home more than 1200 anatomical preparations of the sea fauna which he had carefully categorized and studied.

As a tribute to his original observations, at least four anatomic or pathologic structures bear his name: the ganglion Bochdaleki in the maxillary nerve plexus, a fold of the choroid plexus called Bochdalek's basket, the valves of Bochdalek on the lachrymal duct, and finally, and perhaps most importantly, the hernia Bochdaleki in the foramen of the same name, occupying the posterior part of the diaphragm. The latter finding, first reported in 1848, was accompanied by a description of a child who had died of the hernia and the prediction by Bochdalek that some day surgical treatment to correct this lethal anomaly would be successful.

Apparently, a number of Bochdalek's family lived in the village of Litomerice, located in the beautiful rolling hills northwest of Prague, about 35 miles outside the city. It was here that he came to retire and eventually died in 1883. He was buried there in the village graveyard.

In his paper, containing the first description of the posterior diaphragmatic defect that came to bear his name, Bochdalek discussed the findings of a child who had died of this abnormality. He then went on to reconstruct the pathologic anatomy of this anomaly and inferred that it represented some type of congenital

[1] Division of Pediatric Surgery, The Johns Hopkins University School of Medicine, Baltimore, Maryland 21205, USA

Progress in Pediatric Surgery, Vol. 20
Ed. by P. P. Rickham

malformation occurring in utero. He postulated that this resulted from a rupture of a previously intact membrane through an area of the diaphragm referred to as the trigone of Bochdalek.[2] Others have subsequently questioned the exact anatomy of this diaphragmatic hernia defect, since subsequent information of much greater accuracy has become available regarding the embryologic development of the diaphragm. Nevertheless, he clearly described a lethal case of newborn congenital diaphragmatic hernia which occurred through a posterior defect, and this is properly referred to as Bochdalek's hernia. John J. White has suggested that this is not an appropriate name unless one wishes to remember the inital case and Bochdalek's description of it because this hernia does not actually protrude through the trigone of Bochdalek. White would prefer congenital posterolateral diaphragmatic hernia as a more accurate term for the abnormality, but I am persuaded that such a signal observation made more than 135 years ago should not be lost in minor details and that the embryologic pleuroperitoneal sulcus, which is probably the basic site of this congenital defect, should be permitted to carry the colors of the Prague pathologist. The term pleuroperitoneal hiatus or canal was not used until much later and therefore could not have been familiar to Bochdalek.

It is of great interest that Bochdalek predicted the eventual surgical correction in a newborn baby, but this was not fulfilled until 1946, when Robert Gross first reported the successful operative management of a congenital posterolateral diaphragmatic hernia in a newborn infant. With the rapid development of pediatric anesthesia and pediatric surgery during the 25 years following World War II, many successes in the management of the Bochdalek hernia have been noted, but an equally large number of failures have been recorded. During this time, several management principles have been established: (a) It is imperative to use endotracheal intubation in the newborn baby with a diaphragmatic hernia and not to insufflate with a mask because the oxygen will be driven into the stomach and up into the bowel loops within the chest, causing a further shift of the mediastinum; (b) a nasogastric tube is necessary to prevent further distention of the stomach and intestine; (c) an abdominal incision is preferable to a thoracic incision for at least four reasons. First, it is easier to return the intestine to the abdomen by pulling rather than pushing it. Secondly, associated malformations of rotation of the intestine can simultaneously be corrected transabdominally, but not transthoracically. Thirdly, from below the diaphragm, the hernial defect can be closed and then a decision made as to whether the abdominal wall can be safely closed without putting undue pressure on the diaphragm; this important clinical observation cannot be made satisfactorily with a thoracic incision. Fourthly, forceful expansion of the ipsilateral unexpanded lung must be avoided to prevent rupture of the

[2] Based on L. J. Wells' study of the embryologic development of the human diaphragm, the common congenital posterolateral diaphragmatic hernia *without* a sac (± 90%) results from the herniation of the abdominal viscera through the unused pleuroperitoneal hiatus or canal, while the rarer congenital posterolateral hernia *with* a sac results from a failure of muscle development in the lumbocostal triangle (foramen of Bochdalek), which leaves only the serous pleural sac above and the peritoneum below. Thus to be precise, *only* the posterolateral diaphragmatic hernia with a sac is a *pure* Bochdalek Hernia

contralateral lung, the compliance of which is better. Despite many documented advances in operative management, anesthesia, postoperative monitoring, and intensive care, the mortality in newborn infants with the Bochdalek hernia has remained at about 50%.

In an attempt to understand the pathophysiology of the congenital diaphragmatic hernia of Bochdalek, one should look carefully at two divergent postoperative courses which are quite distinct in this entity. Correction of the tension problem within the chest is accomplished by moving the abdominal organs into the abdomen and closing the diaphragmatic defect. The mediastinal structures return to the midline, and usually, good ventilation and oxygenation accompany this correction. This dramatic response is referred to clinically as the "honeymoon period." It is followed in about one-half of the babies by a smooth postoperative recovery; except for the usual care required by a newborn infant and with due attention to details of the unexpanded lung on the side of the hernia, these babies do well. The other 50% of the patients complete the honeymoon period in 6–12 h and embark on a downhill course characterized by increasing hypoxemia and development of resistant metabolic acidosis, despite adequate ventilation documented by normal arterial PCO_2 levels at reasonable ventilatory pressures. This hypoxemia results from intracardiac shunts from right to left through the foramen ovale and through the patent ductus arteriosus. The majority of the shunt has been shown to be through the patent ductus arteriosus, right to left, from the pulmonary artery to the descending aorta. This has been documented by comparing simultaneous values for PaO_2 from the preductal sampling line at the right.

Of great interest is the recent observation that prostaglandin D may be the primary substance responsible for the normal transition of fetal to newborn circulation specifically by lowering the pulmonary vascular resistance and enhancing closure of the patent ductus arteriosus. An additional and surprising piece to the puzzle is the finding that the richest source of prostaglandin D in the term fetus is the lung. Release of prostaglandin D is likely related to initial lung inflation; therefore, uninflated and immature lungs, i.e., the hypoplastic lung of an infant with congenital diaphragmatic hernia and the underdeveloped lung of a small premature infant, may not release adequate prostaglandin D to trigger the lowering of the pulmonary artery pressure. It remains to be seen whether this is the specific final common pathway for the transition to the newborn circulation.

Much emphasis has been placed on the lung hypoplasia that is invariably present with a congenital diaphragmatic hernia apparent at birth. However, most babies with congenital diaphragmatic hernias who subsequently die because of persistent fetal circulation have adequate pulmonary parenchyma bilaterally. This is reflected in good initial oxygenation and, more importantly, in good clearance of carbon dioxide. The "honeymoon period" after repair is characterized, as noted above, by excellent oxygenation and eucapnia. Therefore, lung hypoplasia per se is probably *not* the main cause of death, although it may contribute indirectly to subsequent pulmonary artery hypertension. A causal relationship between pulmonary hypoplasia and persistent fetal circulation is therefore not established and remains unconfirmed.

Experimental animal models of congenital diaphragmatic hernia have produced lung hypoplasia, but not persistent pulmonary artery hypertension. By using Silastic balloons to simulate abdominal viscera in the chest of fetal lambs, several investigators have produced lung hypoplasia and then deflated the balloons in utero to allow subsequent further lung maturation and survival at birth. On this basis, Harrison has suggested that better survival in babies with congenital diaphragmatic hernias might be possible if intrauterine correction were carried out. Because of the added risk to the expected baby's mother (who would thus require two cesarean sections) and a lack of evidence in lambs and primates that intrauterine correction would prevent persistent pulmonary artery hypertension even while improving pulmonary hypoplasia, no human intrauterine correction for the Bochdalek hernia has as yet been reported.

The next few years may witness increased sonographic diagnosis of this congenital defect with concomitant transport from the uterus to the operating room followed by aggressive ventilatory support of the baby and early, continuous prostaglandin D infusions. Hopefully, this plan of management will improve the unacceptable 50% mortality associated with this abnormality. Bochdalek envisioned only the suturing of the anatomic defect; he could not have predicted the complex pathophysiology or the evolving therapy of the congenital diaphragmatic hernia that appropriately bears his name.

Summary

An account is given of Professor V. A. Bochdalek's life, and special consideration is given to his work on the pathological anatomy of the diaphragmatic hernia which bears his name. The development of the management of congenital diaphragmatic hernias since 1946, when Robert Gross performed the first successful operation on this condition, is briefly outlined.

Résumé

Cette biographie du Professeur Bochdalek traite tout particulièrement de ses travaux sur l'anatomie pathologique de la hernie diaphragmatique qui porte son nom. Ce chapitre fait aussi le point sur l'évolution du traitement des hernies congénitales de 1946 (date à laquelle Robert Gross mena à bonne fin la première intervention chirurgicale) à nos jours.

Zusammenfassung

Es wird aus dem Leben und Wirken von Bochdalek berichtet, unter besonderer Berücksichtigung seiner Arbeit über die pathologische Anatomie der Zwerchfellhernie, die nach ihm benannt wurde. Ferner wird ein Überblick gegeben über die Entwicklung der Behandlung der angeborenen Zwerchfellhernien seit 1946, als Gross die erste erfolgreiche Operation durchführte, bis zu unserer Zeit.

Paediatric Urology 1000 Years Ago

R. E. Abdel-Halim[1]

It is noticeable that, in any contemporary article on medicine, the more than 1000 years between Graeco-Roman times and the modern era are commonly overlooked, giving the appearance that during this period nothing worthy of mention happened in medicine. In Europe, this period is usually referred to as the Dark Ages, in which the great era of the Graeco-Roman medicine came to an end and no progress in medical science was made until the Renaissance [7, 11, 12].

However, in the East, the firm establishment of the Moslem supremacy, coincided with the development of botany, pharmacy and chemistry, branches of science that the Moslem world is given credit for having established [11, 13, 24]. Between the ninth and the sixteenth centuries, the study of medicine and other branches of science revived and acquired a scientific basis [11, 13].

Historical Review of Literature on Paediatric Urology

In this study, we present a brief commentary on four books having to do with urology, with a special view toward aspects of paediatric urology. The books were written by the Moslem scholars ar-Rāzī, Ibn al-Jazzār, al Zahrāwī and Ibn Sīnā, who lived between the ninth and the eleventh centuries.

Al Hāwī

Ar-Rāzī lived in Baghdad between 841 and 926 A.D. [4, 18]. In addition to his treatise *Liber de Variolis et Morbillis* on eruptive fevers [9, 11, 15, 24, 28, 32], which was considered a masterpiece of clinical medicine [8], the 23-volume work al-Hāwī *(Continens),* an encyclopaedia of medicine and surgery, is another major contribution by ar-Rāzī to medicine [9, 11, 24, 28].

Ar-Rāzī critically evaluated the views of the ancients in light of his own experience and practice, a mode of analysis that constitutes basic scientific research. Cumston [11] has stated that the Islamic physician has the merit of having carefully analysed the scattered insights of Greek medicine, extracting from them the most important material and leaving aside everything that was superfluous. According to Ḥusain and al-Okbey, unlike his predecessors, ar-Rāzī followed the original scheme of methodically classifying diseases according to the organs affect-

[1] Urology Unit, King Abdulaziz University Hospital, Jeddah, Saudi Arabia

Progress in Pediatric Surgery, Vol. 20
Ed. by P. P. Rickham

ed [17]. In this, he showed his supreme abilities as a clinician by presenting various pathological conditions, usually starting with the complaint, then analysing its origin and finally describing the signs necessary for diagnosis [9, 25].

Ar-Rāzī was a keen observer, differentiating with great precision among various conditions that produce similar complaints and accurately describing signs necessary for diagnosis. Given the symptom of heaviness in the loin, for example, here is his precise differentiation of renal stones and renal obstruction or swelling: "... and the differentiation between them is that; with inflammation, [there are] mixed fevers, rigors and polyuria with frequency; with obstruction, [there is] oliguria and the urine is clear and with stones, the urine is either clear or not and with sandy sedimentation" [5, part 10, p. 120].

Though Rufus of Ephesus had differentiated between vesical and renal haematuria [12], ar-Rāzī also gave the underlying physio-anatomical reasons for this difference:

> ... Sudden haematuria is due to a ruptured renal vessel as this cannot be the case in the bladder because it cannot be for a vesical vessel to rupture due to plenty of blood coming to it as it happens in the kidney. And this is because blood is not filtered in the vessels of the bladder as it does in the vessels of the kidney. But the amount of blood that comes to the bladder is only enough for its nutrition, while in the kidney because blood is filtered in it and then, large blood vessels and plenty of blood comes to it, far more than its need for nutrition. Also the vessels in the bladder are not close to the interior and unsupported as the vessels which enter deep into the kidney. ... [5, part 10, p. 10].

He also differentiated between renal haematuria due to a ruptured vessel and that due to congestion with increased permeability [5, part 10, p. 10].

His chapter "The Stoppage of Urine" differs from the views of his predecessors Celsus, writing at the start of the Christian era, and Paul of Aegina (625–690 A.D.), both of whom referred only to urinary retention. Ar-Rāzī differentiated between retention and anuria:

> The urine stops either because the kidney lacks it and the sign of this is the stoppage of urine and no heavy pains in the back and not in the loin, ureter and bladder, any discomfort and not at the bladder neck, any cause of obstruction as we will show and together with this, the abdomen is lax and in the body there is swelling and dropsy or profuse sweating.
>
> Or urine is within the kidney which is obstructed and in it the lesion which is swelling or stone or clots of blood or pus. Common to all of them is the pain in the lumbar region with emptiness of the bladder. But if it be a stone, the signs of the stone would appear before that. And if it be a hot swelling, with the pain there is some throbbing. And if it be diseases in the kidney then it is only heaviness. And if it be a solid swelling, the urine does not stop suddenly but gradually and with heaviness only. And if it be clots of blood or pus, then it would be preceded by ulcer.
>
> And if the urine is stopped because of the urinary passages from the kidney, the bladder will be empty and the pain in the ureter along its course with prick-

ing and stitching as the ureteric pain is continuous and pricking, after this, use the previous criteria as in the kidney [5, part 10, pp. 167–168].

In a similar fashion, he discussed clinical observations concerning retention [5, part 10, p. 168].

According to Ḥusain and al-Okbey [17], ar-Rāzī differentiated with great precision between renal or vesical pain and pain due to colitis [5, part 10, pp. 80–81, 105]. He also excelled in differentiating between dormant stones and moving ones, describing the precise location of the latter [5, part 10, p. 92]. Radbill [28] states that ar-Rāzī was the first to describe spina bifida and its relation to incontinence.

From the surgical point of view, ar-Rāzī's procedures for lithotomy were similar to those of Paul of Aegina. However, ar-Rāzī was the first to use enemas as a preparation for surgery and to describe the sign of crepitus on rectal examination in the case of multiple vesical stones. He was also the first to break a large stone by using strong pincers (Fig. 1) to hold the stone firmly and to make it protrude through a perineal cystotomy in order to break it, repeating this procedure at different angles until the stone became small enough to be extracted [5, part 10, pp. 113, 114].

Meatotomy was also first conceived of and practised by ar-Rāzī:

"If a stone is impacted in the tip of the urethra be aware not to force it out by pushing as this causes laceration and subsequent severe pains and infections, but incise the end of the penis and remove the stone" [5, part 10, p. 166].

Risāla Fi Siyāsat Aṣ-Ṣibyān Wa Tadbīrihim

Ibn al-Jazzār, or al Gizar, lived in Qairawān between 895 and 980 A.D. [3]. His book *Siyāsat aṣ-ṣibyān Wa Tadbīrihim,* comprising 22 chapters, is considered a continuation of ar-Rāzī's tradition of distinguishing diatric from other diseases. As far as urological disorders are concerned, he devoted a whole chapter to a discussion of bladder stones, including their aetiology, sex incidence, symptoms and signs. Ibn al-Jazzār's book sums up most of the knowledge of his predecessors.

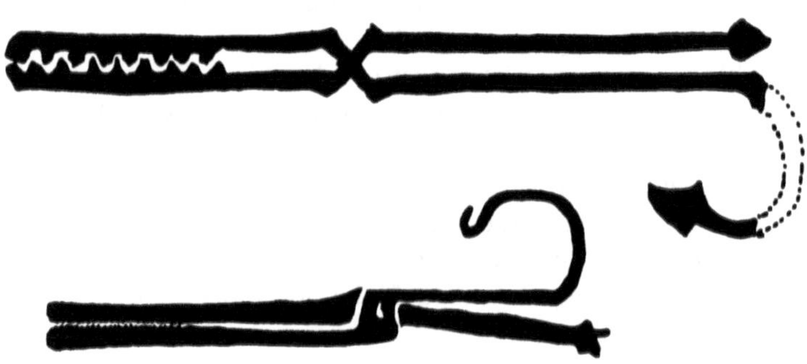

Fig. 1. Pineers devised by ar-Rāzī to grasp vesical stones [31]

At-Taṣrīf

Al Zahrāwī, also known as Albucasis, Abulcasis, Bucasis or al Zahravius [2, 9], lived in Cordoba (al Andalus) between 930 and 1013 A.D. [32].

His book at-Taṣrīf Kitāb at-Taṣrīf li-man ᶜajiza ᶜan at-ta ᶜlif (The disposal of medical knowledge to he who is not able to compile it by himself) constitutes his largest work on medicine. Consisting of 30 volumes it is an encyclopaedia of medicine and surgery [2, 9, 11, 18].

Al-Zahrāwī summed up all the surgical knowledge of his time in the 30th volume of this large medical encyclopaedia [31]. A number of historians have described this volume as giving the first rational and complete illustrated treatment of its subject, and the many surgical procedures and instruments described in it do not appear in any other work of the time [2, 9, 11, 15, 26, 30–32].

According to Cumston [11], Spink and Lewis [31] and El Faquih and Wallace [14], al-Zahrāwī's device of drilling a hole in an impacted urethral stone by a special drill called al Mis̲h̲ᶜab, made of the finest steel, may be considered as the foundation of true lithotripsy:

> ... Now if the calculus be small and be impacted in the opening of the urinary passage, preventing the exit of the urine treat it with the means I am about to describe before you go on to make your incision, for often I have found this treatment sufficient without incision; I have experience of this. You take a drill of the finest steel of this shape. It should be triangular at the point and sharp with a wooden handle. Then take a thread and with it bind the penis beneath the calculus to prevent the stone from returning to the bladder. Then introduce the iron of the drill gently into the meatus until the drill reaches the stone itself and then very, very gently revolve the drill upon the stone with your hand, and try to perforate it, till you pierce it through to the other side. Then the urine will at once be released. Then, with your hand outside the penis, squeeze the remains of the stone and they will crumble and be washed out by the urine and the patient will be cured (Fig. 2) (cited by [31, pp. 416–417]).

Al-Zahrāwī also designed a special forceps he called Kalālīb (Fig. 3), which he used for crushing a large vesical stone through a perineal cystotomy. It was in fact a primitive lithotrite:

> "... But if the stone be very large, it is foolish to make a great incision down upon it, for the result is that the patient either dies or has a chronic urinary fistula because the place will not heal at all. Try rather to manipulate it so that it

Fig. 2. Steel drill used by al-Zahrāwī to pierce urethral stones [31]

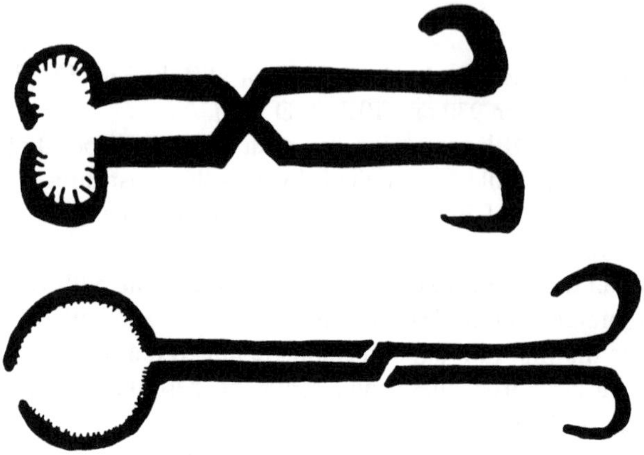

Fig. 3. Forceps designed by al-Zahrāwī to crush vesical stones [31]

protrudes, or else attempt to break it up with the forceps so that you can extract it piecemeal" (cited by [31, pp. 414–415]).

Circumcision was not described by either Celsus or Paul of Aegina. The latter described only the excision of blackened prepuce in gangrenous infections. Therefore, as related by Spink and Lewis, al-Zahrāwī was the first to describe the dissection technique of circumcision performed with scissors (Fig. 4), an instrument he was the first to make use of in surgery [31].

His chapter on bladder irrigation with its numerous illustrations of syringes and other instruments is of utmost originality [31]. In contrast to the Greek S-shaped catheter, al-Zahrāwī used catheters of his own design, which resembled modern ones in that they were straight [24, 31]. For operating on children, he stressed that small versions of the instruments designed specially for this purpose should be used.

From the observations made by al-Zahrāwī with regard to his personal experience and the care with which he warns the reader of the dangers of injury that can be incurred during surgery, he was not a mere compiler, but also a very skillful surgeon [9, 11, 12, 15, 24, 26, 30–32].

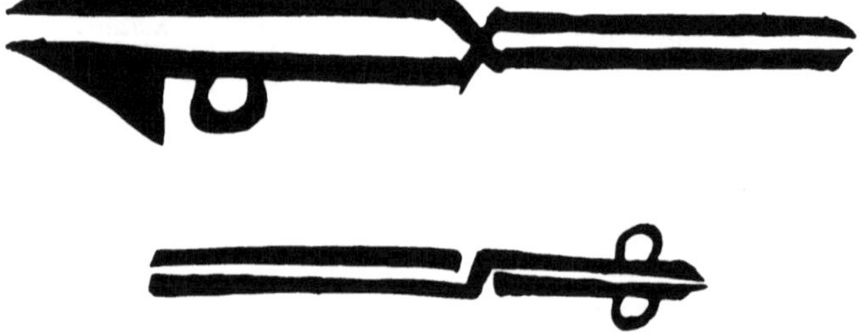

Fig. 4. Scissors inveated by al-Zahrāwī to perform circumcision by dissection technique [31]

Al-Qānūn (The Canon of Medicine)

Ibn Sīnā, or Avicenna [2] lived in Hamaḏān and Jurjān from 980 to 1037 A.D. [18] and acquired great fame in mediaeval European medicine [11, 16, 21, 28, 29].

In *al-Qānūn,* Ibn Sīnā basically followed the methodical, analytical line originated by ar-Rāzī. *Al-Qānūn* was, however, more broadly conceived than the *Continens* [11] and included all branches of medical science [11, 16, 21].

According to Desnos, most of the disesaes of the kidneys and bladder can be recognized in the systemic classification of renal diseases and the accounts of bladder diseases given by Ibn Sīnā in *al-Qānūn* [12, 20]. He was also the first to point out the fact that haematuria may be due to causes outside the urinary system, for example, blood diseases [20, vol. 2, p. 529].

Apart from the methodical classification and precise descriptions of aetiological factors and signs in his chapter on urinary disturbances, Ibn Sīnā pointed out the role of psychological factors in the treatment of certain cases of nocturnal enuresis [20, vol. 2, p. 526].

Both Ibn Sīnā and ar-Rāzī warned against catheterization in the presence of inflammation, as it increases the swelling and pain. To ensure gentle catheterisation, Ibn Sīnā designed catheters with rounded, firm tips and many side holes from the skin of certain marine and other animals [20, vol. 2, p. 522].

The *al-Hāwī, at-Taṣrīf* and *al-Qānūn* were translated into Latin as early as 1150 A.D. by Gerard of Cremona [32] and greatly influenced the European mediaeval schools of medicine well into the eighteenth century [9, 11, 12, 15, 16, 24, 26, 28, 29, 32].

Summary

In this paper we present a commentary on four books from the paediatric urology point of view; *al-Hāwī* (Continens), *R. fi Siyāsat aṣ-Ṣibyān wa tadbīrihim, at-Taṣrīf* and *al-Qānūn* by the Moslem scholars ar-Rāzī, Ibn al-Jazzār, al Zahrāwī and Ibn Sīnā who lived within the period of the ninth to the eleventh centuries.

In these books the supreme abilities of the authors as clinicians and their role in the creation of clinical medicine are shown by: The presentation of the various pathological conditions usually starting with the complaint then describing the origin of the disease and enumerating the accurate signs necessary for diagnosis. Differential diagnosis between various conditions which produce similar complaints is precisely described. For example, retention of urine and different types of anuria, types of renal haematuria, dormant and moving renal stones and their precise localisation, renal or vesical pain and pain due to colitis. Finally the methodical classification of the diseases according to the organs affected is discussed.

The description of the pathology and the knowledge of new diseases was an important advance made by these scholars. From the urological point of view, spina bifida and its relation to incontinence was first described by ar-Rāzī and most of the diseases of the kidney and bladder can be recognized in the systemic classification of the diseases of these organs given by Ibn Sīnā who pointed out the psychological role in some cases of nocturnal enuresis. Though ar-Rāzī was the first to think of and practice meatotomy, introduce enema in the pre-operative preparation for lithotomy and break large vesical stones piecemeal the bladder, the merit of having integrated surgery into scientific medicine must go to al-Zahrāwī. The many operative procedures and instruments described in the thirtieth volume of his encyclopaedia of medicine and surgery *(at-Taṣrīf)*, such as the Kalālīb "a primitive lithotrite", the Mis̲h̲ᶜab to drill a hole in an impacted urethral stone forming the foundation of true lithotripsy, the scissors used in the dissection technique of circumcision, straight catheters and the numerous instruments and techniques for bladder irrigation, do not appear in any other classical writing.

These books were translated into Latin as early as 1150 A.D. and greatly influenced the European mediaeval schools of medicine up to the eighteenth century.

Résumé

Ce chapitre traite de 4 manuels du point de vue de l'urologie infantile, écrits par les savants musulmans ar-Rāzī, Ibn al-Ǧazzār, al-Zahrāwī et Ibn Sīnā qui vivaient entre le IXᵉ et le XIᵉ siècle.

Ces ouvrages témoignent de l'extraordinaire compétence des auteurs et de l'importance de leur rôle lors de la naissance de la médecine clinique. Ils décrivent d'abord les symptômes présentés par le patient, indiquent la cause de la maladie et les signes qui conduisent au diagnostic. Ils connaissent aussi le diagnostic différentiel, par exemple pour les rétentions d'urine dans les cas d'anurie, d'hématurie, de calculs vésicaux, de néphrites ou de colites. Ils discutent aussi des mérites d'une classification méthodique des affections d'après les organes touchés.

Ces savants ont aussi fait progresser les connaissances en pathologie et dans le domaine des maladies nouvelles. Dans le domaine de l'urologie par exemple, ar-Rāzī décrit pour la première fois le spina bifida dans le contexte de l'incontinence. Ibn Sīnā énumère la plupart des affections rénales et vésicales. Il mentionne aussi l'aspect psychologique de l'énurésie. Ar-Rāzī effectua la première méatotomie, utilisait des clystères comme préparation à une lithotomie et broyait de gros calculs vésicaux mais c'est al-Zahrāwī qui fit vraiment entrer la chirurgie dans le domaine de la médecine scientifique. Les diverses méthodes opératoires et les instruments qu'il décrit dans le volume 30 de son encyclopédie de la médecine et de la chirurgie (at-Taṣrīf) tels que le "Kalālīb" un broyeur de calculs primitifs, le "mišᶜab" avec lequel il perçait un trou dans un calcul bloqué dans l'urètre (le début de la lithotritie), les ciseaux pour la circoncision, le cathéter et les nombreux autres instruments pour le lavage vésical ne sont mentionnés dans aucun autre ouvrage classique.

Ces ouvrages ont été traduits en latin dès 1150 et ont eu une grande influence sur la médecine européenne au Moyen-Age et jusqu'au XVIIIᵉ siècle.

Zusammenfassung

Dieser Beitrag ist eine Besprechung von 4 Lehrbüchern vom Standpunkt der pädiatrischen Urologie; das *al-Ḥāwī* (Continens), *R. fī Siyāsat aṣ-Ṣibyān wa tadbīrihim, at-Taṣrīf* und *al-Qānūn* von den moslemischen Gelehrten ar-Rāzī, Ibn al-Ǧazzār, al Zahrāwī und Ibn Sīnā, die zwischen dem 9. und 11. Jahrhundert lebten.

Diese Bücher zeugen von den außerordentlichen Fähigkeiten der Autoren als Kliniker und von ihrer Bedeutung bei der Entstehung einer klinischen Medizin: die Beschreibung der verschiedenen pathologischen Zustände fängt mit der Beschwerde des Patienten an, dann wird die Ursache der Krankheit genannt, dann die genauen Anzeichen, die für die Diagnose von Bedeutung sind. Es wird auch genauestens auf die Differentialdiagnose eingegangen, wie z. B. im Fall der Urinretention bei den verschiedenen Arten von Anurie, bei Hämaturie, bei ruhenden und beweglichen Nierensteinen (und wie man sie genau lokalisiert), bei Nieren- oder Blasenschmerzen oder auch Dickdarmentzündung. Es wird auch die methodische Klassifizierung der Krankheiten nach den betroffenen Organen diskutiert.

Diese Gelehrten haben die Kenntnisse über Pathologie und neue Krankheiten vermehrt. Vom Standpunkt der Urologie wurde die Spina bifida im Zusammenhang mit Inkontinenz zum ersten Mal durch ar-Rāzī beschrieben, und die meisten Nieren- und Blasenkrankheiten wurden in der systematischen Klassifizierung von Ibn Sīnā aufgeführt. Er erwähnt außerdem den psychologischen Aspekt in einigen Fällen von nächtlicher Enuresis. Obwohl ar-Rāzī als erster eine Meatotomie durchführte, Klistiere einführte zur Vorbereitung auf die Lithotomie und große Steine in der Blase zertrümmerte, ist es das Verdienst von al-Zahrāwī gewesen, die Chirurgie zu einem Teil der wissenschaftlichen Medizin gemacht zu haben. Die verschiedenen Operationsmethoden und Instrumente, die er in Bd. 30 seiner *Enzyklopädie der Medizin und der Chirurgie* (at-Taṣrīf) beschreibt, wie z. B. das Kalālīb, „ein primitiver Steinzertrümmerer", das Mišᶜab, um ein Loch in einen eingekeilten Stein in der Harnröhre zu bohren (der Anfang der wirklichen Steinzertrümmerung), die Schere, die für die Beschneidung verwendet wurde, die Katheter und die zahlreichen Instrumente und Methoden für die Blasenspülung, werden in keinem anderen klassischen Werk beschrieben.

Diese Bücher wurden bereits im Jahre 1150 ins Lateinische übersetzt und hatten großen Einfluß auf die europäische Medizin des Mittelalters und bis ins 18. Jahrhundert hinein.

References

1. Abdel-Halim RE, Mohammad Y (1983) Kinderheilkunde vor 100 Jahren: Blick in die arabisch-islamische Medizin. Kinderarzt 14:61–63
2. Abouleish E (1979) Contributions of Islam to medicine. J Islamic Med Assoc (US) 28:45
3. Al-Haila, Muhammad al-Ḥabīb (ed) (1968) Risāla fi aṣ-ṣibyān wa tadbīrihim (Ibn al-Jazzār). Al-Dār at-tūnisiya lin-nashr. Tunis (About management and direction of the youth)
4. Al-Nadīm (1970) The fihrist of al-Nadīm, a tenth century survey of muslim culture. Columbia University Press, New York, vol 2

5. Ar-Rāzī (1955–1969) Kitāb al-Ḥāwī fi ṭ-ṭibb (The book of the collector of medicine) (Rhazes, Liber Continens), 1st edn. Osmania Oriental Publications, Osmania University, Hyderabad, vol 10
6. Deleted in production
7. Bickers W (1969) Adventures in Arabian medicine. J R Coll Surg Irel 5:5–14
8. Browne EG (1962) Arabian medicine. Cambridge University Press, New York
9. Campbell DC (1974) Arabian medicine and its influence on the middle ages, 1st edn (reprint). Philo Press, Amsterdam
10. Celcus (1938) De Medicina. Heinmann, London; Harvard University Press, Cambridge, vols 1–3
11. Cumston CG (1978) An introduction to the history of medicine from the time of the pharoahs to the end of the XVIII century. Dawsons of Pall Mall, London
12. Desnos E (1972) The history of urology up to the latter half of the nineteenth century. In: Murphy LJT (ed) The history of urology. Thomas, Springfield
13. Dickinson EH (1875) The medicine of the ancients. Holden, Liverpool
14. El Faquih S, Wallace DM (1978) Ultrasonic lithotriptor for urethral and bladder stones. Br J Urol 50:255–256
15. Freind J (1727) Histoire de la médecine, depuis Galien, jusqu'au commencement du seizième siècle, part 3. Langerak, Leyden
16. Gruner OC (1930) A treatise on the Canon of Medicine of Avicenna incorporating a translation of the first book. Luzac, London
17. Ḥusain MK, al-Okbey MA (1977) Ṭibb ar-Rāzī, Dirāsa wa tahlīl li kitāb al-Ḥāwī. Dār al-Shorūg, Cairo (The medicine of ar-Rāzī, Studies and researches in al-Ḥāwī)
18. Ibn Abī Uṣaybiᶜa (1965) ᶜUyūnal-Anbā' fi tabaqāt al-aṭibbā. Dār maktabat al-Hayāt, Beirut (The sources of the knowledge of classes of doctors)
19. Ibn al-Jazzār (1968) Risāla fi Siyāsat aṣ-ṣibyān wa tadbīrihim. Ad-Dar at-tunisiya lin-nashr, Tunis
20. Ibn Sīnā (1877) Kitab al-Qānūn fi t-tibb. Dar Sadir, Beirut (The conon of medicine)
21. Iskandar AZ (1967) A catalogue of Arabic manuscripts on medicine and science in the Wellcome Historical Medical Library. Wellcome Historical Medical Library, London
22. Jan MY, Abdel-Halim RES (1983) Ibn Al Gazzar und sein Werk: die Führung von Kindern und ihre Betreuung. Kinderarzt 14:643–646
23.
24. Margotta R (1968) In: Lewis P (ed) An illustrated history of medicine. Hamlyn, Feltham
25. Meyerhof M (1935) Thirty-three clinical observations by Rhazes (circa 900 AD). Isis 23: 321–393
26. Montagnani CA (1983) Paediatric surgery in Islamic medicine from Middle Age to Renaissance. Greek Association of Paediatric Surgeons, 8th annual international meeting, Chios
27. Paulus Aegineta (1844–1847) The seven books of Paulus Aegineta, translated by F Adams. Sydenham Society, London, vols 1–3
28. Radbill SX (1971) The first treatise on paediatrics. Am J Dis Child 122:369–376
29. Shah MH (1966) The general principles of Avicenna's Canon of medicine. Naveed Clinic, Karachi
30. Sprengel K (1815) Histoire de la médecine, depuis son origine jusqu'au dix-neuvième siècle, vol 2. Deterville Libreure, Paris
31. Spink MS, Lewis IL (1973) Albucasis on surgery and instruments (a definitive edition of the Arabic text with English translation and commentary). Wellcome Institute of the History of Medicine, London
32. Ullmann M (1978) Islamic medicine. Islamic surveys series no 11. Edinburgh University Press, Edinburgh

Sketches of Surgical Cases Drawn in 1884–87 at The East London Hospital for Children, Shadweel

V. A. J. Swain, F.R.C.S.[1]

The majority of these cases were under the care of Robert W. Parker (Fig. 1). Born in 1842, he qualified as a surgeon in 1869 and, after appointments at the London Hospital and the West Ham and Stratford Dispensary, he volunteered to serve with the Anglo-American Ambulance in the Franco-Prussian War in 1870–1871 [1]. Having a good knowledge of French and German, his medical services were indispensable. After his distinguished and active service, he was awarded the Albert Commendation Order of Saxony and made a Knight of the Military Order for Merit of Bavaria.

After the war, in 1872, he became resident medical officer at the Children's Hospital, Great Ormond Street. In 1876, he was appointed assistant surgeon at

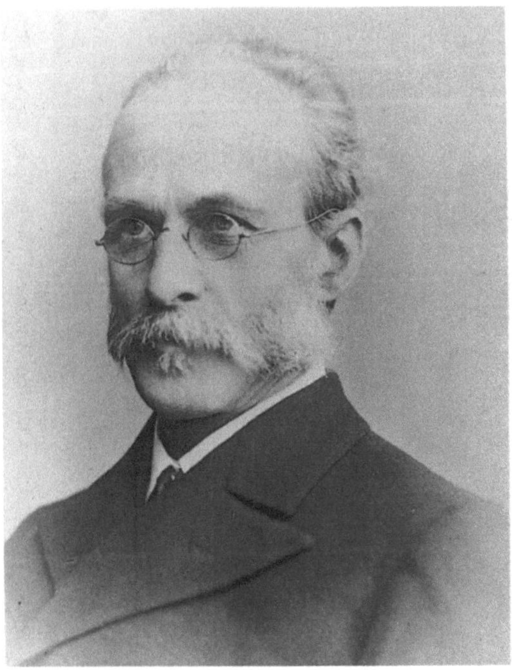

Fig. 1. Robert William Parker (1842–1913)

[1] The Old Cottage, Rolls Park, Chigwell, Essex, 1G7 6DJ. Honorary consulting surgeon, The Queen Elizabeth Hospital for Children, London E2 8PS, United Kingdom

Progress in Pediatric Surgery, Vol. 20
Ed. by P. P. Rickham

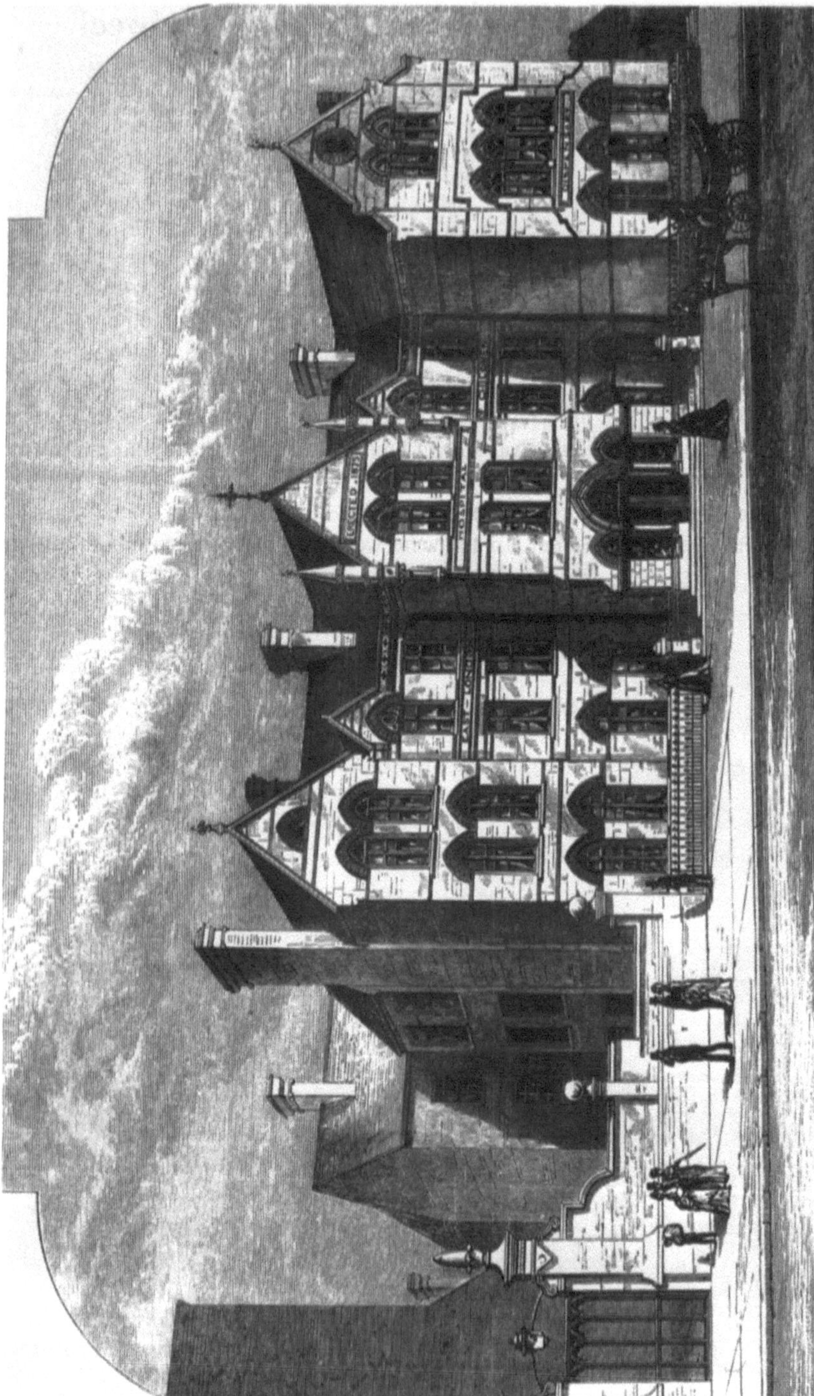

Fig. 2. The East London Hospital for Children, Shadwell. The building was completed in 1877, and replaced the original small hospital in Ratcliff Cross founded in 1868 by Dr. Nathaniel Heckford. In 1881 another floor was added to the hospital

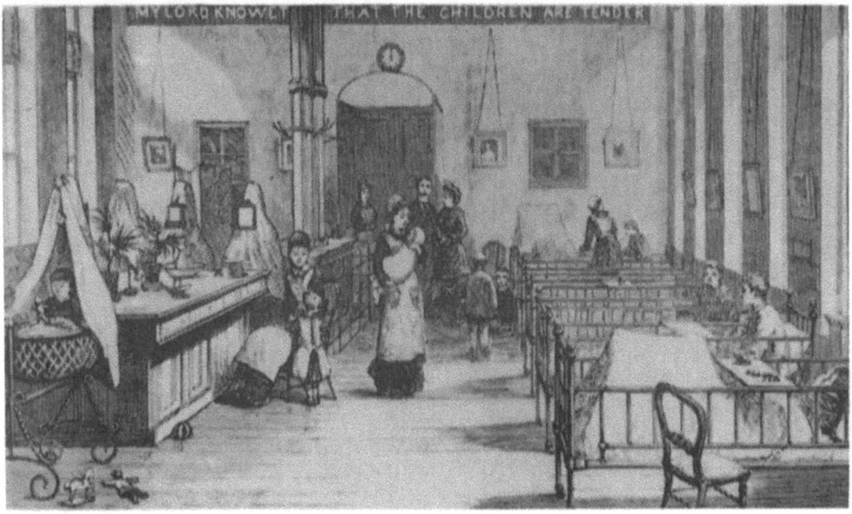

Fig. 3. One of the wards in the New Hospital at Shadwell in 1878

the East London Hospital for Children, Shadwell (Figs. 2, 3) and became senior surgeon in 1887, a position he retained until his retirement in 1902 [2]. In his later years, he married one of the Shadwell nurses in 1882. They had two sons, who were educated first in England and later abroad. Robert Parker died in 1913 in Freiburg, Baden, after 26 years of active work at the Children's Hospital. He was one of "Shadwell's Worthies".

During his professional life, he made many contributions to children's surgery in addition to caring for the many surgical cases sketched by a Nurse Reeve about 100 years ago (Fig. 4). At Shadwell Hospital, he was known for his "wonderful notebooks", but most of these have vanished except for the few drawings portrayed below.

As he was an active member of several London medical societies, such as the British Medical Association, the Clinical Society, the Pathological and Anatomical Societies, their transactions present many of his paediatric cases.

As a linguist, he translated many surgical works from European languages. His skill in treating croup and club foot in infants earned him international recognition [3, 4].

The Sketches of Surgical Cases 1884–1887

These original cut-out sketches on white paper were pasted down on *both* sides of tinted pages, and in most instances a descriptive clinical note accompanied the drawings. For clarity photographs only of the actual drawings are reproduced; with a few exceptions the note is recorded separately.

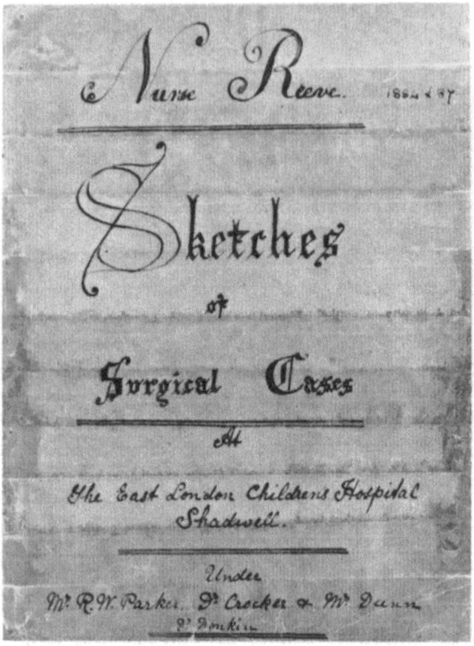

Fig. 4. Frontispiece of Nurse Reeve's sketches 1884–1887.

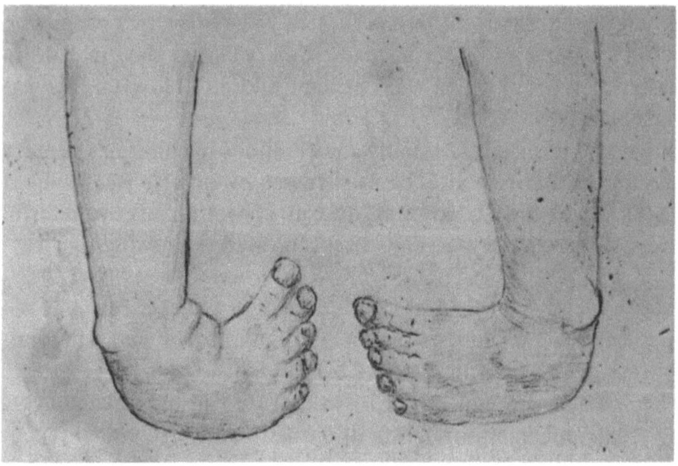

Fig. 5. "Talipes Equino-Varus Fred. Bardell 5 months.
Admitted January 1885. January 18th. Under chloroform Mr. Parker separated Achilles and Tibialis Anticus tendons. Feet put in plaster of Paris.
26th. To have the feet worked in water and rubbed every morning. Flexible splints applied.
February 10th. Great improvement, feet in very good position. Sent home in plaster to be removed in a fortnight.
August. Feet much improved and pair of boots ordered."

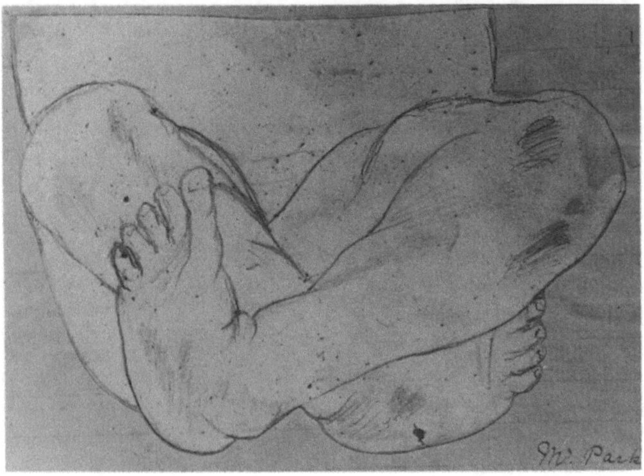

Fig. 6. "Talipes-Varus (double) Francis Adcock. 3 weeks. Illustrating mode of causation" O.P. August 1885.
Right much less severe than left. Flexible splints worn for 3 weeks. Tendo-Achilles divided in both feet. Plaster bandages applied.
October 1886. Feet nearly straight, can walk well.

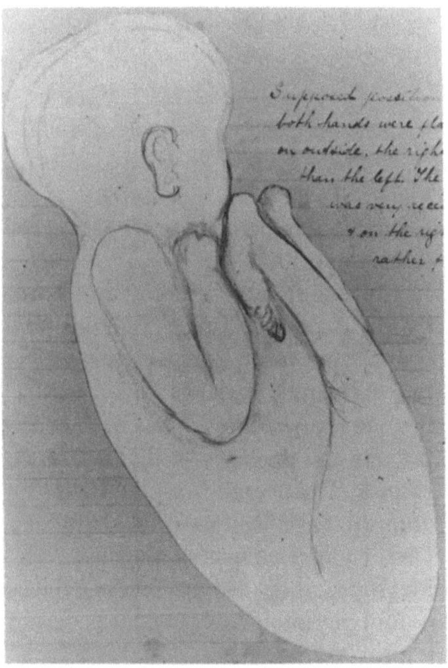

Fig. 7. Genu Recurvatum. "Supposed position – both hands were flattened on outside, the right more than the left. The chin was very receding and on the right side rather flat."

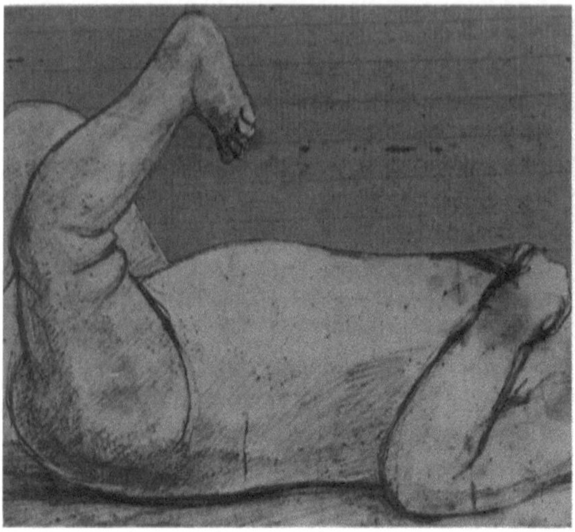

Fig. 8. Genu Recurvatum. "A good sized patella can be felt. The deformity appears to depend on an unusual length of the posterior ligament of the joint. The limb appears to have been extended on the abdomen the leg being hyperextended – Leg put up on an outside straight splint. ...
May 1886 – Fine healthy child, leg quite straight."

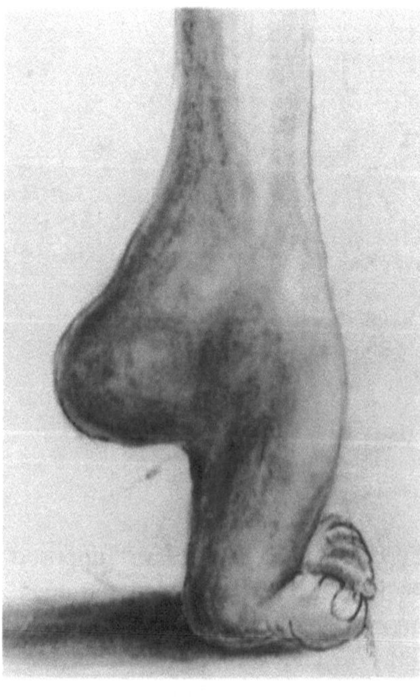

Fig. 9. "Talipes Equinus (Left).
Elizabeth Lampard. 10 years. Admitted October 9th 1885.
In 1881 the *Right* foot was operated on by Mr. Parker for Talipes Equinus (and 'irons' worn for two years) apparently due to infantile paralysis.
For the last year the *left* has been contracting and the leg is smaller in every respect. The operation on the right foot seems to have been most successful.
Cocaine injected hypodermically.
Mr. Bathams divided the Tendo-Achilles – foot put into plaster bandages. Great improvement."

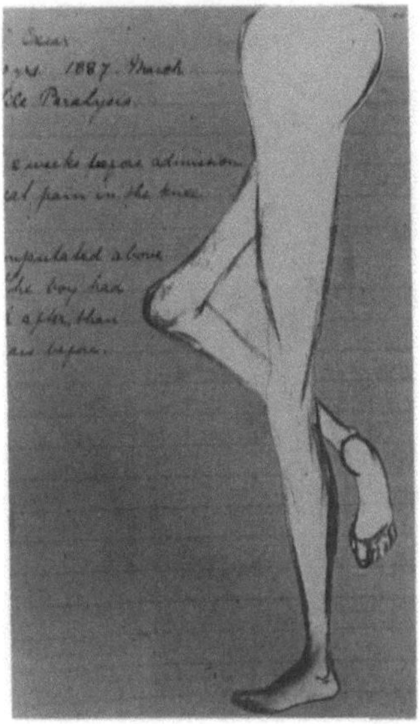

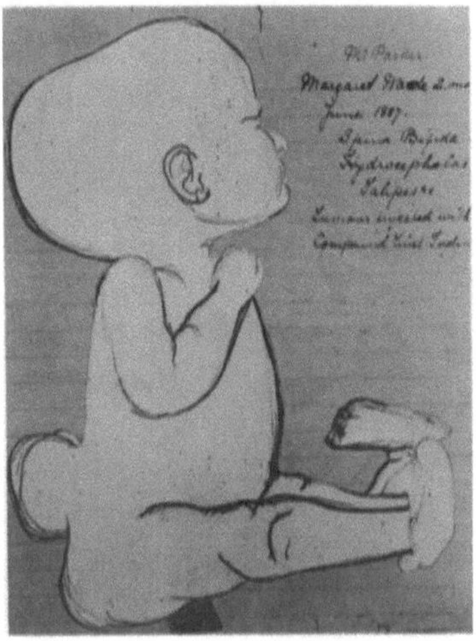

Fig. 11

Fig. 10

Fig. 10. "Mr. Caesar. A boy of 10 years. 1887 March. Old infantile paralysis. Had a fall 2 weeks before admission and had had great pain in the knee since. Mr. Walsh amputated above the knee. The boy had better health after than some years before."

Fig. 11. "Margaret Wade. 2 months. June 1887. Spina Bifida. Hydrocephalus. Talipes etc. Tumour injected with compound tinct iodine."

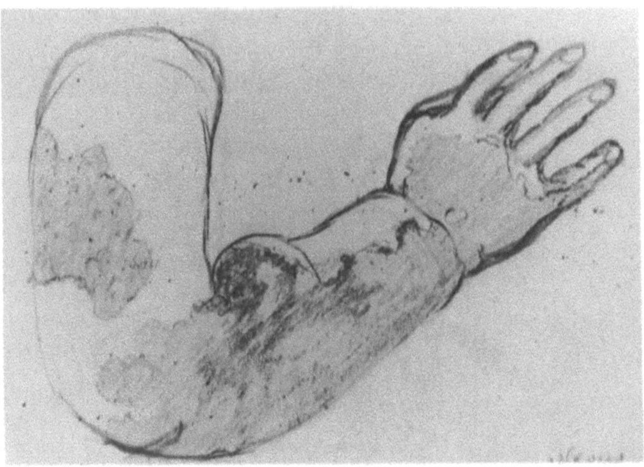

Fig. 12. "Child of 1 year. O.P. May 1887.
Had been touched with nitric acid when the patient was a few months old, but had been growing again, on the darkest parts indicated, the lighter shading is merely deep staining, and had not been touched. Was again painted with ethylate of sodium."

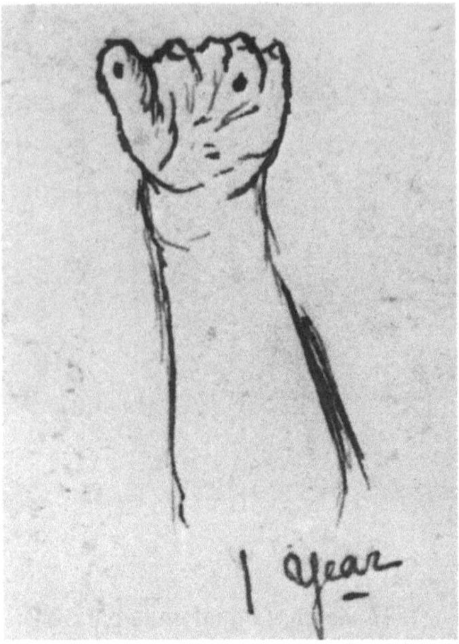

Fig. 13. "Congenital Absence of Hand. Elizabeth Bradshaw. 1 year. October 1884."

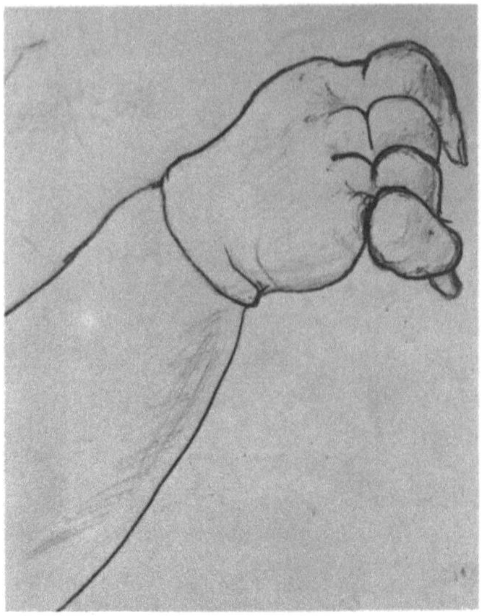

Fig. 14. "Anne Elizabeth Griffiths. 3 months. Out-patient 1885. Congenital Amniotic Band. Amniotic constriction around base of R. little finger and markings over dorsum of 2nd and 3rd and less also of the first fingers."

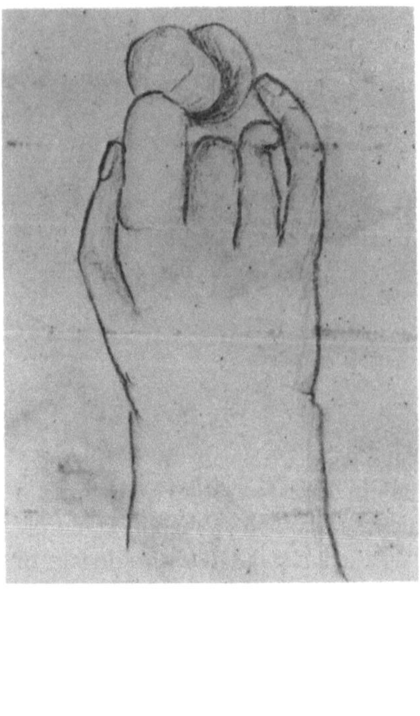

Fig. 15. "Arthur Brown. 12 days. O.P. May 1885. Congenital deformity of left hand – amniotic bands. Nails on thumb and little finger only. Round mass from top removed."

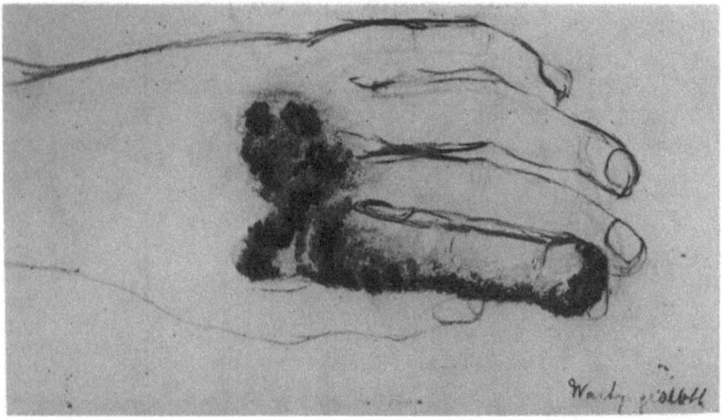

Fig. 16. "Warty growth. Dr. Crocker.
A boy of 12 yrs. April 1887.
The patient came up to see Dr. Crocker, had been some years before for the same thing, and was treated with – plaster, which apparently cured it.
The same treatment was used again round the second joint of the finger for one week, which had quite healed up when the plaster was taken off. The darkest shading shows where the skin was formed into hard black scales."

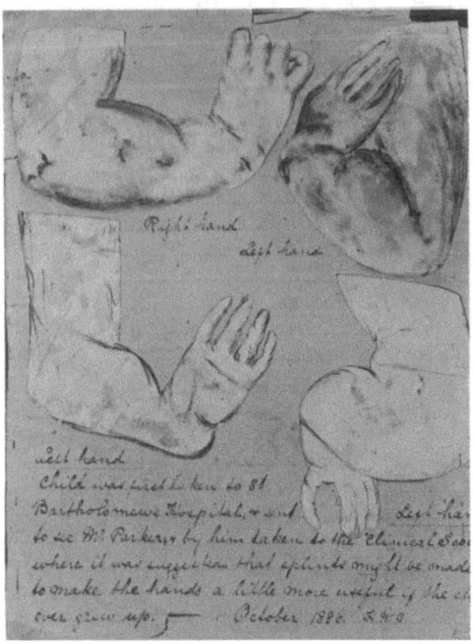

Fig. 17. "Congenital absence of radius and thumbs.
Child was first taken to St. Bartholomew's Hospital and sent to see Mr. Parker and by him taken to the 'Clinical Society' where it was suggested that splints might be made to make the hands a little more useful if the child ever grew up. October 1886."

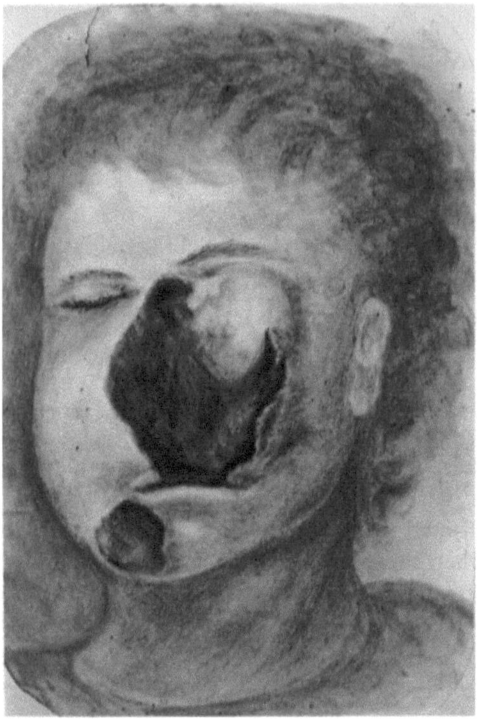

Fig. 18. "Cancrum oris after measles.
March 1887 – lived only 6 days."

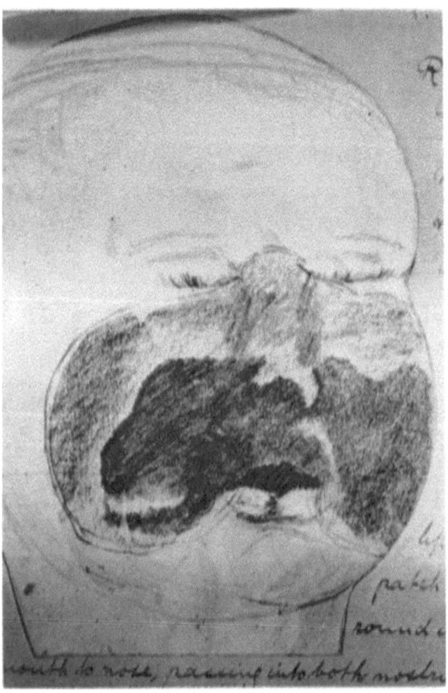

Fig. 19. "Mr. Parker.
Rosina Mann. 3½ yrs.
Admitted May 16th died May 20th 1885.

Began above left angle of the mouth and spread rapidly over almost whole of face. Acid nitric of mercury had no effect whatsoever. The day before admission a small black spot appeared on the lip which was swollen. On admission left half of upper lip was occupied by a large black patch the size of a ½p. with a blue rim round. Reaching from the angle of the mouth to nose, passing into both nostrils. Above right angle of mouth a blue patch a little larger than 6d. Upper lip very much swollen, surface cracked and bleeding. Nose and cheeks also swollen. The gangrene is seen also inside the mouth, on upper gums, hard palate and inside lip. Breath extremely foul. Edges of gangrene were well rubbed with acid Soln. of hyd: nit: Mouth washed over with glycerine and acid carbol.-Spray kettle.
Temp. rose once to 103°, generally 100°.
On P.M. examination found to be a fairly well nourished and healthy. The cheeks were over an inch in thickness. The tissues hard and brawny."

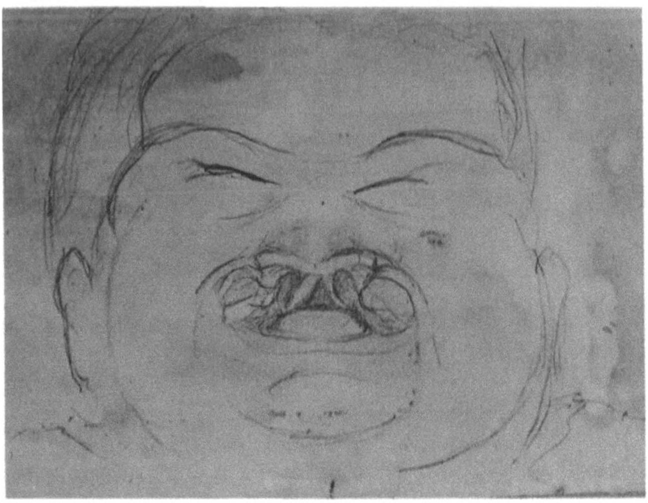

Fig. 20. "Rose Garland – September 1886.
Child was brought to the Hospital when only one hour old, was admitted at two days, as the woman in charge could not get it to take food. Fine healthy child with dark curly hair. Was fed with a glass syringe which had a piece of drainage tubing on the nozzle long enough to reach to the back of the mouth. Child lived about 14 days."

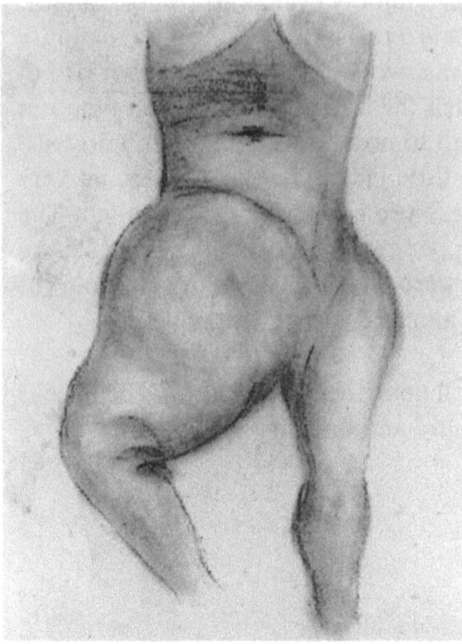

Fig. 21. "O.P. October 1884. Sarcoma.
John. 2 years.
When first brought to O.P. slight fullness noticed on the right side of face and small lump in the right groin, was admitted the next week. Both became gradually more marked. Child had a good deal of pain at night but was very quiet during the day. Became very much wasted and died about the middle of February 1885."

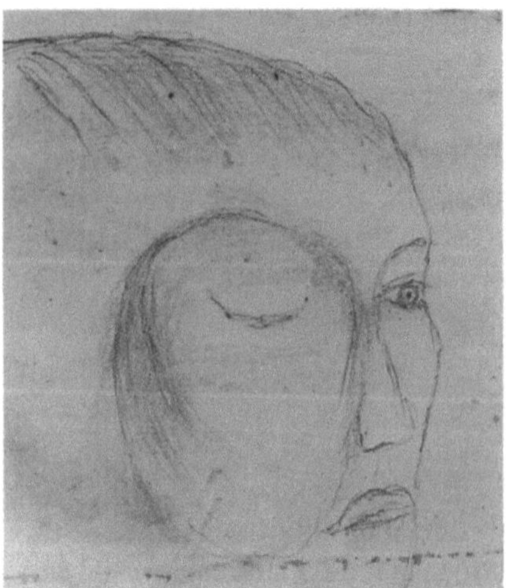

Fig. 22. "In March 1887 the younger brother was brought for a swelling in his right side. Right chest an inch larger than left one slightly flattened."

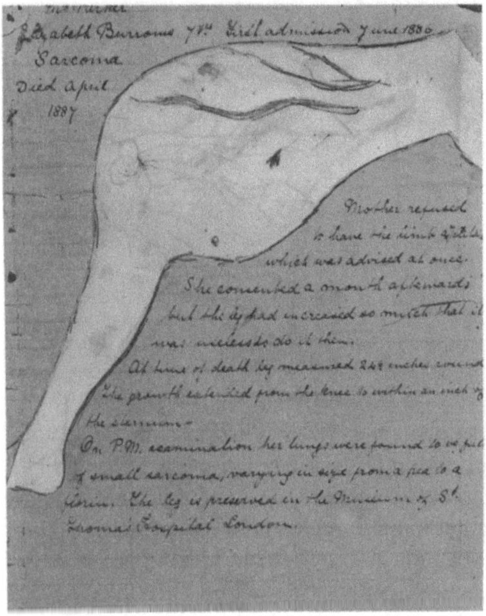

Fig. 23. "Elizabeth Burrows. 7 years. First admission June 1886.
Sarcoma. Died 1887.
Mother refused to have the limb amputated which was advised at once. She consented a month afterwards but the leg had increased so much that it was useless to do it then. At time of death leg measured 24½ inches round. The growth extended from the knee to within an inch of the sternum. On P.M. examination her lungs were found to be full of small sarcoma varying in size from a pea to a florin. The leg is preserved in the Museum in St. Thomas' Hospital, London."

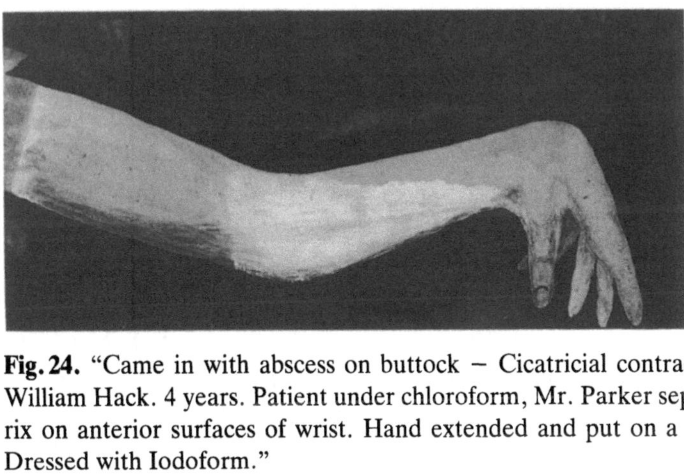

Fig. 24. "Came in with abscess on buttock – Cicatricial contraction after burn. William Hack. 4 years. Patient under chloroform, Mr. Parker separated the cicatrix on anterior surfaces of wrist. Hand extended and put on a straight splint – Dressed with Iodoform."

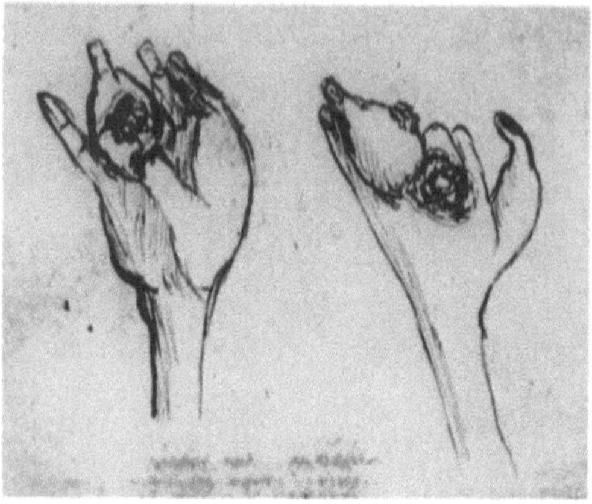

Fig. 25. "Mary Ann Edmunds.
9 years.
Admitted Nov. 25 1885.
Struma. Multiple Dactylitis.

R. hand, fourth shaft, first and second phalanges swollen and egg-shaped. Superficially ulcerated on palmer surface, circumference 3⅝ inches – Second shaft, first phalanx enlarged and bulbous circumf. 3 inches – *L.* hand 4th shaft similarly enlarged with same circumf. as the other hand; but ulcerated on *outer* side of *third* shaft at metacarpophalangeal joint. Thumb, first and second phalanges enlarged and bulbous.
(Ordinary circumf. of finger is 1½ inches.) Dressed with Ung. Hyd. Acid Rubra. Scraped twice, not much improvement. Sent to Braintree Convalescence Home, in May; general health improved, but hands much the same. Attended as O.P. for some months. She dressed at home by district nurse. Neck, cheeks, elbows, arms, groins, legs, heels, toes, and back all more or less ulcerated."

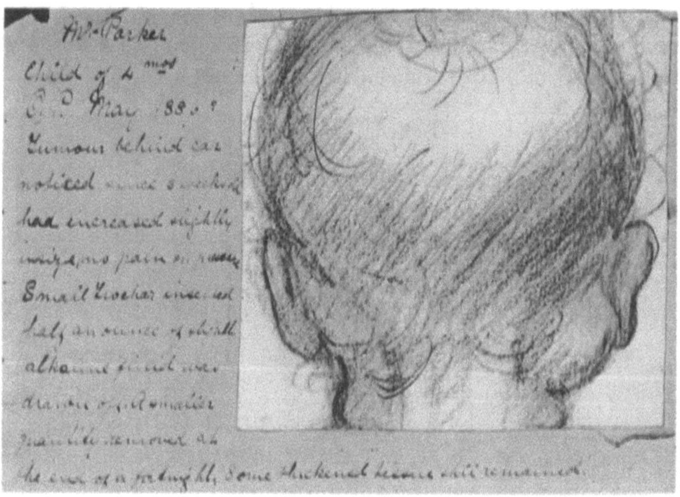

Fig. 26. "Child of 4 months.
O.P. May 1886.

Tumour behind ear noticed since 3 weeks old – had increased slightly in size; no pain on pressure. Small trochar inserted half an ounce of slightly alkaline fluid was drawn off. A smaller quantity removed at the end of a fortnight. Some thickened tissue still remained."

Summary

Most of the surgical cases were under the care of the Surgeon Robert William Parker, who was on the staff of the East London Hospital for Children, Shadwell. He was born in 1842 and qualified in 1869, and after working at the London Hospital he served with distinction as a volunteer with the Anglo-American Ambulance in the Franco-Prussian War 1870–1871. Then he became Resident Medical Officer at the Children's Hospital, 49 Great Ormond Street, and later in 1876 joined the staff of the Shadwell Hospital and was an active member of several London medical societies at which he presented surgical topics and cases of paediatric interest. Also, having a knowledge of German and French, he translated several surgical works from the continent.

This miscellany of sketches drawn by a Nurse Reeve in 1883–1887 consists of the following:

first, talipes and genu recurvatum. Each supposed to be caused by their intrauterine position; flexion contractures of the knee and equinus deformity due to poliomyelitis; lesion, such as amniotic band of the fingers, naevus of the forearm and warty lesion of the finger; skin contracture of the wrist following burns; absence of the lower ends of the radiui; two fatal cases of cancrum oris (noma) following measles; one of cleft palate and lip; three drawings of malignant disease of the thigh and face; finally strumous dactylitis and cyst of the neck.

Résumé

La plupart des cas dont il est question dans ce chapitre ont été traités à l'"East London Hospital for Children", Shadwell, par le chirurgien Robert William Parker. R.W. Parker est né en 1842 et commença à exercer en 1869, d'abord au "London Hospital" avant de s'engager comme volontaire des services ambulanciers anglo-américains pendant la guerre de 1870–71. Après un bref passage au "Children's Hospital", 49, Great Ormond Street, il entra, en 1876, au "Shadwell Hospital". A l'époque, il faisait partie de plusieurs associations médicales dans le cadre desquelles il faisait des conférences et présentait des cas de pédiatrie. Ce chapitre mentionne aussi deux des ouvrages qui lui valurent une réputation mondiale. Comme il parlait le français et l'allemand, il sut se rendre indispensable pendant la guerre franco-allemande. Plus tard, il traduisit plusieurs ouvrages de chirurgie.

Les cas décrits dans les notes prises par une infirmière de 1883–1887 sont les suivants:

pied-bot et genu recurvatum dus, à son avis, à la position du foetus dans l'utérus; contracture de flexion du genou, équinisme dus à une polyomyélite, syndactylie, naevus verruqueux; contracture du poignet due à une brûlure; apylasie de l'extrémité inférieure du radius; deux cas mortels de stomatite gangréneuse; fente palatine et fente labiale; tumeurs malignes de la cuisse et du visage; dactylite strumeuse et lymphangiome kystique.

Zusammenfassung

Die meisten chirurgischen Fälle wurden am East London Hospital for Children, Shadwell, von dem Chirurgen R. W. Parker betreut. Er wurde 1842 geboren und erhielt 1869 die Approbation. Nach kurzer Zeit am London Hospital erwarb er sich große Verdienste als freiwilliger Mitarbeiter der Anglo-American Ambulance im Dt.-Frz. Krieg 1870/71. Danach wurde er Resident Medical Officer am Children's Hospital, 49 Great Ormond Street, und später, 1876, wechselte er zum Shadwell Hospital. Zu dieser Zeit war er aktives Mitglied mehrerer ärztlicher Gesellschaften, für die er Vorträge über chirurgische Themen hielt, wobei er auch pädiatrische Fälle vorstellte. Es werden 2 seiner Bücher besonders hervorgehoben, die seinen internationalen Ruhm begründeten. Da er auch Deutsch und Französisch sprach, waren seine Kenntnisse während des Dt.-Frz. Krieges unentbehrlich. Danach übersetzte er mehrere Werke von Chirurgen vom Kontinent.

Die Aufzeichnungen, die von einer Krankenschwester mit Namen Reeve zwischen 1883 und 1887 angefertigt wurden, beschreiben folgende Fälle:

Zuerst Klumpfuß und Genu recurvatum. Von beiden wird angenommen, daß sie auf die Stellung im Uterus zurückzuführen sind; Beugekontrakturen des Knies und Spitzfuß, die auf Kinderlähmung zurückzuführen sind; Läsionen wie z.B. Syndaktylie, Unterarmnävus und warzenartige Läsion des Fingers, Hautkontraktion am Handgelenk nach Verbrennung; Aplasie des unteren Radius; 2 tödliche Fälle von Noma des Mundbereichs nach Masern; Gaumenspalte und Lippenspalte; 3 Zeichnungen von bösartigen Tumoren am Oberschenkel und im Gesicht; schließlich kropfförmige Fingerentzündung und Halszyste.

References

1. Swain VAJ (1970) Franco-Prussian War 1870–71. Voluntary aid for the wounded and sick. Br Med J 3:511–514
2. Swain VAJ, Woodall L (1968) East London Hospital for Children 1868–1963. Br Med J 4: 696–699
3. Parker RW (1885) Tracheotomy in laryngeal diptheria, 2nd edn. Lewis, London
4. Parker RW (1887) Congenital club foot – its nature and treatment with special reference to subcutaneous division of the tarsal ligaments. Lewis, London

Subject Index

MIX
Papier aus verantwortungsvollen Quellen
Paper from responsible sources
FSC® C105338

If you have any concerns about our products,
you can contact us on
ProductSafety@springernature.com

In case Publisher is established outside the EU,
the EU authorized representative is:
Springer Nature Customer Service Center GmbH
Europaplatz 3, 69115 Heidelberg, Germany

Printed by Libri Plureos GmbH
in Hamburg, Germany